Applied Kinesiology
and Biomechanics

06716

McGraw-Hill Series in Health Education, Physical Education, and Recreation

Deobold B. Van Dalen, *Consulting Editor*

This book is dedicated to those
who have achieved excellence in performance
and to the teachers and coaches
who have devoted their lives
to helping others achieve.

Contents

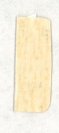

Preface

Through the ages the struggle of human beings to achieve excellence in motor performance has been vigorous and constant. Seemingly, we have always wanted to jump higher, run faster, throw farther, and demonstrate greater strength and skill. We have delighted in challenging opponents and responding to challenges. We are by nature highly competitive, and we search for excellence in performance.

Bit by bit a scientific field of knowledge relative to motor performance has been established, and the field has been divided into phases. One of the most useful phases of this important field is kinesiology, a subject which is now standard in the professional preparation of physical educators, athletic coaches, and physical therapists. While becoming established as a separate subject, kinesiology was associated with several divisions of the college curriculum. It has found its home in physical education and related areas, and it is now offered as a course in almost all colleges and universities in the United States.

Physical education deals with the specific components of performance and methods of improving performance. Through this phase of education, men and women become involved with the improvement of running, jumping, throwing, and other *basic skills*. They also learn *specific skills* which demand great accuracy and precision. Physical educators are especially concerned that human performance be graceful, efficient, and effective.

Because kinesiology has become so strongly identified with this area of education, this text emphasizes the application of the science to dance and sports movement, rather than kinesiology as it relates to occupational skills. The content of the text is especially selected and arranged to help people perform more skillfully and to give teachers, coaches, and therapists additional insight into teaching others how to perform. The book is designed to serve as a college text for undergraduate students.

We believe this book follows the most logical approach to the study of kinesiology at the undergraduate level. It contains the most current and useful information available on the subject. To make the book highly readable, many useful illustrations are included, and to make it more meaningful, numerous practical examples are given. In the latter part of the book practical application is made to the basic performance patterns.

This new edition includes updated information in each of the chapters. Additional emphasis has been placed on the practical application of scientific information. Student laboratory experiences, i.e., projects or problems to be solved, are placed at the end of selected chapters throughout the text. They present scientific aspects of the quantification of human motion, basically in the metric system, and are designed to give students practical experience with each concept to ensure a functional understanding.

The introduction to Part Three contains useful basic physics formulas for motion and force and their various combinations. Appropriate definitions of the symbols used are presented with the formulas. This material is included for the convenience of the student, who may use a pocket calculator, a ruler, and a protractor to solve quantitative problems which bring application to the concepts discussed in the text. While it is recommended that problems be solved using metric units (the international standard), a list of conversion factors is included so that students accustomed to dealing with U.S. customary units may gain a quantitative "feel" for human performance factors.

Portions of Chapter 4 have been adapted from Clayne Jensen and Garth Fisher, *Scientific Basis of Athletic Conditioning*, Lea and Febiger, Philadelphia, 1979, with the permission of the publisher.

The authors express sincere appreciation to Drs. LaVon Johnson and Boyd Call, and to numerous other colleagues who have given sound advice on the book's content. Also, appreciation is expressed to our students who have worked with us in developing the text.

Clayne R. Jensen
Gordon W. Schultz
Blauer L. Bangerter

Chapter 1

Introduction

Kinesiology is a relatively unfamiliar term. The word is derived from the Greek terms *kinesis*, meaning "motion," and *logos*, meaning "word" or "knowledge." Kinesiology, then, was originally defined as the study of motion. The subject contains an organized and systematized body of knowledge, and, therefore, it is referred to as a science. Because it deals with motion involved in human performance, it is precisely defined as "the study of the science of human motion."

Kinesiology today is related to, and draws from, four well-known fields of knowledge: anatomy, physiology, physics, and mathematics. From these fields it takes only facts which relate directly to human performance. Therefore, it may be said that kinesiology is based specifically on biomechanics, musculoskeletal anatomy, and neuromuscular physiology.

The human body, which is very complex, is subject to both *mechanical* and *biological* laws and principles. How effectively and efficiently it performs is dependent upon both its mechanical and biological functions. Kinesiology emphasizes the mechanical aspects, but by necessity it also includes biological functions as they relate directly to performance. Therefore, some of the subsequent chapters deal in a special way with biological functioning, while other chapters deal with mechanics of body structure and movement.

Many performances involve more than movements of the body and its parts. They involve the manipulation of implements such as balls, bats, and rackets. The use we make of these implements and how we handle them influence performance. Therefore, kinesiology must also deal with factors affecting the use of implements, such as force, friction, elasticity, projections, and angles. In summary, then, kinesiology includes a study of human movement and of implements and objects used in performance. We study kinesiology to learn how to analyze performance better and how to apply underlying principles to improve performance.

The foundation on which kinesiology is based is almost as old as recorded history. Aristotle, one of the greatest of ancient Greeks, is often termed the father of kinesiology, for he was the first person on record to study, teach, and write about mechanical principles relating to performance. He is credited as the one whose work on mechanics started the chain of thought that has led us to our present approach to mechanical analysis. Living more than 300 years before Christ, Aristotle demonstrated remarkable understanding of the center of gravity in the human body, laws of gravity and motion, and principles of leverage.

Another great Greek, Archimedes, developed principles of fluid mechanics which govern floating bodies in water. By means of a pulley arrangement, he launched a ship that many men were unable to move. To further emphasize the usefulness of mechanical advantage, he stated, "Give me a place to stand on and I can move the earth."

Claudius Galen (A.D. 131–201), a Roman physician for the gladiators, is considered the first athletic-team physician. He had opportunity to observe and study parts of the human body laid open in mortal combat, and he developed a substantial knowledge of the human anatomy and physiology which underlie kinesiological study. Through the ages of time many other scientists have added bits of knowledge which help to form the subject we now call kinesiology.

Even though kinesiology is based on highly standardized fields of knowledge, it has remained dynamic in nature. The human being in motor performance is a complex and interesting phenomenon. The study of human motion has attracted some of our best thinkers, who have discovered additional knowledge of better methods of teaching, how to apply basic laws and principles to performance, and how to use new devices such as radar guns, minicomputers, pocket calculators, timing apparatus, tensiometers, dynamometers, strain gauges, force platforms, high-speed photography, television replay, the electrogoniometer, and the electromyograph to analyze performance more effectively. This flow of new knowledge has helped to develop kinesiology into a highly practical, useful subject. Additional development of the subject continues, stimulated by the ever-present desire of humans to improve their performance.

Part One

Body Systems Involved in Human Movement

The chapters in Part One are specifically designed to help the reader understand the muscular system and the other body systems which cooperate with it during performance, and to know how these systems can be improved. Chapter 2 describes important facts about muscle tissue and about the structure and function of the muscular system. Chapter 3 explains interrelated actions of the muscular and skeletal systems in movement. Chapter 4 describes the functioning of the nervous system, how it controls muscular function, and its particular role in neuromuscular skill.

To illustrate the complexity and marvel of muscular actions in the human body, the photograph on page 4 shows a complex gymnastic movement. During this performance, the majority of which is completed in about 1 second, well over 100 muscles contract as agonists to cause the desired movements, while the opposite muscles (antagonists) must relax in order to permit the movements. Many additional muscles contract as they play the roles of stabilizers and neutralizers. Practically every motor muscle in the body contributes in some way to this brief but very complex performance. Many of the muscles act in two or more different roles

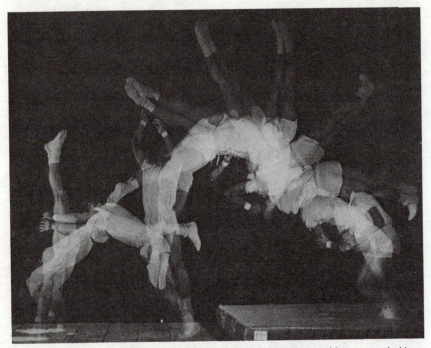

Gymnast doing a back somersault with a full twist in a layout position, preceded by a back somersault and other movements in the routine. This complex performance requires a high level of strength, power, and neuromuscular coordination.

during the performance. For example, at one moment a muscle might be a prime mover; the next moment it might be antagonistic to the desired movement; and a moment later it might play the role of stabilizer or neutralizer. All this may occur within a fraction of a second. Many other performances call for coordinations as complex as those in this illustration.

Chapter 2

Muscular System

Muscle tissue, which constitutes 40 to 50 percent of the adult human body, is one of the most interesting tissues of creation. Its special characteristics are *excitability* (irritability), *contractability*, *extensibility*, and *elasticity*. Excitability means that it is able to receive and respond to a stimulus. Under normal conditions the stimulus is supplied by the nervous system. Contractability means that the muscle changes shape as a result of stimuli, usually becoming shorter and thicker. Extensibility means that the muscle can be stretched (extended) beyond its normal length. And elasticity means that it readily returns to its normal length when the stretching force is eliminated.

All movements in the human body involve muscular contractions. These movements include motor actions, contractions of the heart and vessels, actions in the intestines, and many other specific movements of and within the body. The common acts of walking, picking up food, and breathing all depend directly upon muscular contractions, while such vigorous and complex performances as throwing the discus, pole vaulting, and field running in football depend on a large number of muscles and complex neuromuscular coordinations.

Three different kinds of muscle tissues are responsible for body movements. They are known as *skeletal*, *cardiac*, and *smooth* muscles. The different kinds of muscles have some characteristics in common, but they differ in several ways. For instance, the contractile process is the same in each, but the speed of contraction, duration of contraction, and purposes which they serve differ greatly. Each kind of muscle is especially adapted to the job it is to perform. In fact, each specific muscle of the body is especially suited in both structure and function to its particular task.

Even though cardiac and smooth muscles are essential to life, they are relatively unimportant in the study of human movement, but the actions of skeletal muscles are of prime importance because they attach to the skeletal system and cause it to move. Therefore, this chapter includes only brief points of information about cardiac and smooth muscles, but it expands on the structure and function of skeletal muscle.

CARDIAC (HEART) MUSCLE

Cardiac muscle (Figure 2-1) is the highly durable tissue that forms the walls and partitions of the heart. In the average adult it contracts rhythmically more than 100,000 times per day (72 heartbeats per minute). Like all other muscle tissue, it is composed of thousands of fibers (cells). The most striking characteristics of its fibers are: (1) they are involuntary, meaning that normally we cannot voluntarily prevent them from contracting or cause them to contract; (2) they are striated, similar to skeletal muscle (see Figure 2-3); and (3) they are arranged in syncytia—

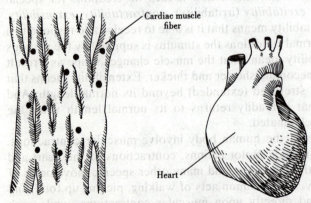

Figure 2-1 Cardiac muscle tissue. Right diagram shows the heart, the only organ composed of cardiac-muscle tissue. Left diagram shows tissue magnified by a microscope. Note how its fibers branch into each other. (*After Catherine Parker Anthony, Structure and Function of the Body, 4th ed., The C. V. Mosby Company, St. Louis, 1972.*)

that is, they appear to be connected with each other. Recent discoveries have shown that the fibers are actually separate in structure but function as syncytia.

The heart is composed of upper and lower syncytia, one forming the wall and septum of the atria and the other forming the wall and septum of the ventricles. When one of the syncytia receives impulses, all the fibers in that syncytium become stimulated. In other words, the whole syncytium contracts as a single unit, meaning that the all-or-none law of muscle contraction applies to the syncytium as a whole. The carefully coordinated alternating contractions of the two syncytia cause the synchronized action of the heart.

Physiologically, cardiac muscle differs from skeletal muscle in two ways: (1) Skeletal muscle normally contracts only when stimulated by nerve impulses, whereas cardiac muscle contracts consistently and rhythmically without receiving impulses from the nervous system. The cardiac contraction is caused by a stimulus which originates within the cardiac muscle. Among adults this occurs about once every $8/10$ second (72 times per minute) under conditions of rest or very moderate activity, and it may be hastened to more than 160 beats per minute with increased exercise demands or emotional excitement. (2) Another striking difference between cardiac and skeletal muscles is the rate of repolarization (time required for relaxation) following contraction. Cardiac muscle remains depolarized for about $3/10$ second, while the depolarization period of skeletal muscle is about $1/500$ second. This simply means that cardiac muscle remains contracted for about $3/10$ second each time it contracts under normal conditions; apparently this prolonged contraction is necessary for the heart to force blood from its chambers.

SMOOTH (VISCERAL) MUSCLE

Smooth muscle is located in the walls of the internal (visceral) organs other than the heart, such as the blood vessels, intestines, alimentary tract, and stomach. Like cardiac muscle, it contracts involuntarily. It is under the control of the involuntary portion of the nervous system, known as the autonomic system. Smooth muscle is characterized by smooth-appearing (nonstriated) muscle cells which are slender and tapered toward both ends (Figure 2-2). The cells are much smaller (0.26 to 0.05 millimeters in length) than those found in most skeletal muscles. Even though smooth muscle is found in almost every internal organ, its specific characteristics and functions vary from one organ to another; for example: (1) smooth muscle around the pupil of the eye is a different type than that in the walls of the stomach and performs quite a different function; (2) contraction of smooth muscle which lines the hollow organs

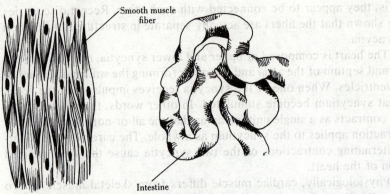

Figure 2-2 Visceral (smooth) muscle tissue. Right diagram shows part of the intestine, one of the many internal organs composed partly of smooth muscle. Left diagram shows muscle tissue magnified by a microscope. Its fibers are "smooth," that is, they do not have cross striations and are shorter than skeletal muscle fibers. (*After Catherine Parker Anthony, Structure and Function of the Body, 4th ed., The C. V. Mosby Company, St. Louis, 1972.*)

causes the organs to empty, as in the case of the intestinal tract, where waves of contractions push the inner content onward; (3) if additional contraction occurs in the smooth muscle of the blood vessels, circulation is impeded and blood pressure rises.

Compared with skeletal muscle, smooth muscle possesses (1) greater extensibility, (2) greater sensitivity to temperature and chemical stimuli, (3) greater ability for sustained contraction, and (4) more sluggishness in its movements.

STRIATED (SKELETAL) MUSCLE STRUCTURE

Because of their structure, human beings are able to accomplish a variety of performances that other forms of life cannot accomplish. But certain other species can perform practically every kind of movement better than human beings. The human being tends to be highly versatile, but not highly specialized in motor performance. We can walk, run, hop, climb, jump, swing, throw objects, and manipulate implements. This great versatility is primarily due to the complexity and refinement of our muscular, skeletal, and nervous systems. The skeletal muscle system is the focal point in movement; the nervous system works through the muscles by providing impulses to control their contractions, and the skeletal system provides the levers against which the muscles apply force to cause bodily movement. (Figure 2-3 shows skeletal muscle.)

If we want to be able to move with greater force, we *strengthen* the muscles involved. If we want to continue movement for a longer time, we

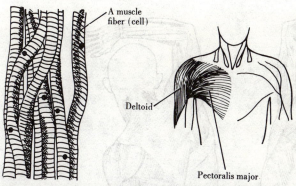

A muscle
fiber (cell)

Deltoid

Pectoralis major

Figure 2-3 Skeletal muscle tissue. Right diagram shows deltoid and pectoralis major muscles. Left diagram shows magnified muscle tissue. Note cross striations of the skeletal muscle fibers. Because they are so long, only part of their length shows on a microscope slide. (*After Catherine Parker Anthony, Structure and Function of the Body, 4th ed., The C. V. Mosby Company, St. Louis, 1972.*)

increase the durability of the muscles and improve the processes that support continued contractions. When we want to perform a movement more efficiently and smoothly, we *increase the coordination* of the muscle action. And if we want to alter body proportions, we may *increase the size* of selected muscles.

In total, there are more than 600 muscles in the human body. Among these are more than 430 skeletal muscles which appear in pairs on the right and left sides. However, most vigorous motor movements are caused by fewer than 80 pairs of muscles. Ordinarily skeletal muscles are voluntarily controlled by nerve impulses transmitted from the central nervous system. As a result of their contractions made in correct sequence with sufficient force, we are able to walk, run, swim, throw objects, breathe, and perform numerous other movements.

Some muscles, such as those involved in breathing, are both voluntary and involuntary; that is, breathing can be controlled at will to a certain extent, but ordinarily it continues without conscious attention of the individual.

Structure of Skeletal Muscle

Muscles vary greatly in size, ranging in length from less than 2 to more than 61 centimeters in adults. Also, muscles vary greatly in shape. Some are long and slender, while others are short, chubby, round, flat, or fan-shaped. Most muscles are *uniceps*, meaning that they taper into only one tendon at each end (one-headed). For example, the *brachioradialis* is a unicep muscle (Figure 6-6). A muscle is called a biceps (two-headed) muscle when it is divided at one end, to form two tapering ends. The

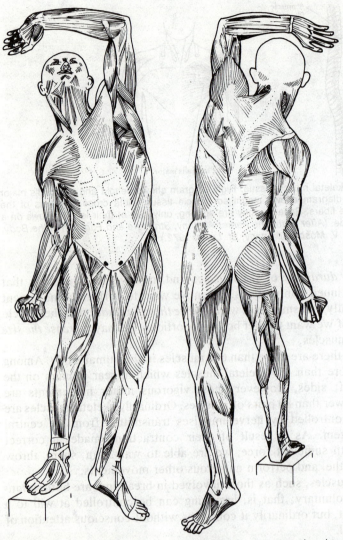

Figure 2-4 Superficial skeletal muscles, anterior and posterior views.

muscle in the front of the arm between the shoulder and elbow (biceps brachii) is an example of a biceps muscle (Figure 6-12). A *triceps* (three-headed) muscle is one that divides into three tapering sections at one end, such as the triceps brachii muscle at the back of the upper arm (see Figure 6-14). (Figure 2-4 shows superficial skeletal muscles.)

Each muscle is composed of a great number of fibers (cells). Fibers are the basic units of muscle structure. The fibers of skeletal muscles are very slender (10 to 100 microns in diameter) and vary greatly in length. Some fibers run the full length of the muscle, whereas others run only part way through the muscle. Each fiber is enclosed by a membrane called the *sacrolemma*, a word which means ·skin. Immediately underneath the sacrolemma is a plasma membrane which has the capacity to transmit nerve impulses throughout the fiber. The fibers are connected by tissue which is penetrated by nerve fibers, through which nerve impulses enter the muscle fibers. Tiny blood vessels carry oxygen and nutrients to the muscle fibers.

In skeletal muscles two kinds of fibers are present, red and white. Generally, rapid movements are performed by muscles in which white cells predominate, while slower, more sustained movements are performed by muscles in which red cells predominate.

Each fiber has cross strips (striations) at right angles to its long axis. The striations, which are visible under a powerful microscope, give the muscle the name *striated* or *striped* muscle. A single muscle fiber contains 1,000 or more long, thin parts called *myofibrils* arranged in bundles longitudinally within the fiber. The myofibrils are composed mainly of two proteins: myosin, which is especially abundant, and actin. The striations in the muscle fibers arise from variations in the density of these proteins at different places along the myofibrils. Apparently these proteins are the actual contractile elements of the muscle (Figure 2-5).

Figure 2-5a illustrates a skeletal muscle made up of many thousands of fibers, a small section of which is magnified in Figure 2-5b. The small branching structures attached to the fibers are *end plates* of a motor nerve fiber branch which conducts signals for the muscle fibers to contract. The lines circling the fibers are striations. A small section of a single fiber is enlarged in Figure 2-5c, giving a better view of the striations and illustrating the myofibrils of which the fiber is composed. In Figure 2-5d a small, greatly enlarged section of a myofibril is shown, and the striation pattern of light and dark bands is illustrated in much greater detail. Figure 2-5e illustrates a single striation and identifies its different parts, the Z lines, I bands, A band, and H zone. Figure 2-5f illustrates how the arrangement of *myosin* and *actin* filaments causes the light and dark zones in the myofibril, thereby giving the muscle fiber a striated appearance. It is rather well established that the thicker filaments are myosin molecules, while the thinner filaments are primarily actin molecules. Notice that the dark A band of the striation is caused by overlapping of myosin and actin (both filaments). The medium-colored H zone consists only of the thicker filaments (myosin), while the lighter I zone is composed of the thinner filaments (actin). Figure 2-9c shows an electromicrographic view of a skeletal muscle in which all the different parts of a striation pattern are apparent (43).

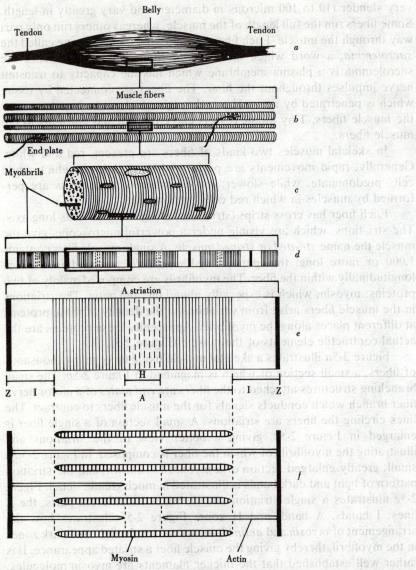

Figure 2-5 Details of the structure of skeletal muscles. (*After Catherine Parker Anthony, Structure and Function of the Body, 4th ed., The C. V. Mosby Company, St. Louis, 1972.*)

Structural Classification of Muscles The structural arrangement of the fibers of a muscle bears an important relationship to the force and distance of its contraction. There are two main kinds of fiber arrangements, the *fusiform* (longitudinal) and the *penniform* (diagonal), but there

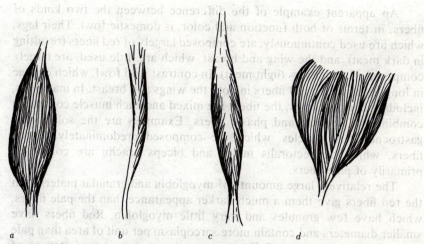

a   b   c   d

Figure 2-6 Variations in the arrangement of muscle fiber. (a) Fusiform—examples of this are brachialis, and brachioradialis of the arm, and the sartorius muscle of the leg. (b) Unipenniform—examples of this structure are the extensor digitorium longus and the tibalis posterior muscles of the leg. (c) Bipenniform—the best example is the rectus femoris. (d) Multipenniform—examples are the deltoid and pectoralis major. In these muscles the tendon runs into the center of the muscle, and diagonal fibers attach to it from all directions.

are several variations from these two basic forms. Even though there is lack of agreement among experts about the variations, the forms illustrated in Figure 2-6 are representative.

The fusiform is structurally simplest. Because the fibers of this kind of muscle run longitudinally along the muscle, there is a one-to-one relationship between shortening of the muscle and the amount of movement it causes. This is an advantage in speed of movement, but it is a disadvantage in the application of force. Conversely, the fibers of penniform muscles are arranged like the structure of a feather, with the tendon in the place of the shaft and the muscle fibers in the place of the barks. With the muscle fibers arranged diagonally to the direction of pull, more fibers can be brought into play, but the range of motion is reduced. Therefore, penniform muscles are designed primarily for the application of force through short ranges of motion, while fusiform muscles are designed for less force through greater ranges of motion.

Red and Pale Muscle Fibers Muscles in the human body are made up of a combination of red and pale fibers, with some muscles having a dominance of red fibers while others have a dominance of pale fibers. Red (tonic) fibers, designed for relatively slow and sustained contractions, are prevalent in the postural muscles. Pale (phasic) fibers are designed for rapid contractions and are less capable of sustained contractions.

An apparent example of the difference between the two kinds of fibers, in terms of both function and color, is domestic fowl. Their legs, which are used continuously, are composed largely of red fibers (resulting in dark meat), and the wing and breast, which are little used, are largely composed of pale fibers (light meat). In contrast wild fowl, which engage in long flights, have red fibers in both the wings and breast. In mammals, including human beings, the fibers are mixed and each muscle contains a combination of tonic and phasic fibers. Examples are the soleus and gastrocnemious muscles, which are composed predominately of red fibers, while the pectoralis major and biceps brachii are composed primarily of pale fibers.

The relatively large amounts of myoglobin and granular materials in the red fibers give them a much darker appearance than the pale fibers, which have few granules and very little myoglobin. Red fibers have smaller diameters and contain more sarcoplasm per unit of area than pale fibers. The pigment in red fibers may serve as a means of storage of oxygen. These fibers depend primarily upon oxidated metabolism, and this is associated with their adaptability for sustained contractions.

Red fibers are innervated by lower thresholds than pale fibers and are therefore used more frequently. Also, red fibers present a high level of electrical activity and contain more protein. A person may, through heredity, have more of one fiber type than the other and as a result will have an advantage in either endurance-type or explosive-type activities.

Muscle Attachments   Muscles are attached to the bones by tough fibrous connective tissue in the form of tendons or aponeuroses (fibrous sheets). When the muscle receives a stimulus, the belly portion contracts, exerting pull on the connective tissues, which in turn pull on the bones to which they are attached. It has been customary to designate the two attachments of a muscle as the *origin* and the *insertion*. The origin is usually at the proximal end of the muscle, meaning that it is the attachment nearest the midline of the body. The origin is attached to the more stable portion of the skeleton, and the belly of the muscle usually lies closer to the origin. On the other hand, the insertion is usually the distal attachment where the skeletal system is more readily movable and the distal tendon is usually the longer of the tendons. The distal tendons are sometimes very long, as in the muscles of the lower arm which control the fingers (Figure 6-5). The tendons actually grow onto bones at locations especially shaped to accommodate the attachments. In some cases the connective tissue is almost nonexistent because the fleshy portion of the muscle grows very close to the bone. An example is the pectoralis major muscle (Figure 6-13) in which only a thin layer of fibrous connective tissue separates the fleshy fibers from the bone at the proximal attachment.

FUNCTION OF STRIATED MUSCLE

Since all forms of animals move by contracting their muscles, muscle contraction is one of the key processes of life. A muscle has the capacity only to contract or not contract (relax). It is said to contract when its fibers respond to a stimulus. When a muscle contracts, tension is applied toward its middle. Muscles can respond in more than one way when they contract, as demonstrated later in this chapter, and they may contract with varying degrees of force. Figure 2-7 shows contraction of the biceps brachii muscle.

When the muscle contracts, it does not pull mostly on the distal

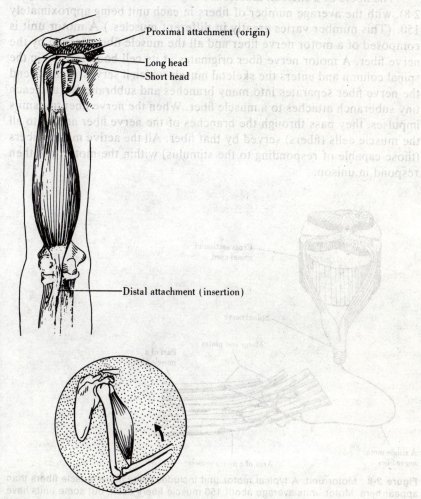

Proximal attachment (origin)

Long head

Short head

Distal attachment (insertion)

Figure 2-7 Attachments of biceps brachii muscle, and the action it causes when it contracts.

attachment, as many people believe. Rather it pulls toward the middle, exerting equal force on the attachments at both ends. The muscle acts like a stretched spring attached to the two ends of a hinge. The spring applies tension toward its middle, and its pull is equal on the two ends. Which body part moves as a result of the muscle tension depends upon the relative stability of the body parts at that particular time. To a large extent stability of body parts at a given time is determined by contractions of muscles acting as stabilizers. For example, from a supine position a person can do either a sit-up or a leg-raise, depending on which part of the body is stabilized.

The fibers of a skeletal muscle are organized into *motor units* (Figure 2-8), with the average number of fibers in each unit being approximately 150. (This number varies greatly in different muscles.) A motor unit is composed of a motor nerve fiber and all the muscle fibers served by the nerve fiber. A motor nerve fiber originates at its cell body located in the spinal column and enters the skeletal muscle which it serves. Near its end the nerve fiber separates into many branches and subbranches, and each tiny subbranch attaches to a muscle fiber. When the nerve fiber transmits impulses, they pass through the branches of the nerve fiber and go to all the muscle cells (fibers) served by that fiber. All the active muscle fibers (those capable of responding to the stimulus) within the motor unit then respond in unison.

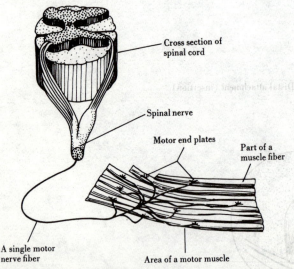

Cross section of spinal cord

Spinal nerve

Motor end plates

Part of a muscle fiber

A single motor nerve fiber

Area of a motor muscle

Figure 2-8 Motor unit. A typical motor unit includes many more muscle fibers than appear here. Motor units average about 150 muscle fibers each, but some units have less than a dozen fibers while others have several hundred fibers.

It is important to note that muscle fibers in a motor unit are not grouped together but are dispersed throughout the muscle. Therefore, if a single motor unit were stimulated, it would appear that a large portion of the muscle contracted very mildly. If additional motor units were stimulated, the muscle would contract with greater force.

Those muscles which control very fine movements and which contract rapidly usually have only a few muscle fibers in each motor unit, meaning that the ratio of nerve fibers to muscle fibers is very high. For instance, muscles which control eye movements have no more than 10 to 25 muscle fibers in each motor unit, while slower-contracting muscles which cause less refined movements, such as the soleus muscle, may have more than 500 muscle fibers in a motor unit.

When the central nervous system provides a stimulus to a particular motor nerve fiber, the fiber either responds or fails to respond, depending on whether the stimulus is strong enough to exceed the threshold of the fiber. If the threshold is exceeded, impulses are transmitted through the fiber to all the muscle fibers which it serves (motor unit).

When the impulses reach the nerve ending (neuromyal junction), calcium ions flow in rapidly, creating an electric potential called the *end plate potential*. This excites the entire muscle fiber and causes it to contract. The contraction actually results from interaction between the layers of myosin and actin filaments, which causes the actin filaments to be pulled inward among the myosin filaments, thus shortening the muscle (Figure 2-9). The exact details of the cause of this interaction between myosin and actin remain unknown.

Once the calcium ions have been released into the interior of the muscle fiber, the contraction will continue until they are removed. Fortunately, within the muscle fiber is a substance called *relaxing factor* which has a natural affinity for calcium ions and combines with them within a few hundredths of a second; this action neutralizes the calcium and causes the muscle fiber to relax.

In short, the nerve impulse causes a pulsation of calcium ions inside the muscle fibers. The calcium concentration goes up very rapidly, causing the fibers to contract, and then it falls to zero within a few hundredths of a second. This total process, including the initiation of the stimulus, transmission of the impulses, contraction of the muscle fibers, and relaxation of the fibers, may occur within a small fraction of a second.

Gradations of Muscle Contractions Everyday experiences show us that the same muscles contract with various gradations of force according to the requirements of the particular act. The leg extensor muscles are able to contract with just enough force to support the weight of the body, or they can contract with much more force, as when they project the body

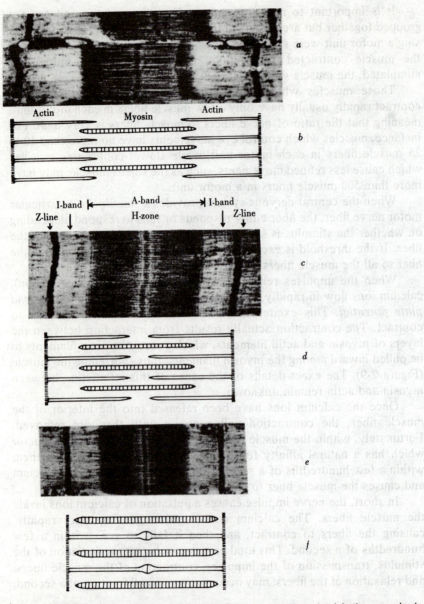

Figure 2-9 Electromicrographic views of skeletal muscles. In (a) the muscle is stretched. In (c) it is in normal extended position, (e) represents partial contraction. (b), (d), and (f) illustrate the relative positions of myosin and actin filaments when the muscle moves from stretch to normal extended length, then to partial contraction (43).

into the air. In the different motor performances, it is essential that a particular muscle or group of muscles contract with various degrees of force at different times. This is controlled by two important variables.

The first variable is the *number of motor units* contracting at once. When a weak contraction is desired, only a few units are activated. When a maximum contraction is needed, as many body motor units as possible are contracted simultaneously. Gradations of muscle contractions between minimal and maximal can be obtained by varying the number of contracting units. The number of motor units that are contracted depends on the number of motor neurons that are activated by the stimuli emanating primarily from the brain and being distributed throughout the central nervous system. Figure 2-10 gives a graphical representation of the effects of various numbers of motor units contracting simultaneously.

The second variable which influences force of contraction is the *summation wave.* Impulses can be sent to the muscle fibers in slow succession, causing the fibers to contract and allowing sufficient time to relax between impulses. If the impulses are close enough, further contraction will occur before the shortening from the previous contraction can allow return to resting length. Therefore, each succeeding contraction will add to the force of the previous contraction. This process is limited, finally, because the actin filaments are physically incapable of sliding any farther. Figure 2-11 illustrates the buildup of the contractile force as the rate of impulses per second (frequency) increases. In large skeletal muscles, when the rate of impulses reaches about 35 per second, the muscle tetanizes, meaning that the responses to individual impulses

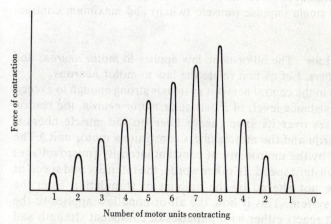

Figure 2-10 Multiple-motor-unit summation illustrating the progressive increase in contractile force caused by increasing numbers of motor units contracting simultaneously. (*After Arthur C. Guyton, Functions of the Human Body, 4th ed., W. B. Saunders Co., Philadelphia, 1974.*)

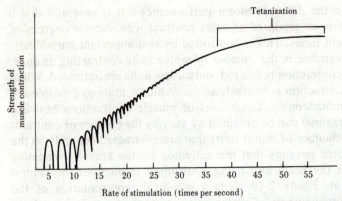

Figure 2-11 Wave summation, showing progressive summation of successive contractions as the rate of stimulation is increased. Tetanization occurs when the rate of stimulation reaches approximately 35 per second, and maximum force of contraction occurs at approximately 50 per second for large skeletal muscles. (*After Arthur C. Guyton, Functions of the Human Body, 4th ed., W. B. Saunders Company, Philadelphia, 1974.*)

are no longer detectable, and the contraction becomes smooth and continuous. Maximum contractile force occurs at about 50 impulses per second in large muscles. However, in smaller muscles which cause highly precise and rapid movements, such as those controlling the eyelid, maximum contraction comes at 400 to 600 impulses per second. Tetanization produces about three to four times the contractile force that occurs from a single nerve impulse. By varying the frequency of impulses to the motor unit, the amount of force can be varied to any amount between that produced by the single impulse (muscle twitch) and maximum contraction.

All-or-None Law The all-or-none law applies to *motor neurons* and also to *muscle fibers*. Let us first relate the law to motor neurons.

If a stimulus in the central nervous system is strong enough to exceed the threshold (resistance level) of a particular *motor neuron*, the neuron will carry impulses over its axon (nerve fiber) to the muscle fibers it serves. (The neuron and the muscle fibers constitute a motor unit.) The impulses carried by the neuron are of constant intensity (microvoltage) and travel at a constant speed. In other words, the intensity and speed of the impulses are not altered by the amount of stimulation from the central nervous system. This is how the all-or-none law applies to the motor neuron. It reacts either with impulses of consistent strength and speed, or not at all. However, it should be remembered that the frequency (number of impulses per second) can alter at the will of the performer to suit the task at hand.

When impulses reach the individual *muscle fibers*, those fibers which are capable of contracting (some fibers are dormant) do so in accordance with the all-or-none law. In other words, if a fiber contracts, it contracts to its present maximum ability. The all-or-none law does not imply that the strength of the contraction is the same each time the fiber contracts, because sometimes the contractile elements of a fiber are weaker than at other times owing to fatigue, lack of nutrients, or other causes. In essence then, the all-or-none law means that when a muscle fiber is excited, the entire fiber contracts to the full extent of its immediate ability to contract. The effect of the summation wave is the buildup in contraction that results from a high-frequency stimulation through the wave-summation process.

Kinds of Muscle Contractions

The term *contraction* means that a muscle responds to a stimulus. When a muscle responds, tension, which may cause shortening, develops. Following are different ways a muscle can contract.

Concentric Contractions When stimulated muscles develop tension sufficient to move a body segment, the muscles shorten, and the body segment moves. The muscles are then said to have contracted *concentrically*. For example in flexing the elbow in the anatomical standing position, the biceps brachii (and other muscles) contract, causing the elbow to bend, thus drawing the hand close to the shoulder. In vigorous motor movements, such as in athletics, most of the apparent contractions are concentric, but many of the less apparent contractions are either eccentric or static in nature.

Eccentric Contractions A muscle contracts *eccentrically* (Figure 2-12) when it responds to a stimulus and applies tension which is overcome by the external resistance, thus causing the muscle to lengthen instead of shorten. Eccentric contractions are demonstrated by moving slowly from a standing to a squatting position. To allow this movement, the leg extensor muscles must lengthen while their contractions tend to oppose lengthening. In other words, these muscles apply tension which is less than the force of gravity pulling the body downward. However, the tension is sufficient to control the speed at which the body lowers. Eccentric contraction is also demonstrated in the actions of the latissimus dorsi when the body is lowered from a pull-up position, and in the actions of the triceps in lowering the body from the push-up position.

In all eccentric contractions, the movement is directly opposite the action ordinarily assigned to the muscle. In lowering the hand from the shoulder, the movement is elbow extension, but the active muscles are

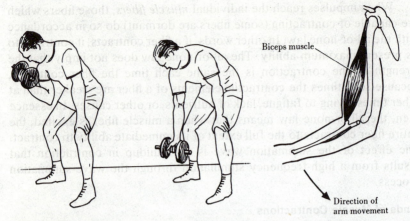

Biceps muscle

Direction of
arm movement

Figure 2-12 Muscles contracting eccentrically as weight is lowered. The elbow *extends*, but the *elbow flexor* muscles contract (eccentrically) to control the rate of extension.

the elbow flexors. Eccentric contractions are common in wrestling and football, where force applied by the opponent often causes muscles to lengthen while in contraction, and in gymnastics, where the body, in arm-supported positions, is often lowered slowly. When the body lands, or when a heavy object is received, the muscles contract eccentrically to absorb the shock of the force. It should be noted that the lengthening of a muscle in a relaxed condition (no tension) due to contraction of opposite muscles is not considered eccentric contraction.

Isotonic (Dynamic or Phasic) Contraction   Both concentric and eccentric contractions are *isotonic* in nature, meaning the body segment *moves* as the muscles shorten or lengthen. All motor movements involve isotonic contractions.

Isometric (Static or Tonic) Contraction   A muscle contracts *isometrically* when it attempts to shorten (applies tension) but does not overcome the resistance; therefore, shortening of the muscle and movement of the body segment fail to occur. Isometric contraction occurs when a person pushes or pulls against a fixed object, or when the muscular tension equals the opposing force. Such contractions are used frequently in stabilizing the body or portions of the body during performance.

Important Characteristics of Skeletal Muscles

If skeletal muscles are to perform their functions effectively, they must possess certain characteristics in sufficient amounts. Most important are the abilities to (1) contract forcefully to cause strong movements, (2) contract rapidly to cause fast movements, (3) endure repeated contractions, and (4) remain in good tone.

Contractile Force Every muscle, unless totally paralyzed, has ability to contract with some force (tension). This ability varies greatly among the different muscles of the body and in the same muscles of different individuals. This quality changes considerably in a particular muscle at different times, depending on the state of conditioning. The force with which a muscle can contract is related to and influenced by the following:

Size (cross-sectional measurement) of the muscle The ability of a muscle to contract forcefully varies approximately in proportion to its cross-sectional measurement. That is, if a muscle develops until its cross-sectional area doubles, its strength will approximately double. Increased muscle size results primarily from increased size of individual fibers, while the number of fibers might remain constant. An increase in muscle size results from either (1) normal growth during the formative years, or (2) consistent and systematic overloading of the muscle (contracting it against greater resistance than it is accustomed to).

Proportion of active fibers Only a portion of the fibers in a muscle is capable of contraction, and this portion increases as the condition of the muscle improves. As a result of training, inactive (dormant) fibers are reactivated. As they are reactivated, they increase in size, as do the active fibers, and thus contribute to the increased size of the total muscle. If the percentage of active fibers in a muscle can be increased by about 10 percent, then obviously the contractile force of the muscle will increase.

Speed of Contraction Certain muscles are able to contract with much greater speed than other muscles because they are designed to perform functions requiring fast contractions. Similarly, muscles in different individuals vary in their ability to contract rapidly. Speed of contraction can be increased by training techniques which emphasize fast contractions. Such training increases the efficiency of the total contractile process. Maximum power, as required in putting the shot, throwing a fast ball, or jumping for maximum height, results from the best combination of speed of contraction and application of force.

Endurance of Muscles Every muscle is able to contract repeatedly against a given resistance; in other words, it has a certain ability to resist fatigue. Endurance of a muscle is influenced primarily by (1) contractile force (strength) of the muscle, (2) efficiency of the circulorespiratory functioning (most important is internal respiration), and (3) ability of the nervous system to continue to provide sufficiently strong stimuli. To illustrate:

1 If muscles of varying strengths were called upon to contract against an equal resistance, the weaker muscles would have to contract near maximum, while the stronger muscles could repeat the action considerably more times than the weaker muscles before being overcome by fatigue.

2 Circulorespiratory functioning directly influences a muscle's ability to endure because the muscle fibers depend on the circulorespiratory system to keep them supplied with oxygen and nutrients and to clear them of waste products which contribute to fatigue. If circulorespiratory functioning is insufficient, muscle fatigue occurs.

3 Muscle fibers contract only when they receive a stimulus. When partial failure occurs in the transmission of impulses to muscle fibers, those fibers fail to contract, resulting in a weaker total muscle contraction. In such a case, the point of fatigue is in the nervous system, but the result is a weaker muscle contraction, and it appears as though muscle fatigue has occurred.

Muscle Tone   Tone is the quality which gives firmness and proper shape to muscles. Skeletal muscles have a certain amount of tone, depending on their state of conditioning. Well-conditioned muscles possess good tone, while poorly conditioned muscles are poorly toned or flabby.

IMPORTANT CONCEPTS

1 The working structure of skeletal muscles is the motor unit. Most skeletal muscles are composed of thousands of motor units.

2 Muscle contraction ordinarily occurs in response to volleys of nerve impulses originating primarily from the brain.

3 Muscle contraction is a process by which protein elements within each muscle fiber slide closer together in a way that shortens the fiber, creating a tension or force toward the middle of the muscle.

4 Contractile force creates tension where tendons attach, and if the tension is sufficient motor movement occurs.

5 The location and position of the contracting motor units determine the exact direction of movement.

6 The relative stability of the body parts on either side of a joint determines which body part moves.

7 Gradations of muscle contraction occur in two ways:

    a *Recruitment*—selection of fewer or more motor units.

    b *Wave summation*—control of nerve-impulse frequency, which can vary the contractile force of each selected motor unit.

8 Three kinds of contractions are possible: *concentric*, *isometric*, and *eccentric*. Which kind occurs is dependent upon the contractile force in relation to the resistance.

a If the contractile force dominates, concentric contraction results.

b If an external force (resistance) dominates, eccentric contraction results.

c If an external resistance cannot be overcome or an external force is equal to the contractile force, isometric contraction results.

9 Potential for muscle contraction can be improved in regard to:

a *Strength*—amount of contractile force available.

b *Speed*—quickness in generating contraction.

c *Endurance*—ability to repeat or maintain contractions of a given force.

Chapter 3

Skeletal Action

It would be impossible for skeletal muscles to perform their functions without the assistance of the skeletal system (Figure 3-1), for this system provides levers to which the muscles apply force and provides joints (axes) around which movements occur. Amazing versatility is displayed in the human skeleton. It is a complex network composed of several kinds of bones, joints, and connective tissues, designed to serve particular purposes. The skeletal system is another marvel of the human structure, and students of kinesiology must visualize its role clearly to understand human performance.

The skeletal system is composed of 208 named bones and more than 200 joints (articulations) between bones. Most of the bones and joints appear in pairs, with one on the right side and one on the left side of the body. When the skeleton is classified into major divisions, the number of bones in each division is: cranium, 8; face, 14; ear, 6; hyoid, 1; spine, 26; sternum and ribs, 25; upper extremities, 64; and lower extremities, 64.

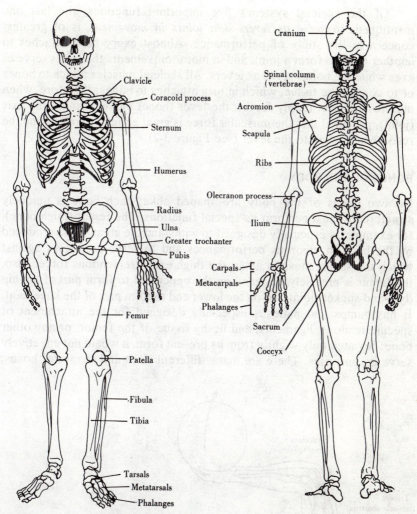

Figure 3-1 Front and back views of the human skeletal system.

FUNCTIONS OF THE SKELETON

The skeletal system serves five important functions: (1) to give form and structure to the body, (2) to protect internal organs, (3) to produce blood cells, (4) to store calcium and phosphorus, and (5) to serve as levers and joints in body movements. Visualize what the body would be like without this system. It would have no definite shape and could not stand upright; vital organs would be almost totally unprotected, and motor movements would be impossible.

Of the skeletal system's five important functions, the last one mentioned, *to serve as levers and joints in movement*, is of greatest concern in the study of performance. Almost every bone attaches to another bone to form a joint, and in motor movements the joints serve as axes while the bones serve as levers. All skeletal muscles attach to bones or to connective tissue, which in turn attaches to bones; therefore, when muscles contract (apply force), the lever (bone) moves around the axis (joint), provided that the muscular force is great enough to overcome the resistance applied to the lever (see Figure 3-2).

BONES OF THE BODY

No two bones of the body are shaped alike; each bone is uniquely structured to best perform its special functions. The femur (thigh bone), for example, is especially designed to withstand the great stress produced by the body in vigorous performances and to serve as a lever against which the strong muscles about the thigh exert tremendous force. Also, the femur is precisely designed on the upper end to form part of the hip (ball-and-socket) joint and on the lower end to form part of the knee joint. It has bumps and plateaus especially designed for the attachment of specific tendons, ligaments, and fleshy tissue. If the femur, or any other bone, deviated only slightly from its present form, it would not effectively serve its purposes. There are many different sizes and shapes of bones,

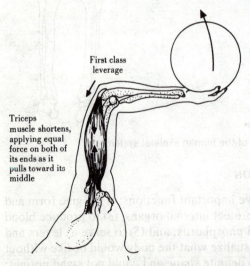

First class
leverage

Triceps
muscle shortens,
applying equal
force on both of
its ends as it
pulls toward its
middle

Figure 3-2 The movement of a body lever as a result of muscular force. In this case the mechanical ratio is about one to ten, meaning that the muscle contraction must be about ten times as great as the resistance at the hand (see explanation in Chapter 11).

and they are classified as *long*, *short*, *flat*, and *irregular*. Several of each type can be readily identified in Figure 3-1.

Long Bones

Long bones consist of slender shafts which are usually thicker toward both ends where tendons and fascia sheets attach, and thinner toward the middle. The two ends of a long bone are especially shaped to form portions of the joints which they help to compose. The proximal end is the head, and the distal end is the foot of the bone. Typically, both ends display protrusions called *tuberosities* which are located to serve as attachments for ligaments and tendons. The shaft of the bone is hollowed and filled with marrow, and the hollow is surrounded by compact bone. The thickness of the compact bone layer varies to accommodate the amount of stress the bone is expected to bear at any particular point. The bones seem to be designed to conserve weight (tubular and hollow) and still withstand heavy stress. Long bones are found in the arms and legs. Examples are the femur, radius, and humerus bones (Figure 3-3). Long bones are designed for sweeping-type movements of great speed and long range, and their muscle attachments are usually located to enhance speed of movement.

Short Bones

Among the short bones are the carpals, the tarsals, and the patellae. These bones are composed of spongy-type tissue with a thin, hard surface. Their shapes tend toward roundness as opposed to flat, irregular, or shaftlike structures. Even though they contribute significantly to movement, their role in movement is much less dramatic than that of long bones.

Flat Bones

Flat bones are those with broad and smooth surfaces, such as the sternum and the bones of the cranium. They are composed of two thin layers of hard surface tissue, with variable amounts of spongy tissue enclosed between the layers. Except for the scapulae and pelvis, flat bones serve little purpose in movement. They exist primarily in the skull and face, and their main function is to protect vital organs.

Irregular Bones

All bones that do not fit into one of the above three categories are classified as irregular. Examples of irregular bones are vertebrae, ear bones, and bones of the face. Vertebrae form the spinal column, and they are among the most used bones in body movements. Practically every vigorous motor movement involves the spinal column.

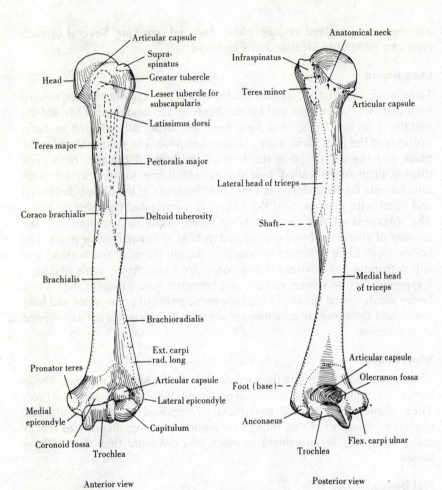

Figure 3-3 Parts of a long bone (the left humerus) with positions of muscle attachments indicated. (*After C. M. Goss, Gray's Anatomy, 29th ed., Lea & Febiger, Philadelphia, 1973.*)

BODY JOINTS

A *joint*, which is one of the most specialized and perfectly formed structures in the body, is a point in the skeletal system where two or more bones meet (articulate). The bones are usually attached to each other by connective tissue, but this is not always the case. Joints vary considerably in the amount of movement they allow and are classified generally as *immovable*, *slightly movable*, and *freely movable*.

Immovable Joints

An immovable joint is an articulation of two bones that have been fused together. Such joints are not capable of movement by muscular force. For all practical purposes, they could as well not exist, except that they do serve a protective function. When external force is applied, slight movement might occur in the joints, resulting in a cushioning effect. For example, if a blow is struck on the head, the *immovable* joints of the cranium will permit slight movement.

Slightly Movable Joints

Slightly movable joints are not firmly fixed as are immovable joints, but the structure of bones and connective tissues in and around the joints restricts the range of motion to only a few degrees. Examples of slightly movable joints are those located in the spine. Every two vertebrae are separated by a disk which is compressible, allowing the vertebrae to be moved a very limited amount in any direction. However, the combined movements of all the joints in the spine result in extensive spinal action. Slightly movable joints are also found between the sacrum and ilia, and at the front and back attachments of the ribs.

Freely Movable Joints

Freely movable joints have a relatively large range of movement and are of prime importance in motor performances. They are located in the upper and lower extremities. Examples of freely movable joints are the shoulder, elbow, wrist, hip, and knee joints (Figure 3-4).

JOINT STRUCTURE

The structure of each joint is best for the functions of that joint. The structure determines the actions and range of motion of which the joint is capable.

The structure of an *immovable* joint amounts to two bones fused together with a thin layer of fibrous tissue between them, such as the joints in the cranium and face. These are true joints in the sense that they form articulations of bones. Even though they are nonfunctioning in motor movements, they often serve protective functions.

Slightly movable joints are of two kinds: ligamentous and cartilaginous. A ligamentous joint is two bones bound together by ligaments in such a way that only a meager amount of movement results and no disk is present within the joint. Examples are the midradioulnar joint near the wrist and the joint at the back attachment of each rib. A cartilaginous joint is two bones bound together by ligaments and separated by a cartilage-type disk. Examples are the joints of the spinal column and the joints that connect the ribs to the sternum. In this kind of joint, movement results from the pliability of the disk.

Freely movable joints are especially structured to allow for great sweeping and rapid motor movements. In these joints the articulating

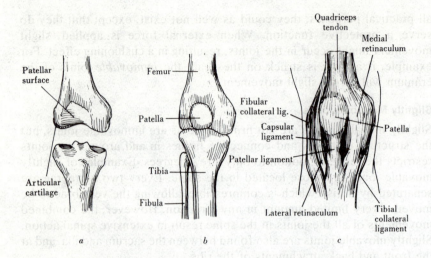

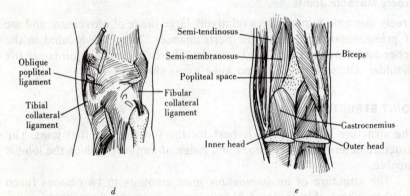

Figure 3-4 Structure of a freely movable joint (the knee joint). (a) The joint spread apart, showing the articulating surfaces. (b) Bone structure of joint. (c) Front view showing ligaments. (d) Back view showing ligaments. (e) Back view of muscles and tendons which cross over the joint and add support to it.

surfaces are covered with a layer of cartilage known as articular cartilage (Figure 3-4a) which prevents direct wearing on the bones and helps to absorb shocks. The bones are bound together by ligaments, and a ligamentous sleeve (capsular ligament) completely encloses the joint and attaches firmly all the way around both bones of the joint (Figure 3-4c). The interior of this sleeve-type ligament is lined with a membrane which secretes fluid into the interior of the joint to keep it lubricated. In most freely movable joints several additional ligaments assist the capsular ligament in binding the two bones together (Figure 3-4c and 3-4d).

Muscles or their tendons extend across most movable joints (Figure 3-4e) and assist the ligaments by holding the joints closed and preventing them from dislocating. Added muscular strength and tone will add stability to the joints, because stronger muscles hold the joints more tightly intact.

Freely movable joints are of six different structural types, each especially designed to accommodate the movements of the particular segment of the body.

Gliding Joints

Gliding joints permit only gliding movements, as the joints between the carpal bones of the wrist or between the tarsal bones of the ankle. The gliding surfaces of these bones are nearly flat, or one may be slightly concave and the other slightly convex. During movement the surfaces simply slide across each other.

Hinge Joints

These joints are similar to a door swinging on its hinges. Examples of this type are the elbow and the first and second joints of the phalanges. Hinge joints allow movement in only one plane; in other words, they allow only flexion and extension.

Condyloid Joints

This type of joint is characterized by an oval-shaped head (condyle) of bone fitted into a shallow cavity, such as the joints between the metacarpals and phalanges (except the thumb). Movements permitted in these joints are extension, flexion, abduction, adduction, and circumduction. The movements are through two planes. Condyloid joints are similar to ball-and-socket joints, except that they are shallower, and the muscle arrangements around them do not usually allow rotation.

Saddle Joints

These joints function very much like condyloid joints, but their structure is different. From one angle the articular surfaces appear convex, and from the opposite angle they appear concave. This type of joint consists of two saddlelike structures fitted into each other. The movements in saddle joints are the same as in condyloid joints. The carpal-metacarpal joint of the thumb is an example of the saddle type.

Pivot Joints

Pivot joints allow only one kind of movement—rotation around the longitudinal axes of the bones involved. The articulating surfaces in this kind of joint consist of a ring-shaped bony structure rotating around a pivotlike process. An example of a pivot joint is the proximal articulation of the radius with the capitulum of the humerus and the radial notch of the ulna.

Ball-and-Socket Joints

Characterized by a ball-shaped bone structure inserted into a concave socket, ball-and-socket joints afford a greater variety of movements and a larger range of movement than any other kind of joint. They permit angular movement in all directions in addition to rotary movements. Examples of ball-and-socket joints are the shoulder and hip joints. For practical purposes the articulation of the clavicle at the sternum acts as a shallow ball-and-socket joint.

RANGE OF MOTION

Range of motion is the amount of movement through a particular plane that can occur in a joint. It is expressed in degrees. Range of motion in any joint is dependent upon three factors: (1) bone structure of the joint itself; (2) amount of bulk (muscle and other tissue) near the joint, which may restrict movement; and (3) elasticity of the muscles, tendons, and ligaments around the joint. The following examples illustrate how each factor may restrict range of motion.

Example A The range of motion in the elbow joint is restricted by the bony structure which allows the arm to extend no farther than the straight position. It can bend and then straighten, but because of the joint structure, it cannot bend in the opposite direction. Owing to its bone structure, the thoracic spine can do little more than rotate, and most spinal rotation is from that portion of the spine. In contrast, the lumbar spine provides considerable flexion, extension, hyperextension, and lateral flexion, though hardly any rotation. Meanwhile, the cervical spine (neck) is capable of all these movements.

Example B As the biceps of the arm increases in size, extreme flexion at the elbow is restricted. If the biceps becomes excessively large, range of motion at the elbow may be reduced considerably. Also, a person's ability to bend the trunk forward and downward might be restricted by too much bulk in the abdominal region.

Example C It may be impossible to bend over and touch the toes with the hands while the knees are straight, because the muscles and connective tissues of the lower back and upper legs are not elastic (flexible) enough to allow this much movement. In such a case, inadequate elasticity of muscles and connective tissues restricts range of motion.

Inadequate range of motion in certain joints may restrict one's ability to perform. Often range of motion can be increased by regular exercises which stretch muscles and connective tissues in opposition to the particular movement. Inflexibility acts as a resistance or a "brake" to both speed and strength of movement. Continual overcoming of such resistance hastens fatigue and thus reduces endurance. Also, inflexibility of muscles may contribute to injury of those muscles when they are forced to stretch beyond the customary length. However, it is important to recognize that increased flexibility reduces joint stability, and this may contribute to joint injuries in such sports as football, soccer, and wrestling. In some instances, stability of the joint is more important than additional range of motion.

KINDS OF JOINT MOVEMENT

Some joints permit only two movements, flexion and extension, whereas other joints permit several additional movements. A few joints such as the shoulder and hip allow a large variety of movements. The following are descriptions of all the movements that occur in the body joints. The descriptions are based on the assumption that the body is in the standard anatomical position, that is, the erect position with the palms forward. The skeleton in Figure 3-1 demonstrates this position except for the right hand, which is turned inward. The specific movements that can be performed at each joint are given in Chapters 6, 7, and 8.

Flexion (*bending*) is movement of a segment of the body causing a decrease in the angle at the joint, such as bending the arm at the elbow or the leg at the knee. The trunk and neck can flex forward or sideways. Bending sideways is *lateral flexion*, and it can occur to both the right and the left. Sometimes a body segment flexes through the horizontal plane: this is called *horizontal flexion* (or *horizontal adduction*). For example, the arm moves through horizontal flexion at the shoulder joint in throwing the discus or in the sidearm pitch. When the ankle is flexed, causing the top of the foot to draw closer to the tibia, it is said to *dorsiflex* (or *dorsal flex*). The opposite movement is *plantar flexion* (actually extension) at the ankle.

Extension (*straightening*) is movement in the opposite direction of flexion which causes an increase in the angle at the joint, such as straightening the elbow or the knee. *Horizontal extension* (or *horizontal abduction*) occurs when the body segment extends through the horizontal plane. In putting the shot, the opposite arm moves through horizontal extension. *Hyperextension* is extension of a body segment to a position beyond its normal extended position, such as arching the back or extending the leg at the hip beyond its vertical position. (Movement is limited by the strong anterior cruciate ligament.)

Abduction is movement of a body segment in the lateral plane away from the midline of the body, such as raising the leg or the arm sideways.

Adduction is movement of a body segment toward the midline, as moving the arm from the outward horizontal position downward to the vertical position.

Rotation is movement of a segment around its own longitudinal axis. A body segment may be rotated inward (medially) or outward (laterally). The scapula may be rotated upward or downward and the spine may rotate to the right or the left. *Pronation* is rotation of the hand and forearm downward, resulting in a "palm-down" position. *Supination* is rotation of the hand and forearm upward, resulting in a "palm-up" position. *Inversion* is rotation of the foot turning the sole inward. *Eversion* is rotation of the foot turning the sole outward.

Circumduction is a circular or conelike movement of a body segment, such as swinging the arm in a circular movement about the shoulder joint. This kind of movement is also possible in the wrist, trunk, neck, hip, shoulder girdle, and ankle joints.

The shoulder girdle is capable of movements that are somewhat different from other body movements. *Elevation* of the shoulder girdle results when the shoulder is lifted upward as in shrugging the shoulders. *Depression*, the opposite of elevation, results in lowering of the shoulder girdle. *Protraction* (*abduction*) is movement of the shoulder girdle away from the midline of the body, resulting in broadening of the shoulders. *Retraction* (*adduction*) is movement of the shoulder girdle toward the midline of the body, resulting in narrowing of the shoulders. The clavicle is capable of some rotation at the sternum and accompanies scapular upward and downward rotation.

The scapular portion of the shoulder girdle is capable of upward rotation and downward rotation. In *upward rotation* the lower tip of the scapula moves away from the spinal column. *Downward rotation* occurs when the lower tip moves close to the spinal column.

Abduction and adduction at the wrist are based upon the anatomical position (hands at the sides with the palms forward) and are confusing because movements are rarely made from that position. More convenient terms are *radial flexion* (bending toward the thumb side—actually abduction) and *ulnar flexion* (bending toward the little finger—actually adduction).

IMPORTANT CONCEPTS

    1   Bones serve as levers with the joints as axes or pivotal points about which the levers move.

    2   The greatest ranges of motion can be achieved in the most freely movable joints.

3 Limitations on range of motion are primarily due to:
  a Bone structure at the joints
  b Excessive soft tissue (mostly muscle or fat)
  c Nonelastic connective tissue (inflexibility)

4 Various kinesiological terms have been devised to afford a common language for the description of the kinds of movements possible at each of the various movable joints. These terms occur in pairs of opposites (i.e., flexion-extension, abduction-adduction, etc.). Terms account only for movements in certain planes, and not for the many possible directions between the planes. Such "in-between" movements might be described, for example, as flexion-abduction at the shoulder joint, signifying that the upper arm moved in neither direct plane but in a course somewhere between the two.

5 In some cases it is useful in the recognition of specific movements within skills to isolate the joint being considered. To isolate is to concentrate on the body parts on either side of the joint and to exclude the influences of all other parts. In other cases it is preferable not to isolate but to view the skill in its entirety.

STUDENT LABORATORY EXPERIENCES

1 Identify the different bones of the body (excluding the head) and indicate the type (long, short, flat, or irregular) of each bone. Treat the following bones as groups rather than list them individually: phalanges, metacarpals, carpals, ribs, vertebrae, tarsals, and metatarsals.

2 Identify the various joints of the body (excluding the head), indicate the type of joint (ball-and-socket, hinge, etc.), and name the movements of which each joint is capable. Group certain joints as the bones were grouped in project 1.

3 Practice identifying the various kinds of movements as you observe yourself and others in daily activities.

4 Dressed in an activity costume and working with a partner, make and name all of the possible actions at the following joints.

  a Shoulder girdle (look for seven actions)
  b Shoulder joint (look for ten actions)
  c Elbow and forearm (look for four actions)
  d Wrist (look for five actions)
  e Fingers (look for five actions)
  f Thumb (look for seven actions)
  g Trunk (look for four actions)
  h Neck (look for four actions)
  i Pelvis on trunk (look for three actions)
  j Thigh on pelvis (look for ten actions)
  k Knee (look for three actions)
  l Ankle (look for two actions)
  m Foot (look for five actions)
  n Toes (look for four actions)

Chapter 4

Neural Control of Movement

Skilled movement cannot be understood without a basic understanding of the function of nerve tissue. All body activity, both obvious movement and unseen internal movement, is controlled by nerve impulses, chemical stimuli, or both. Normally, without nerve impulses, the muscles are unable to contract, and consequently, the organism is unable to function—or even survive. Other impulses (inhibitory in effect) prevent unwanted contractions or reduce the strength or length of contractions. The timing with which impulses arrive at particular muscles determines skill (coordination of movements). Physiologically, the establishment of coordinated movement patterns is a highly complicated process. Gaining insight into this process is difficult, but it is a mark of a well-prepared physical educator.

NERVOUS-SYSTEM DIVISIONS

The nervous system is conveniently divided into two parts according to function (Figure 4-1). The *autonomic system* is most aptly described by a

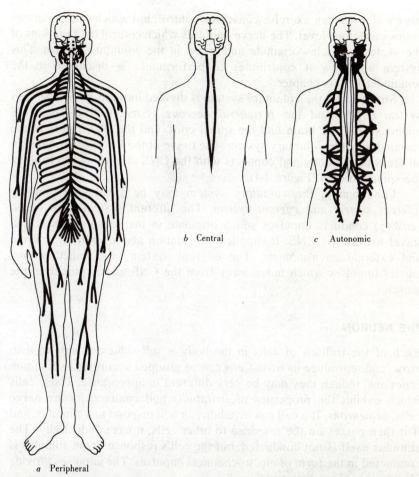

b Central

c Autonomic

a Peripheral

Figure 4-1 Divisions of the human nervous system simplified. All these systems are interconnected and integrated. (*a*) The peripheral nervous system reaches out to the end organs, such as the retina of the eye and nerve endings on the surface of the skin. As shown above, the nerve trunks originating from the central nervous system have been cut off before branching out and reaching the end organs to which they go. Many fine, complex branches are not shown. (*b*) The central nervous system includes the brain and spinal cord. (*c*) The autonomic nervous system, which parallels but lies outside the spinal cord, includes both sympathetic and parasympathetic nerves and their junctions (ganglia). This system "automatically" controls many body functions, such as breathing and digestion.

similar word, *automatic*. There is no conscious control over autonomic functions. Mostly, this system governs vegetative responses which keep us alive; and while of utmost importance to us, it is beyond the scope of this discussion. The *voluntary system* is that part of the nervous system over which we can exercise conscious control, but which often operates below conscious level. The nerve impulses which control the functions of the skeletal muscles originate and travel in the voluntary system. This system and how it contributes to performance is discussed in the remainder of this chapter.

Structurally, the voluntary system is divided into the *central nervous system* (CNS) and the *peripheral nervous system* (PNS). The CNS includes only the brain and the spinal cord, and the PNS refers to the remainder of the voluntary system. The tissue of the PNS is distributed in all areas of the body and connects with the CNS at various levels along the spinal column (Figure 4-1).

Functionally, the voluntary system may be subdivided into the *afferent system* and *efferent system*. The afferent system (also called *sensory*) conducts impulses which originate in the sensory organs and travel toward the CNS. It supplies information about both our internal and external environments. The efferent system (also called *motor*) carries impulses which move away from the CNS and terminate in the muscles.

THE NEURON

Each of the trillions of cells in the body is self-sufficient, able to live, grow, and reproduce its own. Cells can be grouped according to common functions, though they may be very different in appearance. Those cells which exhibit the properties of *irritability* and *conductivity* are nerve cells, or *neurons*. If a cell has irritability, it will respond to a stimulus, and if it then passes on the response to other cells, it has conductivity. The stimulus itself is not conducted, but the cell's response to the stimulus is conducted in the form of electrochemical impulses. The impulses provide information about the stimulus.

A neuron (nerve cell) consists of a cell body and appendages. The appendages, which branch out from the cell body, are of two kinds, *axons* and *dendrites*. Each neuron usually has several dendrites which conduct impulses toward the cell body. They serve as receptors. Each neuron has only one axon, which is the appendage that conducts impulses away from the cell body, usually to muscles or other neurons. Axons are bound together into bundles, and a bundle of axons is called a *nerve* (Figure 4-2).

If a neuron of the afferent (sensory) system receives a stimulus, the information usually terminates in a specialized area of the brain. On the other hand, the stimulus may originate in the brain, travel the efferent (motor) system via a motor neuron, and terminate in a muscle, causing the muscle to contract. In addition, some afferent impulses may travel to the

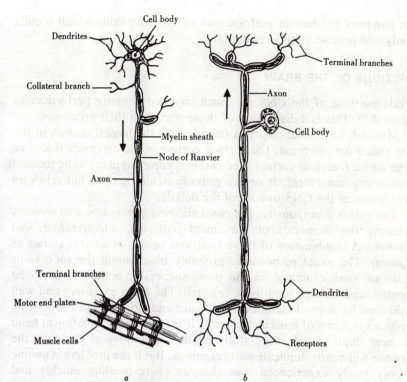

Figure 4-2 Typical spinal neurons. (a) Motor. (b) Sensory.

spinal cord, and there may transfer to the efferent system and arrive at the muscle without brain involvement.

The sensory neurons are quite different from the motor neurons, but they both have the same basic components. Each has a cell body in which all its life functions are centered, and each has its threadlike appendages which perform their specialized functions. There are about three times as many sensory as motor neurons in the human body.

Nerve tissue is either white or gray in color, with the cell bodies gray and the appendages to the bodies white. This difference is functional as well as structural, for the white color of the appendages is due to deposits of a fatty material called *myelin*, which surrounds the appendages. The myelin covering (or *sheath*) serves two functions: (1) insulation, hence the prevention of the dispersion of the impulses to surrounding neurons; and (2) speeding the conduction process. *The larger the fiber and the thicker the myelin sheath, the faster is the conduction of impulses.* An immature CNS will not yet have received its full complement of myelin.

This hampers children in performance of intricate skills which require speedy and precise impulse patterns.

FUNCTIONS OF THE BRAIN

Certain portions of the CNS are much involved in motor performances (Figure 4-3). This is a discussion of those parts and their processes.

Most of the cranial cavity is occupied by the largest section of the brain called the *cerebrum*. The surface portion of the cerebrum is known as the *cortex* (cerebral cortex). The cerebral cortex appears to be the seat of voluntary movement. It orders gross muscular actions but relies on lower levels of the CNS to control the details.

The cortex is responsible for *consciousness*, *perception*, and *memory* (including the memories of movement patterns), *interpretation*, and *reasoning*. A combination of these functions results in what is known as *judgment*. The exact response is probably based upon the success or failure of similar actions in the past; successful actions tend to be repeated, and failures tend to be rejected. The more extensive and well established its store of memories, the faster and more accurate will be its responses in terms of muscular actions. If the particular situation at hand is a near duplicate of successfully handled situations of the past, the response will nearly duplicate past responses. But if the problem is unique or only rarely experienced, the chances of responding quickly and correctly are lessened. In the latter case, the judgment of how to respond will be based on the most nearly related experiences.

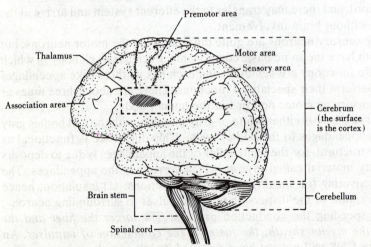

Figure 4-3 Parts of the CNS which have major functions in the control of skeletal muscle actions.

All this indicates that children should be provided with opportunities for experience in a great variety of basic movement patterns before their interests become too specialized. Otherwise, overall skill development will be limited. Extensive experience in motor movements will undoubtedly provide a base from which will result increased success in a variety of motor-movement patterns (skills). The parts of the cerebral cortex directly concerned with motor movements are the *sensory cortex*, *motor cortex*, and *premotor cortex*.

The *sensory cortex* is the terminating area for most of the afferent (sensory) information coming from the various sensory receptors. Interpretation of the sensory impulses takes place in this area. On the basis of the interpretation, action is initiated.

The *motor cortex* provides stimulation to individual muscles and to small muscle groups. A single shock of near-threshold level from an electrode in the motor-cortex area usually elicits a discrete motor movement such as a flick of the finger or a deviation of the lip. The muscle groups of the body are represented in this area according to the discreteness of the movement required. The thumb and forefingers, lips, vocal cords, etc., have large representation, while the areas for postural muscle activities are relatively small. The motor cortex has some coordinating functions, but its primary functions relate to muscle responses in a local area.

The *premotor cortex* produces impulses for complicated patterns of movement (complex coordinations). It has been found that loss of function in this area of the brain destroys the sequence and timing of complex movement patterns. Because many coordinations are basically repetitious, the performance of the premotor area is not as complex as it might seem. But still it is the key area of the brain so far as motor performance is concerned.

The most important differences between the *motor cortex* and the *premotor cortex* are functional. In first learning a skill in which conscious attention must be given to each action, the motor cortex has the greatest involvement. As the skill progresses, the origin of the movements is likely to shift to the premotor cortex. However, the motor cortex still acts as a relay station with fibers passing through it from the premotor cortex.

The *interior of the cerebrum* is composed mostly of white matter which links the cerebrum to all the levels of the spinal cord. This white matter provides fast and often direct impulse conduction from the higher centers of the central nervous system to the various junctions in the spinal cord, and vice versa. The nerve fibers composing the white matter are bundled together according to common functions; the bundles are called *nerve tracts*. The afferent (sensory) bundles are *ascending* tracts and transmit sensory impulses to be interpreted in the sensory cortex. The efferent (motor) bundles are *descending* tracts which conduct impulses from the higher centers to the motor nerves.

In addition to the white matter in the interior of the cerebrum, several clusters of gray matter, called *nuclei*, are present. Little is known about the functions of some of these clusters. However, the largest and probably the most important to motor movement is the thalamus. It serves as an important relay center for both motor and sensory impulses. It has extensive connections with the cortex.

The *cerebellum* is not in the main line of impulse travel between the cerebral cortex and the spinal cord, but it is tied to the main tracts through a series of collateral nerve endings. As far as motor performance is concerned, the function of the cerebellum is to modify motor impulses and thereby contribute to the perfection of the desired movements. A person with a malfunction of the cerebellum will not have the ability to refine a movement or make needed adjustments as the movement progresses. The result will be extreme inaccuracy, overcompensation, and a marked jerkiness in movement. The cerebellum can predict from the present state of the muscles and joints what will occur as the movement progresses and can distribute signals which prevent errors in the movement pattern.

The *brain stem* is the direct connection between the brain and the spinal cord, and thus impulses pass through it in both directions. The functions of the brain stem are more directly concerned with autonomic responses than with responses involving the voluntary nervous system. Part of the stem (the *medulla* and the *pons*) governs the rates of respiration and heartbeat. Some authorities think inhibitory impulses originate in the cerebrum, but most neural experts claim they originate in the brain stem. The inhibitory impulses produce conditions which make it necessary for more facilitative impulses to arrive in order to excite a neuron in the spinal cord. If this phenomenon did not exist with a normal degree of efficiency, we would experience unwanted contractions, and perhaps the inability to stop contractions short of complete fatigue.

Thus, motor activity is influenced by the sum of all the information reaching the motor neuron from both the higher centers and the sensory organs. The descending impulses from the higher centers of the brain, including those voluntarily evoked, are modified on the basis of information from the receptor organs because of the many possible alternatives available through the synaptic system of interneurons within the spinal cord. This coordination of motor information makes possible the movement patterns associated with athletic performances.

Brain and Skill Development

In general, the lower the involvement is in the CNS, the more gross, primitive, and stereotyped the movement will be. For example, a walking or running stride can probably be repeated over and over with an involvement of only the cerebellum, brain stem, and spinal cord. But if an abrupt change of direction or speed is required, the more involved coordinations and judgments would probably require the higher involvement of the cerebral cortex, the thalamus, or both.

It has been postulated that as skill develops, the innervation is relegated to lower centers of the CNS. It is probably more accurate to say that the pathways of impulses within the cerebrum develop "ruts" by repeatedly traveling the same paths, and these ruts allow faster impulse travel with fewer detours from the etched pathway. The performance of the act then requires less conscious consideration to keep the impulses on the proper course. This action can develop to a point where the term "conditioned reflex" would apply.

THE SPINAL CORD

The spinal cord is actually an extension of the brain, encased within the vertebral column (backbone) (Figure 4-4). It is composed of both gray and white matter. The central column of gray matter is butterfly-shaped, or roughly forms the letter H (Figure 4-5). The points of the H are referred to as horns, and the two horns on the anterior (front) side of the column are formed by motor-neuron cell bodies. Called *anterior horn cells*, they

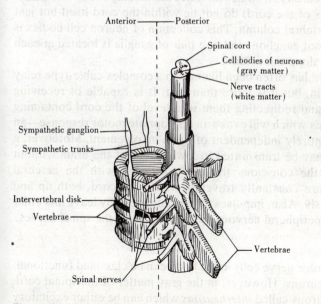

Figure 4-4 Relationship of the vertebral column to the spinal cord, spinal nerves, and sympathetic trunks. (*After Catherine Parker Anthony, Structure and Function of the Body, 4th ed., The C. V. Mosby Company, St. Louis, 1972.*)

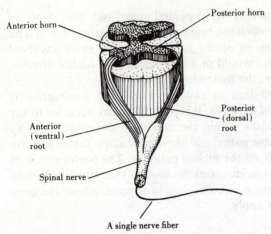

Figure 4-5 Section of the spinal cord showing the anterior and posterior roots of a spinal nerve.

conduct motor impulses. The chief function of the cell bodies forming the *posterior horns* is to serve as connectors from neuron to neuron. This intermediary action becomes important, since the connectors may block signals, pass them on, or distribute them to several levels of the cord or to the brain.

The sensory-neuron cell bodies (at times mistakenly thought to be the posterior horn cells of the cord) do not lie within the cord itself but just adjacent to the vertebral column. This collection of neuron cell bodies is called the dorsal root ganglion, and one pair of ganglia is located at each level of vertebrae along the column.

The spinal cord has often been likened to a complex cable-type relay system to the brain, but it is more than that. It is capable of receiving sensory impulses and redirecting them to a level of the cord containing the anterior neurons which will evoke an appropriate motor response—an accomplishment entirely independent of brain involvement. Moreover, a sensory impulse may be transmitted to lower areas of the brain without involving any of the conscious thought associated with the cerebral cortex. Impulses are constantly traveling within the cord, both up and down simultaneously. Also, impulses may simultaneously leave and enter the cord from the peripheral nervous system (PNS) via the spinal nerves.

Interneurons

All sensory and motor nerve cells in the body can be classified functionally as excitatory neurons. However, in the gray matter of the spinal cord, there are short neurons called *interneurons* which can be either excitatory or inhibitory (Figure 4-6). Some of these neurons, when excited, liberate a

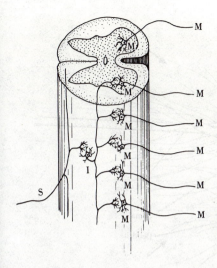

Figure 4-6 An internuncial neuron of the spinal cord: *S*, sensory neuron; *I*, internuncial neuron; *M*, motor neurons. A flexor reflex is distributed in this manner.

chemical which excites other nerve cells by depolarizing the membrane. Others inhibit nerve-cell transmission by hyperpolarizing the cell membrane. The obvious importance of an interneuron system which can inhibit as well as excite is that information from other areas can be modified to suit the needs of the organism by either passing it along the pathways or stopping it from being transmitted. For example, the inhibition or blocking of nerve impulses to those muscles in opposition (antagonistic) to a desired movement is of utmost importance to the efficiency and speed of that movement. The process of inhibiting contractions is mostly automatic and is done at the subconscious level. However, it can also be done consciously to some extent. Ordinarily, with additional practice of a movement the inhibition of the antagonistic muscles becomes quicker and more complete, and the movement becomes more efficient and effective. Thus, the nervous system can either excite or inhibit muscle activity, depending on information received from the higher centers or from receptor organs.

Synapses

A synapse is a junction between two or more neurons. These junctions operate much like the motor end plates, with a release of a chemical that causes depolarization of the fiber to which the message is being passed. Information is passed from one neuron to another via the synapse which connects them (Figure 4-7).

The body is able to regulate the activity of motor neurons by the amount of chemical released at the synapses. For instance, if enough of the vesicles (small glandlike organs, Figure 4-7) at the end of one neuron

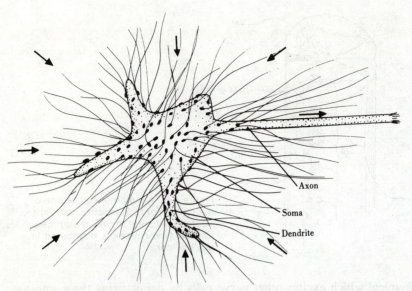

Figure 4-7 A typical synapse, showing many terminals that originate in other neurons.

release their chemical, the membrane potential of the connecting neurons will be reduced to a critical value, and depolarization will occur. However, sometimes the amount of chemical liberated is insufficient to cause depolarization, but it does lower the membrane potential. This is called *facilitation*, and it prepares the neuron to fire more readily if a second volley of impulses arrives while the membrane is still facilitated. If this occurs because of repeated impulse volleys from the same synapse, it is called *temporal summation*. If several synapses are in proximity to each other, their combined effort is called *spatial summation*.

THE PERIPHERAL NERVOUS SYSTEM

It is important not to confuse neurons and nerve fibers with nerves. In review, a neuron is a nerve cell which includes the cell body and all its appendages. Each appendage (usually one long one) is a nerve fiber. When nerve fibers are bound together side by side in a cablelike arrangement, the resulting bundle of fibers is a nerve. The larger nerves are those which connect to the spinal cord; they are called spinal nerves. Spinal nerves have many smaller collaterals (side branches) which become more numerous and smaller as the distance from the spine becomes greater.

All nerve tissue outside the CNS is classified as part of the PNS. Motor neurons originate at the spinal cord and terminate in the muscle tissue which they innervate. Sensory neurons arise in some specialized sensory receptor and terminate at the spinal cord. Both sensory and motor neurons make connection with the spinal cord, and the cord connects to the brain. Very near its entrance to the spinal cord, each spinal nerve branches into two connections (Figure 4-5). One branch goes to the front of the cord (anterior roots), and the other goes to the back of the cord (posterior roots). At this branch the mixed spinal nerve (impulses are conducted in both directions in a mixed nerve) is no longer mixed. The anterior roots conduct only efferent (motor) impulses away from the cord, and the posterior roots conduct only afferent (sensory) impulses toward the cord.

Spinal Nerves

A human being has 31 pairs of spinal nerves (see Figures 4-1, 4-4, and 4-5). One of each pair is on the right side of the body, and the other is on the left side. In general, the spinal nerves of the upper spinal cord innervate the neck and arm muscles, and those of the lower cord innervate the hip and leg muscles. Each of these spinal nerves is about as thick as a pencil and is composed of thousands of individual nerve fibers, each about as thick as a human hair. These fibers vary in length, with the longest ones several feet and the shortest hardly measurable. As previously stated, the larger the fiber and the thicker the myelin sheath, the more quickly the impulse will travel along the fiber. The larger fibers are capable of conducting over 2,000 impulses in 1 second.

Motor Neurons

Special attention is devoted to motor neurons because they carry impulses to muscles. The motor neuron, like other cells, is surrounded by a cell membrane which is metabolically very active, and which provides a barrier between the intracellular and the extracellular fluid so that a membrane potential of electrical difference between the inside and outside of the cell can be maintained. The potential difference between the inside and outside of a typical motor neuron has been measured at about -70 millivolts. When the membrane potential is reduced to a critical value (about -60 millivolts), the sodium ions rush through the membrane and it becomes *depolarized.*

The axon of a motor neuron is enclosed in an insulated sheath called the *neurolemma* or *sheath of Schwann*, and the larger axons also have a *myelin sheath*. It is the myelin sheath that is responsible for the white color of the nerve tissue in the brain, spinal cord, and many peripheral nerves. The sheath of Schwann and the myelin sheath are interrupted at regular intervals by structures called *nodes of Ranvier*, which are small uninsulated areas almost 500 times as permeable as the membranes of some unmyelinated fibers. Since the myelin sheath is an excellent insulator which prevents almost all flow of ions from the cell membrane, the depolarization of myelinated fibers occurs at the nodes of Ranvier, instead of continuously along the entire fiber. This conduction from node to node is thought to be the explanation for the high transmission rate of myelinated fibers, and it probably conserves energy for the axon since only the nodes need to depolarize. It is this property which allows information to be transmitted the length of the axon at the speed of up to 100 meters per second.

Neuromyal Junction

The neuromyal junction is the place where a branch of a motor-nerve fiber reaches the muscle fiber which it innervates. Each of the motor-neuron cell bodies (located in the anterior horn cells of the spinal cord) has its nerve fiber (axon) that conducts impulses to a muscle. Although there is only one conducting fiber (axon) per neuron, the end of this fiber is frayed into a large number of endings. Each of the endings (branches) will innervate one muscle fiber, and all the muscle fibers innervated by one neuron receive the same signal. Each ending of the nerve fiber makes a connection called the *motor end plate.* There are at least as many motor end plates in a muscle as there are muscle fibers (many thousands), and each muscle fiber has one, and sometimes several, motor end plates. The neuromyal junction is that junction between the end plate and muscle fiber (Figure 4-8).

The neuromyal junction should not be confused with a synapse, which is a junction between the appendages of two different neurons. It enables impulses to be transmitted from one neuron to another.

Sensory Receptors

Sensory receptors are all located in the afferent (sensory) nervous system. They are divided into the three following general groups. *Exteroceptors,* which provide information about the external environment, are stimulated by temperature, pressure, light, vibrations, or chemicals. These

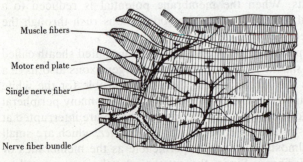

Muscle fibers —

Motor end plate —

Single nerve fiber —

Nerve fiber bundle —

Figure 4-8 Motor nerve endings of intercostal muscle fibers of a rabbit. *(After Bremer, A Textbook of Histology, 6th ed., The Blakiston Company, New York, 1944, p. 201.)*

receptors initiate the impulses for the interpretation of the classic five senses (touch, taste, smell, sight, and hearing). The impulses travel the cranial (within the skull) nerves. *Interoceptors* are mainly receptors which initiate sensory impulses in the visceral organs. Impulses from this group are conducted by the spinal nerves. *Proprioceptors* are of the most direct concern to this discussion. They provide the organism with information about skeletal muscle and joint awareness, which is called the *kinesthetic sense*. These impulses are also conducted by the spinal nerves.

All these receptors are very specific in nature, reacting only to the type of stimulation for which they were designed and rejecting all other types of stimulation under normal conditions.

Proprioceptors are of greatest concern in the study of kinesiology. They are sensory receptors located in the muscles, joints, and connective tissues, and they provide information based upon conditions existing in the areas of their location. These receptors provide information about position, direction, and rate of movement, as well as the amount of muscle tension in a locality. In truth, then, we have a muscle sense as real as the external five senses which can be demonstrated when one or more of the exteroceptive senses—sight, for example—are prevented from functioning. The organism is still aware of movements and positions of body and limb. *Kinesthesis* is the term given to this muscle sense. A performer who states that executing a skill "felt right" is referring to the kinesthetic perception of the action. The sense becomes keener as the act is repeated a sufficient number of times. However, this does not necessarily mean that the skill is performed correctly; often the performer has an incorrect mental picture of the action, or an erroneous concept of a correct performance.

THE IMPULSE: EXCITATION AND CONDUCTION

The nerve fiber is nearly cylinder-shaped. Under rest conditions, an electrical potential exists across the fiber from its outside to its inside. The fiber's outer area is electrically positive, and its interior is electrically negative. This condition results from an abundance of positively charged sodium ions located in the fluids on the outside of the fiber's membrane. The positive ions strive to enter the fiber through the membrane in an effort to establish equilibrium (neutral electrical state). It is as if a spring were compressed and its tension awaits release. The sodium ions are prevented from entering the interior of the fiber because of the impermeability of the fiber's membrane. Two other conditions, which may appear unimportant at this time, need to be noted: (1) a much smaller number of potassium ions (also carrying a positive charge), which are *not* restricted by the impermeability of the membrane, pass freely between the outside and inside of the nerve fibers but are incapable of causing an impulse (no resistance to passage—no tension); and (2) all points along the nerve fiber are electrically the same, meaning that no difference exists in potential between any two points along the length of the fiber.

Conduction of Impulses

The nerve impulse is actually a reversal of the electrical charge of the nerve fiber. As the impulse progresses along the fiber, it somehow affects the permeability of the membrane to sodium ions, and a very minute amount of sodium quickly rushes in, providing a momentary change in electrical potential. At this moment, the outside of the fiber is electrically negative to the inside. The electrical difference between the nerve fiber at this point and at other points is called the *action potential*, and its strength is between 50 and 100 microvolts (100 microvolts = 0.0001 volt). The impulse moves along the fiber by removing the membrane's resistance to sodium ions, thus allowing some of them to enter the fiber at another point. The passage from one point on the nerve fiber to the next is much like the successive action of a falling row of dominoes—when one falls, each adjacent one is knocked over in succession. One impulse may travel as fast as 90 to 120 meters per second, depending on the particular fiber and its condition (Figure 4-9).

Speed of Impulse Conduction

Reaction time is the interval of time between the signal to respond (stimulus) and the beginning of the response, not including the time it takes to accomplish the task. The latter is *movement time*. Reaction time reflects the lag in the functions of an individual's nervous system. Variations in this time occur as a result of the distance the impulse must travel, the number of synapses it crosses over, the irritability of the receptors and synapses, the intensity of the stimulus, the chemical state and composition of the innervated tissues, and perhaps other factors. When a reaction involves nothing more than an automatic reflex, the terms "reflex time" and "reaction time" are interchangeable. But often the reaction demands involvement of the cerebrum, in which case it may be desirable to call this "thought delay" and distinguish it from the time it takes for the signal to travel the rest of the system. This "thought time"—also termed *analysis*, *interpretation*, or *judgment* time—is separable from reflex time, but not from reaction time.

Thought time means that the performer consciously analyzes the situation and then selects the proper response with the greatest haste. Reaction time includes a combination of reflex time and thought time, if thought is required. In most cases, the teacher or coach can have more influence on judgment (thought) time than on reflex time; however, it has been shown that reflex time can be improved somewhat in *specific* tasks. When a response is new to an individual, the reaction is usually slow,

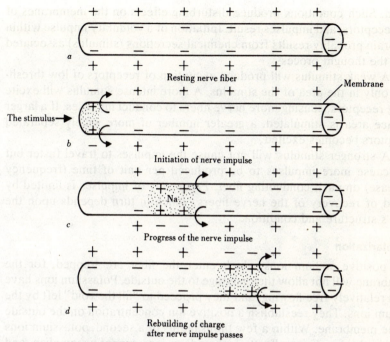

Figure 4-9 The progress of the nerve impulse along the nerve fiber. (a) The resting nerve fiber, with positive charge on the outside of the membrane and negative charge within. (b) The initiation of the nerve impulse; for a fraction of a second the charges on the membrane are reversed. (c) The nerve impulse passes rapidly along the nerve fiber. (d) The charge on the membrane returns to normal after a brief refractory period. *(After Russell Myles DeCoursey, The Human Organism, 4th ed., McGraw-Hill Book Company, New York, 1974.)*

allowing great potential for improving reaction time. As the response is repeated many times, it becomes more automatic, reaction time becomes shorter, and the potential for improving reaction time is lessened. It should be remembered that a small change in reaction time may often have significant influence on performance. Reaction time is highly specific to a particular movement. Therefore, it seems that the current popularity of reaction drills, called *quick cals*, for increasing athletic quickness has little justification unless the movements duplicate those used in the contest, in which case both reaction and movement times may be reduced.

Excitation

Impulses result from a stimulus caused by environmental changes near or about (1) special sensory receptors, (2) free nerve endings, or (3) neurons located in various areas of the brain. Impulses can be initiated by temperature changes, pressure changes, and electrical or chemical stimulation. Such conditions produce disturbing effects on the membranes of the receptors, and impulses result. Initiation of a voluntary impulse within the brain probably results from chemical secretions (stimulus) associated with the thought process.

A weak stimulus will produce excitation of receptors of low thresholds only in the area of the stimulus. A more intense stimulus will excite more receptors, causing more nerve fibers to conduct impulses. If a larger surface area is stimulated, a greater number of more widely separated receptors becomes excited.

A stronger stimulus will not cause the impulses to travel faster but will cause more impulses to be produced per unit of time (frequency increase) on each conducting fiber. Frequency of impulses is limited by speed of recovery of the nerve fibers, which in turn depends upon the fiber's structure and condition.

Repolarization

The positive sodium ions which enter the fiber are trapped, for the membrane will not allow their passage to the outside. Potassium ions have been relatively free flowing, and they proceed to "fill the void" left by the sodium ions. They reestablish a positive ion concentration on the outside of the membrane. Within a few thousandths of a second, potassium ions provide the equalizing effect which sodium ions cannot accomplish, and the nerve fiber is again ready to conduct an impulse. Repolarization trails directly behind each impulse. This process can continue for 100,000 successive impulses in some fibers because very few of the total number of sodium ions cross the membrane with each impulse, and many more are still available. When the fiber is no longer receiving impulses, the sodium ions are returned to the outside by a metabolic action called the *sodium pump*. The normal range of impulse frequencies is between 10 and 500 per second.

Reflexes

An innate (inborn) reflex is a predictable response to a given stimulus which is accomplished below the level of conscious control. Such reflexes must originate in the afferent system, and the efferent (motor) response will occur before the organism is consciously aware of the stimulus. If the organism is aware of the stimulus, the reflex response may occur without interference, or it may be consciously inhibited or intensified.

Reflexes which are learned (not innate) are called *conditioned reflexes*. If the performer learns to respond in the same manner to the same stimulus, this is a conditioned reflex. A conscious movement can be superimposed on a reflex, either innate or conditioned, by consciously adding nerve impulses.

Three innate reflexes seem most pertinent to human performances. The first and simplest of these is the *stretch reflex*. It depends upon the muscle spindles to initiate the impulse volley when the muscle is stretched. For the human being to remain erect, the posture muscles (mostly extensors) must be active to support against the pull of gravity. If there were no muscular contraction, the body would collapse. An example of a stretch reflex occurs when one falls asleep while sitting, and the head nods (the neck flexes), causing a stretch to be placed on the neck extensors. The stretch reflex responds, returning the head to the erect position with a jerk (see Figure 4-10).

The stretch reflex is primarily a postural reflex, but the principle of it is used to aid contractions in voluntary movements. If a performer wishes to throw, the muscles that will be used in the action phase are placed on sudden stretch from the windup. The result is that the throwing muscles receive impulses originating in their own spindles (stretch reflex), in addition to impulses initiated in the CNS. Thus, the contraction is stronger than it would be without impulses from the reflex.

Pressure on the bottoms of the feet initiates the *extensor thrust reflex*, which produces contraction of extensor muscles. This reflex results in extension at all the weight-bearing joints, and is especially important in maintaining balance and in preventing too much flexion upon landing from a jump or landing while in locomotion. Its extension pattern can be altered at one or several of the joints by the stretch reflex or by voluntary impulses. The importance of this reflex is that it causes the performer to automatically dissipate the shock of landing, and conscious thought can be devoted to other problems at hand.

The *withdrawal* (flexor) *reflex* is somewhat more complicated than the stretch reflex. The flexor muscles ordinarily respond to pain stimuli. If a person touches a hot stove, for example, the receptors will send a sensory impulse volley to the spinal cord, where a synapse response is made with an internuncial neuron. From here the impulse volley is distributed to the appropriate levels of the spinal cord (higher, lower, or both), which house the motor-neuron cell bodies that connect to the flexor muscles, causing withdrawal of the injured part (Figure 4-6). Apparently, this response is accomplished before the impulse reaches the brain because spinal animals (brain destroyed) perform the task with the same ease as intact specimens.

ESTABLISHMENT OF SKILL PATTERNS

Skill is the ability to perform a combination of specific movements smoothly and effectively. It is the coordination of all the different muscles involved, whether they are agonists, antagonists, neutralizers, or stabiliz-

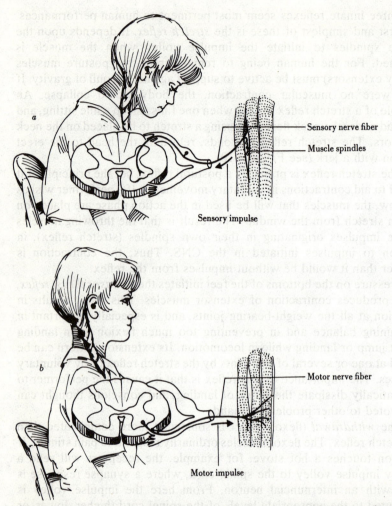

Sensory nerve fiber

Muscle spindles

Sensory impulse

Motor nerve fiber

Motor impulse

Figure 4-10 A postural stretch reflex. (a) represents relaxation of trunk muscles causing an increase in length of muscle fibers, which acts to stimulate the neuromuscular spindles (sensory receptor in muscles). The resulting impulse is transmitted to the spinal cord by way of sensory neuron. (b) represents a motor impulse being transmitted to the muscle originally lengthened by relaxation. The muscle contracts and regains its former length so that the posture is also regained. (*After Sigmund Grollman, The Human Body, 3rd ed., The Macmillan Company, New York, 1974.*)

ers. In other words, skill is the ability to use the correct muscles at the correct time, with the exact force necessary to perform the desired movements in the proper sequence and timing.

Coordinated movements occur as a result of muscle contractions, and muscles contract only in response to nerve impulses. Therefore, coordinated movement occurs if nerve impulses reach the proper muscles at the correct time.

Even though skill is a result of the teamwork of the nervous and muscular systems, it is primarily a function of the nervous system, since the muscles contract at specified times and with certain amounts of force as dictated by the nervous system. Of course, there are some conditions of the muscles themselves, such as strength and speed of contraction, which influence skill. But even these factors are partially determined by the functioning of the nervous system.

It is generally agreed that skillful acts are accomplished without conscious thought, except for the thought needed to initiate the act. Consequently, highly skillful acts are mostly *conditioned reflexes*. For example, we can perform the skill of walking while we are occupied in deep thought or conversation. Actually, we may walk more skillfully under these conditions than if we concentrate on the movements. The movements involved in walking result from conditioned reflexes. During active contests, it is often necessary for the performer to concentrate on external cues, and any preoccupation with specific body movements will destroy effectiveness. In such cases, while the general idea of the desired response is conveyed by the cerebrum, lower centers of the central nervous system work out the details.

In the final analysis, the resulting movements are dependent upon three factors: (1) which neurons conduct impulse volleys, (2) the frequencies of the impulses, and (3) exactly when these impulses reach the muscle fibers. Another important factor is which muscles are prevented from contracting because of neural inhibition.

As a certain skill is developed, its specific movements tend to become less variable and more exact, because the selected patterns of impulses become more easily duplicated. This is because the impulse volleys tend to follow previously established pathways within the nervous system. As stated earlier, the impulses are conducted along the paths of least resistance. Nerve pathway possibilities are inherited, but it is *use* that determines the development of the pathways. As certain synapses are used repeatedly, their thresholds are lowered, and the chance of repeating that pattern under like conditions is increased. Conversely, it is difficult to blaze new pathways for the same act once the pathways have been established. As in walking through deep grass, the more often a certain path is taken, the deeper the pathway becomes. Paths not repeated tend to become obscure, but they are not completely eliminated.

When one begins to learn a skill, many pathways are possible. But gradually, pathways are selected which have resulted in successful performances, and the other pathways are rejected. The more often a pathway is repeated, the more firmly ingrained the pattern becomes and the more difficult it is to avoid. Gradually the path is used with greater ease and smoothness, and superfluous movements are eliminated. Unproductive paths are rejected, and the act becomes "skillful."

Certain obstacles exist, such as the following: (1) Conditions, both of the internal and external environments, are never exactly the same from one time to the next. (2) Most skills are complex enough to involve several joints and many muscles, and even though the skill may appear correct, variations in only a few movements may detract from success. (3) The performer may incorrectly judge the performance as successful and continue to perform incorrectly. For instance, a performer may throw with the wrong foot forward and assume this is the correct procedure because of a degree of success. Or a young basketball player who is a head taller than the opposition may use an undesirable shooting technique with much success until an opponent of equal height appears.

From Basic to Refined Skills

The acquisition of refined skills necessitates prior learning of gross skill patterns (basic skills). Highly refined skills are usually only slight modifications of basic patterns. For example, if a child learns a basic throwing pattern by throwing objects of all sorts under a variety of conditions, the addition of a forearm rotation and a wrist snap in the direction of the little finger can result in a curve ball. Similarly, a tennis player who has learned the basic tennis strokes can add slight modifications which result in spin (english) on the ball. In golf, the basic stroke patterns are learned rather quickly, but the refinement of them and the learning of stroke variations require much time and practice. In every athletic activity there is a set of basic skills, and there are refinements and variations of the basic skills which make the difference between *mediocrity* and *excellence*.

Instructional Techniques

In theory, skill development is a simple matter, but in actuality it is very difficult. One key is *repetition*. But, it is necessary to repeat the skill pattern *correctly*. Otherwise, lack of skill or incorrect technique will result.

In order to ensure correct practice, the learner must know what is correct. This means practice must be preceded by information about the correct technique. The information may be obtained from *instruction* by one who knows correct technique, from *reading*, *watching film*, or *observing a skilled performer*. Once the learner understands the elements of correct technique and has had some opportunity to practice the skill, *error detection and correction* become an effective tool for the instructor. As the learner practices the skill over and over, the instructor detects imperfections and prescribes methods for correcting them. Bit by bit, as a result of practice and correction, the skill is perfected.

A key role of the teacher or coach is to recognize incorrect techniques and prescribe drills which will cause improvement. The younger the performer, the easier, quicker, and more precise will be development, assuming the nervous system has matured adequately to develop the skill in question.

Reciprocal Inhibition

The inhibition or blocking of nerve impulses to those muscles in opposition (antagonistic) to a desired movement is of utmost importance to the efficiency of that movement. It appears that the antagonistic muscles are automatically inhibited. Thus, one may wonder why it should even be discussed. It must be recognized that with the practice of a movement, the inhibition of the antagonistic muscles becomes quicker and more complete. Obviously, antagonistic tension interferes with the effectiveness of a performance, and by reducing tension, effectiveness is increased, and the onset of fatigue is postponed.

Anxiety or other emotional involvement can limit the effectiveness of reciprocal inhibition. Thus, such heightened emotions tend to hinder performances where fine muscle coordinations are required. Golf is an activity that is adversely affected by anxiety. Another example is a basketball player who misses a crucial free throw when the pressure is on. Conversely, activities not requiring a high degree of fine muscle control may benefit from heightened emotions. For example, the performance of a football lineman or a shot-putter may be enhanced by anxiety. But if the football player must handle the ball, his performance is likely to suffer. Many so-called "sophomore mistakes" are attributable to the inability to contend with emotional stress because it has a detrimental effect on refined neuromuscular coordinations.

PRACTICAL APPLICATIONS

Because the nervous system is very complex and its functions are not visually obvious, people often fail to recognize its importance in performance. The strength, speed, and duration with which muscles contract all depend directly upon the nervous system. Following are some specific examples of how knowledge of the functioning of the nervous system may influence performance.

1 The preparatory stage of a throwing or striking action, such as the backswing in golf or tennis, exists only to achieve the most advantageous forward swing. It is known that if a muscle is stretched approximately one-third beyond its resting length, it is best prepared for a forceful contraction. This is partly because the muscle is under greater tension (like a towrope, the slack has been removed) and can effectively shorten

through a greater distance and partly because impulses, in addition to the voluntary impulses, result from the stretch reflex, adding to the force of the contractions.

To avoid stimulation of inhibitory impulses and to maximize the efforts of the stretch reflex, the backswing must be fairly rapid. This negates the use of an extremely slow backswing, especially stopping the action at the height of the backswing. On the other hand, too fast a backswing generates a momentum in the direction *opposite the action*. This momentum must be overcome by contractions of the muscles which produce the forward swing.

The conclusion is to select that speed of backswing which is fast enough to utilize the stretch reflex, but not too fast. Typically, a performer tends to select a backswing which is too fast, in which case he should be taught to slow it down. However, occasionally the backswing is too slow, resulting in loss of force application. Similar examples could be given in batting actions, jumping actions, and other performances where the stretch reflex contributes.

2   To improve flexibility in an area of the body, movement must be consistently performed to stretch the muscles and connective tissues which tend to resist the movement. In this case, inhibitory impulses to the muscles which resist movement are essential. It is wise to avoid jerky movements which cause the stretch reflex. Slow stretching results in the blocking of impulses and the release of tension in the muscles, consequently allowing a greater degree of stretch. Also, too fast an action may produce enough momentum to stretch tissues too far and cause injury. Slow and steady stretching is safer and more effective for increasing flexibility, although some flexibility may be achieved by bouncing at the end of the range of motion.

IMPORTANT CONCEPTS

1   Neurons possess the properties of *irritability* (response to stimulation) and *conductivity* (the ability to transmit impulses). Because of these properties the stimulation of muscle tissue and ultimately the control of movement lies in the nervous system.

2   Children are unable to perform intricate skills with the same quickness of response and precision as adults, because their immature nervous systems have not accumulated their full complement of *myelin*.

3   Much of the brain plays a role in skilled performance, but the *premotor cortex* appears to store and direct the emission of preestablished volleys of nerve impulses which constitute the stimuli for timed and coordinated skills. These "computer tapes" of impulses are subconsciously emitted in response to an "order to act" and are subject to modification from both conscious and subconscious neural sources.

4   The skill-learning process advances to less and less conscious control with appropriate practice, allowing the performer to concentrate on necessary cues. Finally, this results in *conditioned reflexes*.

5 Skilled movements require both *facilitating* and *inhibiting* impulses affecting the synapses of motor neurons, causing their motor units to contract, or blocking contraction, respectively.

6 The *kinesthetic sense* provides the "feel" for a movement and is due to responses of sensory receptors (*proprioceptors*) located within muscles, tendons, and joints.

7 *Reaction time* may be improved with practice of the specific task.

8 The correct use of inherent reflexes, especially the *stretch reflex*, may induce superior performances.

9 *Skill* implies efficient and effective performance. It includes: (*a*) coordination and timing of muscular actions, (*b*) control of the power (strength and speed) of the contractions, (*c*) accurate direction of all joint movements (selection of particular motor units), and (*d*) prevention of antagonistic and extraneous muscular tension. All the foregoing occur in response to the dictates of nerve-impulse volleys. Variations in external and internal environments make it all but impossible to accomplish exact duplication with each repetition.

10 Heredity establishes one's skill-learning potential, and certain skill patterns are inherently more natural than others. All skills must be learned, however.

11 Skill performances are learned by repeating successful actions and rejecting those considered unsuccessful. In one sense, all skill is learned through "trial and error," since each individual must experience it to form personal impulse volleys. Teaching can help eliminate unproductive trials from consideration and thus avoid errors.

12 A variety of *basic skills* established in youth permits ease of attainment of more refined skills later.

13 Appropriate control of the anxiety associated with competition may aid performance. Without appropriate control, anxiety may partly destroy certain kinds of skills.

14 The keys to successful skill development are *correct repetition* and *specificity* of the performance. *Any* variation from competitive conditions will reduce the effectiveness of the practice.

Muscular Actions— Key to Human Movement

The muscular system is the focal point in movement. If we want to be able to move with greater force, we strengthen the muscles. If we want to continue movement for a longer time, we increase the endurance of the muscles. When we want faster movements, we attempt to speed the rate of muscle contractions. If we want to perform movements more efficiently and smoothly, we increase the coordination of the muscles. If we want to alter body proportions, we may increase the size and alter the contour of muscles.

Part Two tells many interesting things about muscles. Chapter 5 explains the great versatility of muscles—how they may be used in a variety of ways during performance. Chapter 6, 7, and 8 give explanations and many illustrations of the locations and the specific actions of the individual muscles and muscle groups. However, the complete anatomy of skeletal muscles is beyond the scope or intent of these chapters. Chapter 9 tells how to improve the effectiveness of muscle contractions in performance. Chapter 10 is an example of how to perform a muscle analysis of a particular skill.

Chapter 5

Specific Muscle Uses

A muscle can only contract or relax, and under normal conditions contraction results only from a series of nerve impulses. A muscle may contract fully or partially, with maximum force or less. A muscle may contract isometrically or isotonically, singly (in rare instances) or as a member of a group. Because muscles can contract in these different ways, they have the ability to act in different roles and to change quickly from one role to another.

ROLES OF MUSCLES

At any given time a particular skeletal muscle may play the role of *agonist*, *antagonist*, *stabilizer*, or *neutralizer*. It may change from one role to another instantly, and during a motor performance, a particular muscle may function in all the different roles at different times. The role of a muscle is determined by its particular function at a given time during performance.

Agonist (Mover) Role

A muscle is a mover (agonistic to the movement) when its concentric contraction contributes to the desired movement of a segment of the body. For instance, in flexion at the elbow, the biceps brachii is a mover, as are seven other muscles in this case. Some muscles are movers for more than one action in a particular joint, and some cause movements in more than one joint, For instance, the biceps brachii may cause elbow flexion, shoulder flexion, or lower-arm supination, depending on the simultaneous actions of other muscles. If the biceps contracted singly, all three of its movements would occur simultaneously. If only one or two of the movements are desired, the other movements may be omitted by the coordinated contractions of other muscles. When this is done, the other muscles are said to neutralize part of the functions of the biceps.

Mover muscles are classified as *prime movers* and *assistant movers*. A prime mover is a muscle whose chief function is to cause the particular movement, and one which makes a strong contribution to that movement. An assistant mover is a muscle which has the ability to assist in the movement but is of only secondary importance to the movement. An example is the triceps brachii, a prime mover in elbow extension but only an assistant mover in shoulder extension. In shoulder extension, the latissimus dorsi and teres major muscles are the prime movers; when the load is heavy, the triceps muscle (along with others) is called upon for assistance. There is usually more than one prime mover in a particular joint action, and there are often several assistant movers. There are prime-mover muscles for all the movable joints, and there are assistant movers for most of the joints.

Antagonist Role

A muscle is antagonistic to a movement when it must relax to allow the movement to occur. Antagonist muscles cause actions opposite those caused by the agonist muscles. The triceps brachii is antagonistic to flexion at the elbow; therefore, the triceps must relax in order to allow flexion to occur efficiently. It is possible to achieve flexion against triceps opposition if the force of the flexors exceeds that of the triceps. However, this is inefficient unless a controlled movement is needed. In elbow extension the triceps becomes an agonist and the biceps an antagonist; in other words, the biceps and triceps are antagonistic to each other. Generally, extensors and flexors are antagonistic to each other, as are abductors and adductors and medial rotators and lateral rotators. In motor performances it is important for antagonistic muscles to experience just the right amount of controlled relaxation to permit smooth and efficient movements. This is an important aspect of neuromuscular coordination (Figure 5-1).

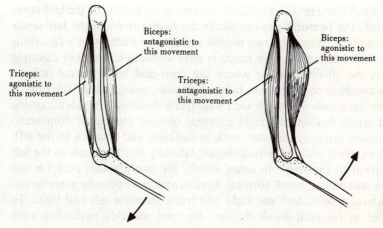

Figure 5-1 Biceps and triceps muscles exchange roles as the arm movement changes from extension to flexion.

Stabilizer (Fixator) Role

In order for a segment of the body to move, the body part on which the segment moves must possess the right amount of stability. For instance, when the arm moves at the shoulder joint, the shoulder girdle must be held firm by the contraction of certain muscles which attach to it. Without being stabilized, the shoulder girdle would move and thus reduce the effectiveness of the force which the muscles of the shoulder joint exert on the arm. The same could be said about movement of the leg around the hip joint (the pelvic region must be stable) or about movement at numerous other joints. When acting as a stabilizer, a muscle usually contracts statically (isometrically) because its role is to hold the body segment motionless or nearly motionless. Therefore, the muscle shortens very little, if any, during its contraction, and it causes very little, if any, movement. A clear example is the action of the abdominal muscles during floor push-ups. If these muscles did not contract statically, the trunk would bow, causing the exercise to be performed incorrectly.

Another important fact to remember is that muscles make major contributions toward stablizing joints. Even though it is ligaments that bind the bones together at a joint, muscles whose tendons cross over the joint contribute much to stability, and thus muscles help to prevent injuries to joints.

Neutralizer Role

A muscle plays the role of neutralizer when it equalizes or nullifies one or more actions of another muscle. To neutralize each other, two muscles must cause opposite movements. For example, the pectoralis major and the latissimus dorsi muscles are both movers in adduction of the humerus; in addition, the pectoralis major flexes the humerus while the latissimus dorsi extends it. When the two muscles neutralize each other's functions of flexion and extension, the result is pure adduction. Another example occurs in the sit-up exercise where the right and left external oblique muscles combine to contribute to trunk flexion, neutralizing each other's functions in trunk lateral flexion and trunk rotation. Besides causing forward trunk flexion, the right external oblique muscle, if contracted singly, would laterally flex the trunk to the right and rotate it to the left. The left external oblique muscle would laterally flex the trunk to the left and rotate it to the right. In other words, the two muscles perform one common movement, trunk forward flexion, and two opposite movements, trunk lateral flexion left and right and trunk rotation left and right. To cooperate in forward trunk flexion, the two muscles neutralize each other's roles as lateral trunk flexors and rotators.

Occasionally, a portion of a muscle must neutralize another portion of the same muscle. An example is the contraction of the deltoid muscle to abduct the humerus (Figure 5-2). The anterior portion of the deltoid also causes horizontal flexion, while the posterior portion also causes horizontal extension. The horizontal extension and flexion movements are neutralized when pure abduction is performed. Further, the anterior deltoid rotates the humerus inwardly, and the posterior deltoid rotates it outwardly. These rotations are also neutralized in pure abduction of the humerus. Often neutralizations are responsible for guiding the direction of movements and thus contributing to accuracy. An underarm action at the shoulder joint such as a bowling delivery, for instance, primarily involves a flexion movement while abductors and adductors balance tendencies to move left or right as the arm proceeds forward.

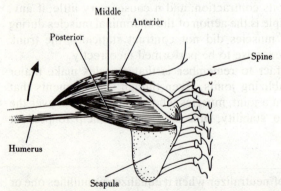

Figure 5-2 The three portions of the deltoid muscle contract to cause shoulder abduction. Middle portion causes pure abduction, while the anterior and posterior portions contribute to abduction and neutralize each other's functions.

Synergist Role

The term *synergist* has been used in so many different ways that it has become confusing and ambiguous. For example, some kinesiologists have used it to describe an assistant mover, and others have used it to describe a neutralizer. Some sources have even implied that a muscle which plays a secondary role in stabilization is a synergist. Because of the confusion associated with the term, it has been purposely omitted from use in this text, except for this explanation.

COORDINATED ACTIONS OF MUSCLES

Motor muscles nearly always act in groups rather then individually; whenever a major motor movement occurs, many muscles contract and numerous coordinations take place (see Figure 5-3). Those muscles which are agonistic to the movement (both prime movers and assistant movers) contract concentrically and must be coordinated with each other in order to produce maximum total contractile force. Those muscles antagonistic to the movement must relax and must be coordinated with the agonist muscles, or they provide unwanted resistance to the movement. Numerous other muscles must contract to stabilize parts of the body on which the active segments move, and these muscles must be coordinated with the agonists and antagonists. Also, many other contractions are required to neutralize undesired actions of some of the active muscles.

Visualize the tremendous number of muscular actions involved in various roles during the common, but very complex, overarm pitch, keeping in mind that the ball is pitched with the whole body, not just the

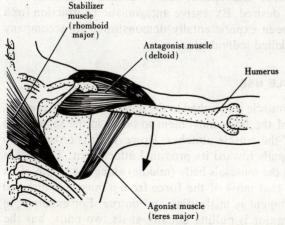

Figure 5-3   Teamwork of three muscles in arm adduction: teres major as agonist, deltoid (middle) as antagonist, rhomboid major as stabilizer of the scapula.

arm. Also, visualize the complex coordinations involved in the pole vault, discus throw, swimming the crawl stroke, or field running in football. It is absolutely amazing that so many muscles can be so precisely coordinated into so many different functions within a brief moment. The extent to which the necessary contractions can be effectively coordinated with each other is the prime element of what is known as *skill*. Hence, when we practice to improve skill, we attempt to perfect the coordinated contractions of the many different muscles in their various roles.

Neuromuscular coordination (or neuromuscular skill) is the act of causing each movement to occur in the correct sequence and timing and with just the right amount of force. When a well-coordinated act occurs, it appears smooth and rhythmical. Of course, body movements normally occur as a result of muscular contractions, and muscles contract when directed to do so by the nervous system. Therefore, when coordinated movements occur, it is because the nerve impulses reach the proper muscles at the correct times. The muscles then cause the movement patterns which constitute skilled performance.

The concept known as reciprocal inhibition means that when motor neurons carry impulses to agonistic muscles, inhibitory impulses are carried to the muscles which are antagonistic to the movement. This prevents them from contracting, which would detract from the speed and force of the desired movement. The extent to which inhibition is accomplished determines the amount of internal resistance to the movement. One of the important aspects of skill is the ability to cause the correct amount of inhibition of antagonistic muscles. When maximum speed and force movements are desired, complete inhibition of antagonistic muscles would be ideal. When controlled movements are needed with less than maximum force and speed, some voluntary resistance by antagonistic muscles is desired. Excessive antagonistic contraction for a given movement has been experimentally demonstrated to accompany performances of less skilled individuals.

MECHANICS OF MUSCLE USE

The proximal end of a muscle is attached to the more stable body portion, and this causes most of the body movement to occur in the segment to which the distal end of the muscle attaches. However, it is erroneous to assume that a muscle pulls toward its proximal attachment. The pull is from both ends toward the muscle's belly (middle) along the length of its fibers. The conception that most of the force from a muscle is directed toward the distal attachment is misleading and untrue. For example, in Figure 5-3, the teres major is pulling equally at its two ends, but the humerus, which is the least stable of the two segments, performs most of the movement.

The amount of movement that occurs in any body segment as a result of muscle contraction is determined by the relative stability of the segment involved. For example, when the deltoid contracts, the arm usually moves on the shoulder girdle because the shoulder girdle is the more stable of the two segments, and other muscles usually contract to stabilize it and reduce its movement further. If the shoulder girdle were less stable than the arm, it would move on the arm because the amount of tension applied to both segments by the deltoid is equal. Following are reasons why some segments are less movable (more stable) than others.

1 *Segment structure.* If a muscle attaches on both the scapula and the humerus (see teres major, Figure 5-3), the pull on the humeral attachment can cause free movement of the humerus at the shoulder joint (ball-and-socket joint). The pull on the scapula can produce a movement of the scapula only over the rib cage, and the scapula is not highly movable and is easily stabilized. Its movement is greatly restricted by the structure of that region of the body. Therefore, when the muscle applies equal force to the scapula and the humerus, the humerus moves the greater amount because it is freer to move.

2 *Stabilizing actions of muscles.* The extent to which muscles are used to stabilize a segment influences its movability. For example, the rhomboid muscle often works in connection with the teres major to stabilize the scapula. The action of the rhomboid is in direct opposition to the movement caused by the teres major on the scapula, and the two forces cancel each other, causing stability of the scapula. As a result of this, all the force of pull by the teres major can now be effective on its attachment on the humerus, making this action more extensive than would be possible if both segments moved freely.

In some instances a muscle will reverse its customary function. This means the proximal attachment becomes the movable part. For example, think of the hip flexors raising the legs in a forward and upward direction as in running. But, when we perform a sit-up, the same hip flexors pull the same way except that the legs are stabilized, causing the trunk to be the movable part. If both the trunk and legs are equally free to move, the result is an exercise called the V-sit, in which both the legs and upper body leave the floor simultaneously and move toward each other.

Another essential consideration is that most muscles act as single units: that is, they are not capable of exerting force in portions. Their pulling force is directed to their attachments, and the forces produced work to accomplish *all* their assigned movements, regardless of which motor units were selected to act. However, a few muscles are subdivided into parts, and any part can be contracted separately to cause an action which the whole muscle cannot cause. Examples of such muscles are the trapezius (Figure 6-15), which is divided into parts I, II, III, and IV; and the deltoid (Figure 6-13), which has three parts—anterior, middle, and posterior. The anterior deltoid causes arm horizontal flexion, among other movements, while the posterior portion causes the opposite movements, and the middle portion abducts the arm. If all three portions were contracted simultaneously, the arm would only abduct.

A muscle, because of its position of attachment, may contribute to more than one movement. It is established that all a muscle can do is contract and relax; therefore, it is apparent that when a muscle contracts, it tends to cause all the movements of which it is capable. The only way any of the movements can be prevented is for another muscle to contract simultaneously and neutralize the undesired actions. For example, the serratus anterior muscle (Figure 6-17) causes abduction and upward rotation of the scapula. It is not possible for that muscle to contract to cause only abduction or only upward rotation. Therefore, when only abduction is desired, another muscle must be called upon to nullify the upward-rotation action. In this case, the most logical choice is the pectoralis minor (Figure 6-17), whose function is to rotate the scapula downward. The two muscles neutralize each other's rotational actions and permit the one desired action, abduction of the scapula.

KINDS OF MUSCLE ACTION

A muscle contraction varies in speed, force, and duration to cause different kinds of movements, which vary in relative importance in different performances.

Maximum-Force Movements

In maximum-force movements the agonist (mover) muscles apply maximum force and contract at maximum speed, resulting in fast and forceful movement. An example is putting a shot, where the agonistic muscles contract maximally and the resistance always exists to some degree. One's ability to coordinate maximum contraction of agonists with minimum resistance by the antagonists is a key factor in the force and speed of that movement. Maximum-force movements may be of two kinds, *continuous-force* and *ballistic*.

Continuous Force

Continuous-force movements occur when near-maximum muscle tension is applied throughout the range of the movement, as in performing a heavy weight lift or a slow pull-up. In such movements the muscles contract at nearly the same intensity all through the movement. Sometimes this kind of movement demands near-maximum contraction over a relatively long time.

Ballistic Movements

A ballistic movement occurs when the body or a segment is put into rapid motion by fast, but very brief, contractions of the mover muscles. After the initial tension has been applied, the remainder of the movement results largely from momentum of the moving parts. Examples of ballistic movements are swinging a golf club, tennis racket, or baseball bat. These are all explosive movements in which the implement is put into motion by vigorous, very brief contractions. After movement has quickly reached the desired velocity, it continues as a result of built-up momentum along with reduced muscle force. When a muscle contraction stops, the velocity of movement gradually diminishes because of (1) internal resistance in the joints, (2) resistance of antagonist muscles, and (3) external resistance. To stop the movement at the desired time, the antagonist muscles must apply resistance through eccentric contractions, during the follow-through phase.

Sometimes ballistic movements occur in repetition, such as movements of the arms during running and movements in the elbow when dribbling a ball. This calls for quick reversal of ballistic movements. In skills requiring ballistic actions, many, but not all, joint movements will be ballistic.

Slow-Tension Movements

When speed and force are not of prime importance, and great steadiness and accuracy are needed, slow-tension movements are used. Examples are threading a needle, slow and graceful movements in modern dance and ballet, and slow, steady, and precise gymnastic movements. In these kinds of movements the forces applied by the opposite muscle groups are almost equal to each other. If the opposite forces were equal, the body part would be stabilized and steady. As the force of one muscle group overcomes that of the opposite group, slow and steady movement occurs. The fact that all opposing muscle groups apply almost equal tension causes the body part to be highly stable and subject to quick adjustment in direction and rate of movement. One's ability to keep the forces of opposing muscles equal is the limiting factor in steadiness, and the effort greatly taxes one's muscular endurance.

MULTIJOINT MUSCLES

As the name implies, a *multijoint* muscle is one that extends across more than one joint and contributes to movement in each joint that it crosses. Examples of such muscles are the biceps brachii, which flexes the elbow and shoulder, and the triceps brachii, which extends both the elbow and the shoulder. The hamstring group, located in the back of the thigh, flexes the knee and extends the hip, while the rectus femoris extends the knee and flexes the hip (Figure 5-4). Several muscles of the lower arm, which contribute to movement of the fingers, act upon several joints. The same is true of the muscles of the lower leg, which contribute to toe movements. Of course, numerous muscles of the back contribute to movement in a series of joints in the spinal column, but this is not a comparable situation because joints of the spine do not usually act separately. Spinal joints work in groups to cause a single movement.

An interesting characteristic of many multijoint muscles is that they do not allow complete range of motion in all joints at one time. For example, the wrist cannot be fully flexed at the same time that the fingers are fully flexed. This is partly because multijoint flexors cannot contract far enough to cause complete flexion in all the joints simultaneously and partly because the multijoint extensors are unable to stretch far enough to allow complete flexion. To demonstrate this characteristic, flex the wrist as far as possible while the hand is gripped tightly; then release the grip and notice that the wrist is able to flex through an additional range of motion. Because the hamstring muscles cross over both the hip and knee joints, the hip cannot be fully flexed at the same time the knee is fully

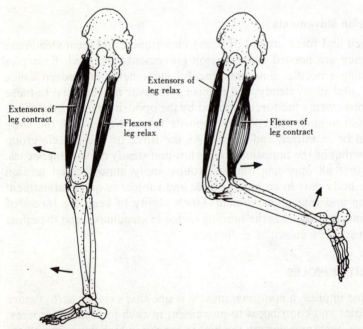

Figure 5-4 Side view of two joint muscles with opposing actions. Rectus femoris (front of leg) extends the knee and flexes the hip; the hamstring group (back of legs) flex the knee and extend the hip.

extended, except in a few individuals who have devoted much time to increasing flexibility (some dancers and acrobats).

When a multijoint muscle contracts, it tends to perform its assigned movements in all the joints on which it acts. For instance, if the rectus femoris contracts, it flexes the hip and extends the knee. If only one of the actions is desired, the other action must be nullified (neutralized) by contractions of other muscles. Through coordination with other muscles, a multijoint muscle can contribute to any portion of the total movements that it is capable of causing.

POSTURAL MUSCLES

There are two kinds of posture: dynamic and static. Both kinds depend primarily upon muscular contractions, and the muscles involved the most are referred to as *postural* (or *antigravity*) muscles. The muscles most obviously involved in posture are the extensors of the legs, back, and neck. These muscles must contract for the body to maintain any kind of erect position. The abdominal muscles contract to prevent sag of the visceral organs. Numerous other muscles are less important but also involved in posture, including the trunk and neck flexors and lateral flexors, leg abductors and adductors, and muscles of the foot. If all the antigravity muscles were to relax, the body would collapse. The collapse would occur in flexion at all the support joints, which indicates why extensors must provide the support against the pull of gravity.

We know that a muscle contracts only when it receives a stimulus; therefore, postural muscles must receive constant stimulation to carry on their functions. Although much remains to be learned about the exact process by which these muscles are stimulated, it is currently believed that the stimulus comes from two main sources: (1) stretch reflexes, which are initiated from within the skeletal muscles, and (2) the five "righting reflexes," which consist of:

1 Optical righting reflexes
2 Body righting reflexes acting on the body
3 Body righting reflexes acting on the head
4 Neck righting reflexes
5 Labyrinthine righting reflexes

Whenever a body segment deviates from the desired postural position, the appropriate reflex mechanisms initiate a stimulus which causes muscle contractions necessary to correct the deviation (see Figure 4-10). The classic illustration is the swaying action of a person attempting to hold a perfectly erect position. The body repeatedly moves in various directions away from perfect balance (even though this is not apparent). When a certain amount of movement occurs in a given direction, the appropriate reflex mechanism is activated, and the imbalance in position is quickly corrected. This process is continuous during the erect position. (Also see the section on reflexes, Chapter 4. pages 54–55.)

IMPORTANT CONCEPTS

1   Skeletal muscles have the ability to function in more than one role at different times, and often muscles function in two or more roles during a performance. The different roles are agonist, antagonist, stabilizer, and neutralizer.

2   One of the important aspects of neuromuscular coordination is the ability to coordinate the agonist and antagonist muscles properly. The inability to do this results in loss of skill and efficiency. In some movements it is desirable to be able to relax the antagonist muscles as completely as possible, while at other times where controlled movements are needed, it is desirable to have just the right amount of tension in the antagonist muscles.

3   The inability to coordinate the agonist and antagonist muscles properly during vigorous performance is one source of muscle injury. In fact, it is probably the predominant cause of muscle strains and pulls.

4   The stabilizing role of skeletal muscles is not always apparent but always exists in a complex motor skill and is fundamental to success of the skill.

5   Practically all motor movement requires neutralizing actions, because the muscles which cause the desired movement usually contribute to other movements which are unwanted in the particular case. The only way to eliminate the unwanted movements is to contract muscles which nullify (neutralize) those movements, thus causing only the desired movements.

6   Neuromuscular coordination (skill) is the act of causing each movement to occur in the correct sequence and timing and with just the right amount of force.

7   Reciprocal inhibition is relatively unapparent but very important in skilled performances. It is the process primarily responsible for causing the appropriate amount of relaxation in antagonist muscles.

8   A muscle has the ability only to contract or not contract (relax). When the muscle contracts, it has the ability to apply tension only toward its middle, thus applying equal force at both ends (attachments). The part of the body that moves as a result of the muscular force is the part that is the most free to move, and usually this is the body part farthest from the midline of the body (the portion where the distal end of the muscle attaches).

9   When a multijoint muscle contracts, it causes movements in all the joints that it normally acts upon, unless some of those movements are

neutralized by the contractions of opposing muscles. By this process, multijoint muscles can be used effectively to cause desired movements in selected joints.

10   Certain skeletal muscle groups are sometimes labeled *postural muscles* because they are involved in a primary way in body support. In erect positions the muscles that most often play a postural role are the leg and back extensors. These muscles are also referred to as antigravity muscles, because if they were relaxed the force of gravity would cause the body to collapse.

Chapter 6

Muscular Actions of the Upper Extremities

The upper extremities (see Figure 6-1) include the hands, arms, and shoulder girdles. In terms of movement these are the most versatile and freely movable of the large portions of the body; they are used in the greatest variety of ways. Visualize, for example, the numerous movements that occur in the upper extremities during an overhead badminton shot, a baseball pitch, or a batting action. Few performances involve the upper extremities alone. In almost all cases, their movements must be closely coordinated with and assisted by movements in the neck, trunk, and lower extremities. More than 40 pairs of skeletal muscles contribute to movement in the upper extremities, and practically all these muscles contribute to more than one movement.

MUSCULAR ACTIONS OF THE HAND

Throughout history the human hand has played a significant role in daily human activities. Its ability to manipulate precisely in a variety of ways is yet unequaled by machines. Of all the specific segments of the body, the hand is the most versatile.

The great mobility of the hand is owed to its many joints and

78

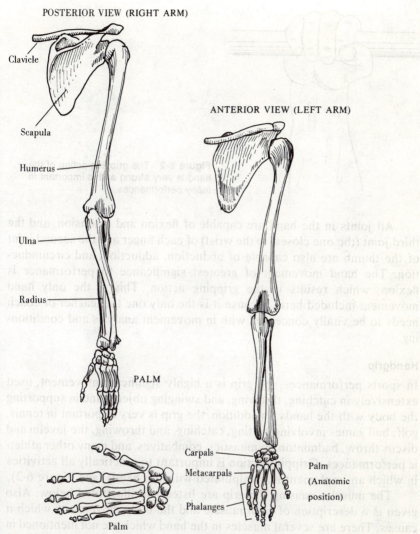

Figure 6-1 Anterior and posterior views of the bone structure of the upper extremity.

elaborate muscular system. There are fourteen joints in the hand alone and several additional joints in the wrist, which contribute directly to the usefulness of the hand. Ten muscles are located in the hand and nine additional muscles, which manipulate the fingers and thumb, are located in the forearm. These nineteen muscles work together in different combinations so that a muscle, through interaction with other muscles, may contribute to more than one movement. Several of the muscles are multijoint muscles.

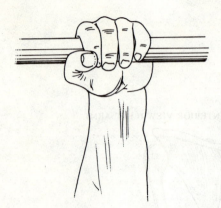

Figure 6-2 The gripping action of the hand is very strong and is important in many performances.

All joints in the hand are capable of flexion and extension, and the third joint (the one closest to the wrist) of each finger and the second joint of the thumb are also capable of abduction, adduction, and circumduction. The hand movement of greatest significance to performance is flexion, which results in the gripping action. This is the only hand movement included here, because it is the only one the teacher or coach needs to be vitally concerned with in movement analysis and conditioning.

Handgrip

In sports performances, the grip is a highly significant movement, used extensively in catching, throwing, and swinging objects and in supporting the body with the hands. In addition, the grip is very important in tennis, golf, ball games involving batting, catching, and throwing, the javelin and discus throw, badminton, gymnastics, combatives, and many other athletic performances. Gripping action is important to practically all activities in which an implement is manipulated with the hands (see Figure 6-2).

The muscles causing the grip are listed and illustrated below. Also given is a description of each muscle and the body movements which it causes. There are several muscles in the hand which are not mentioned in this text, because they contribute to hand movements not considered here.

Muscle	Description and actions
*Flexor digitorum profundus (Figure 6-5)	Attaches proximally on the anterior and medial surfaces of the ulna, approximately halfway up the forearm. It extends down the arm, and its tendons extend across the wrist and hand and attach at the bases of the distal phalanges of the four fingers. It flexes the distal phalanges, contributes to flexion of the other finger joints, and flexes the wrist.

Muscle	Description and actions
*Flexor pollicis longus (Figure 6-5)	Attaches proximally at the anterior surface (middle one-third) of the radius, extends down the anterior of the arm, and attaches to the distal phalanx of the thumb. It crosses three joints and causes flexion of the thumb (both joints) and wrist.
*Flexor digitorum sublimis (or superficialis) (Figure 6-6)	The proximal attachment is on the medial epicondyle of the humerus, the coronoid process of the ulna, and the upper portion of the radius. It extends down the anterior side of the forearm and attaches by split tendons to the second phalanges of the four fingers. It crosses over four joints, causes flexion of the middle and proximal phalanges, and assists in flexing the wrist and elbow.
*Lumbricalis (Figure 6-3)	Proximal attachment is on the tendons of the flexor profundus muscle, located in the palm of the hand. It extends downward and attaches to the tendons of the extensor communis, which attaches to the back of the distal phalanges of the fingers. It causes flexion of the first phalanges and extension of the distal phalanges of the fingers. Also, it aids in finger abduction (radial flexion).
*Flexor pollicis brevis (Figure 6-3)	Proximal attachment is on the trapezium, trapezoid, and capitate bones of the wrist. It extends down the front of the thumb and attaches on the proximal phalanx of the thumb. It flexes and adducts the thumb.
Adductor pollicis (Figure 6-3)	Proximal attachment is on the second and third metacarpal bones on the palm side near the wrist. It extends down the front of the thumb and attaches to the first phalanx of the thumb on the inner surface. It crosses the two joints of the thumb, and it adducts and flexes the thumb.
Abductor digiti quinti (Figure 6-3)	Attaches proximally to the ulna side of the heel of the hand and extends downward to its distal attachment at the first phalanx of the little finger. It abducts the little finger and assists in flexing its proximal phalanx.
Abductor pollicis brevis (Figure 6-3)	Attaches proximally to the navicular and trapezium bones of the wrist and the transverse carpal ligament. It extends downward and attaches distally to the base of the first phalanx of the thumb. It abducts the thumb.

*Throughout this chapter, this device indicates prime-mover muscle.

MUSCULAR ACTIONS OF THE WRIST

The wrist is composed of a cluster of eight small bones with numerous joints at their points of articulation. There are six muscles of the forearm which cause movement in the wrist only. Nine additional muscles, which

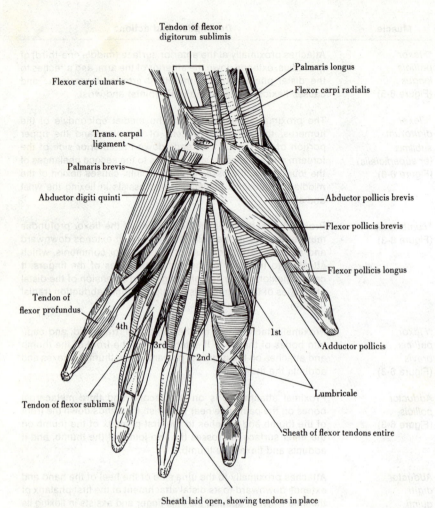

Tendon of flexor digitorum sublimis

Palmaris longus

Flexor carpi ulnaris

Flexor carpi radialis

Trans. carpal ligament

Palmaris brevis

Abductor digiti quinti

Abductor pollicis brevis

Flexor pollicis brevis

Flexor pollicis longus

Tendon of flexor profundus

4th

3rd

2nd

1st

Adductor pollicis

Lumbricale

Tendon of flexor sublimis

Sheath of flexor tendons entire

Sheath laid open, showing tendons in place

Figure 6-3 Muscles of the palm of the left hand.

move the thumb and fingers, also contribute to wrist movements. The wrist, which is highly useful in athletic performance, is capable of flexion, extension, abduction (radial flexion), adduction (ulnar flexion), and circumduction. (The movement that appears to be wrist rotation is actually rotation of the lower arm, involving the ulna and radius.)

Wrist Flexion

Flexion (Figure 6-4) is a very strong movement and one used extensively in throwing, lifting, pushing, pulling, and handling sports implements. Wrist flexion is very important in throwing objects such as a baseball or

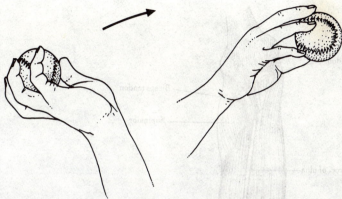

Figure 6-4 Wrist flexion, one of the most important contributing movements in throwing.

softball; striking as in badminton, squash, handball, and the tennis serve; supporting and thrusting the body as in gymnastic movements and pole vaulting; and putting actions as in the shot put. Following is information about the muscles which cause the wrist to flex.

Muscle	Description and actions
*Flexor carpi ulnaris (Figure 6-6)	Proximal attachment of the two heads are at the medial epicondyle of the humerus and the olecranon process of the ulna. It extends down the medial side of the arm and attaches to the fifth metacarpal and the pisiform bone of the wrist. It crosses two joints, and it flexes and adducts the wrist and flexes the elbow.
*Flexor carpi radialis (Figure 6-6)	Attaches proximally on the medial epicondyle of the humerus, extends down the anterior of the forearm, and attaches distally at the base of the second metacarpal bone. It crosses two joints, and it flexes and abducts the wrist and flexes the elbow.
*Palmaris longus (Figure 6-6)	Attaches proximally on the medial epicondyle of the humerus, extends down the anterior of the forearm, and attaches to the carpal ligament in the palm of the hand. It crosses over two joints and contributes to flexion of the wrist and flexion of the elbow.
Flexor digitorum profundus (Figure 6-5)	See Handgrip, page 80.
Flexor digitorum sublimis (or superficialis) (Figure 6-6)	See Handgrip, page 80.

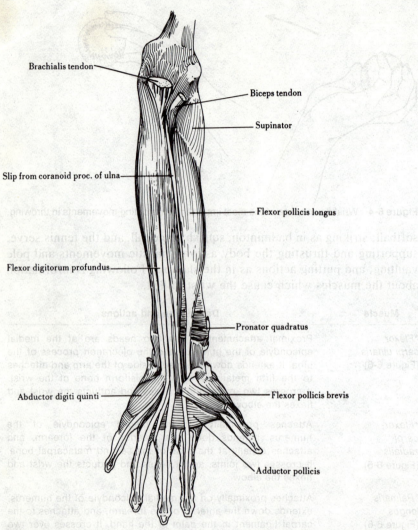

Brachialis tendon

Biceps tendon

Supinator

Slip from coranoid proc. of ulna

Flexor pollicis longus

Flexor digitorum profundus

Pronator quadratus

Abductor digiti quinti

Flexor pollicis brevis

Adductor pollicis

Figure 6-5 Deep muscles of the front of the left forearm. (*After C. M. Goss, Gray's Anatomy, 29th ed., Lea & Febiger, Philadelphia, 1973.*)

Muscle	Description and actions
Flexor pollicis longus (Figure 6-5)	See Handgrip, page 80.

Wrist Extension

Wrist extension (Figure 6-7) is a relatively weak but necessary movement in sports. When wrist extension occurs beyond the straight (180°)

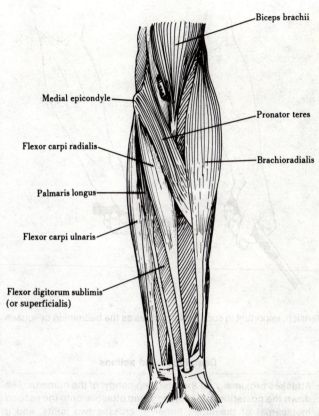

Biceps brachii

Medial epicondyle

Pronator teres

Flexor carpi radialis

Brachioradialis

Palmaris longus

Flexor carpi ulnaris

Flexor digitorum sublimis
(or superficialis)

Figure 6-6 Superficial muscles in the front of the left forearm. (*After C. M. Goss, Gray's Anatomy, 29th ed., Lea & Febiger, Philadelphia, 1973.*)

position, the movement is called *hyperextension*. The wrist extensor muscles are of prime importance in such performances as badminton, raquetball, and squash backhand shots, golf swings, and batting actions. In the tennis backhand drive and other similar performances, the wrist extensors contract to stabilize the wrist in the desired position. If the wrist is to be held in a fixed position, the extensor muscles must be strong enough to equalize a strong contraction by the opposing muscles (flexors). Following are the muscles which cause wrist extension.

Muscle	Description and actions
*Extensor carpi radialis brevis (Figure 6-9)	Proximal attachment is on the lateral epicondyl of the humerus. It lies down the posterior of the forearm and attaches on the posterior surface of the third metacarpal bone. It crosses over two joints, and it extends and abducts the wrist and extends the elbow.

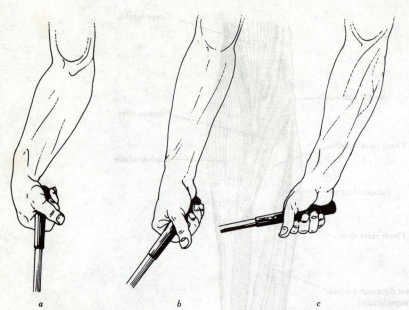

a   b   c

Figure 6-7 Wrist extension, important in such performances as the badminton or squash backhand shot.

Muscle	Description and actions
*Extensor carpi radialis longus (Figure 6-9)	Attaches proximally on the lateral epicondyl of the humerus, lies down the posterior of the forearm, and attaches onto the second metacarpal of the index finger. It crosses two joints, and it extends and abducts the wrist and extends the elbow.
*Extensor carpi ulnaris (Figure 6-9)	Proximal attachment is on the lateral epicondyle of the humerus and the posterior of the ulna at the elbow joint. It lies down the back of the forearm and attaches to the fifth metacarpal. It crosses two joints, and it extends and adducts the wrist and extends the elbow.
Extensor digiti quinti (Figure 6-9)	Proximal attachment is on the tendon of the previous muscle, approximately 8 centimeters above the wrist, along the posterior of the forearm. It extends downward and attaches to the fifth metacarpal bone. It extends the wrist and little finger.
Extensor digitorum communis (Figure 6-9)	Attaches proximally on the lateral epicondyle of the humerus, lies down the posterior of the forearm, and attaches onto the distal phalanges of the four fingers. It crosses over five joints, and it extends the fingers, the wrist, and the elbow.
Extensor indicis (Figure 6-8)	Attaches proximally on the lower posterior surface of the ulna, extends downward, and attaches distally on the second and third phalanges of the index finger. It extends the index finger and the wrist.

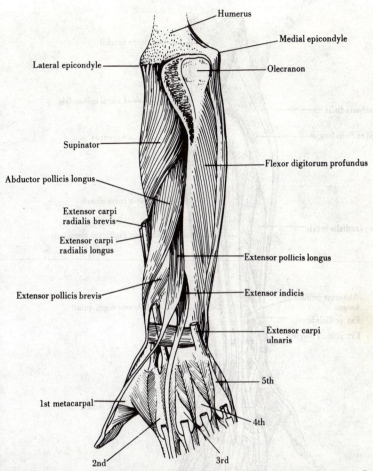

Figure 6-8 Deep muscles of the posterior surface of the left forearm. (*After C. M. Goss, Gray's Anatomy, 29th ed., Lea & Febiger, Philadelphia, 1973.*)

Muscle	Description and actions
Extensor pollicis longus (Figure 6-8)	Proximal attachment is on the lower one-third of the ulna on the posterior surface. It extends down the back of the arm and attaches onto the base of the distal phalanx of the thumb. It crosses three joints, and it extends the thumb and the wrist.

Wrist Abduction (Radial Flexion)

Wrist abduction is a movement of the hand toward the thumb side. It is a relatively weak movement. However, it is important in such skills as the backswing in golf and batting, and the cocking of the wrist for throwing

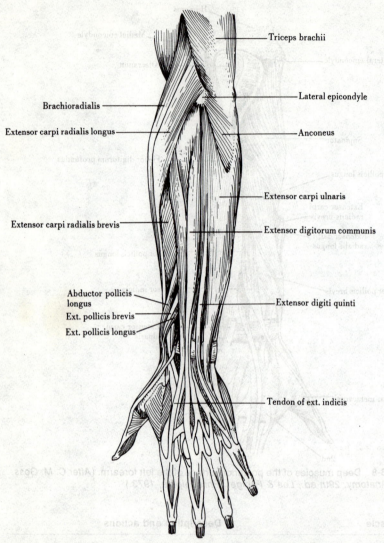

Figure 6-9 Superficial muscles of the posterior surface of the left forearm. (*After C. M. Goss, Gray's Anatomy, 29th ed., Lea & Febiger, Philadelphia, 1973.*)

the football and javelin. Also, it is a very important movement in throwing the discus. Five muscles contribute to wrist abduction.

Muscle	Description and actions
Flexor carpi radialis (Figure 6-6)	See Wrist Flexion, page 82.

Muscle	Description and actions
*Extensor carpi radialis brevis (Figure 6-9)	See Wrist Extension, page 84.
*Extensor carpt radialis longus (Figure 6-9)	See Wrist Extension, page 84.
Abductor pollicis longus (Figure 6-8)	Proximal attachment is on the inside of the radius and the outside of the ulna about halfway up the forearm. It lies diagonally down the front of the forearm and attaches on the radial side of the first metacarpal of the thumb. It abducts the thumb and wrist.
Extensor pollicis brevis (Figure 6-8)	Proximal attachment is on the posterior surface of the radius approximately 4 centimeters above the wrist. It extends down the back of the arm and attaches to the first phalanx of the thumb. It extends and abducts the thumb and abducts the wrist.

Wrist Adduction (Ulnar Flexion)

Adduction of the wrist moves the hand toward the side of the small finger. It is a short-range movement with a fair amount of application in athletics. It is used in the golf swing and in batting actions and is important in the football pass, javelin throw, and some shots in badminton, squash, volleyball, and some hand-supported gymnastic movements. It is also used to give spin to a baseball, causing it to curve. Two muscles are responsible for wrist adduction.

Muscle	Description and actions
*Flexor carpi ulnaris (Figure 6-6)	See Wrist Flexion, page 82.
*Extensor carpi ulnaris (Figure 6-9)	See Wrist Extension, page 84.

Wrist Circumduction

Circumduction is movement in a circular, cone-shaped pattern. It is simply a sequential combination of flexion, abduction, extension, and adduction. Circumduction is caused by the muscles which contribute to the four movements which compose it. Even though it is not a frequently used movement in sports activities, it is used in a limited amount in such performances as the sidearm throw and certain handball shots.

MUSCULAR ACTIONS OF THE LOWER ARM

A segment rotates when it moves in a circular direction around its own longitudinal axis. Because of the ability of the radius bone to turn in the socket of the ulna, the lower arm may be rotated either medially or laterally. These rotary movements are frequently used. Supination is the same as lateral rotation of the lower arm, resulting in the supine position of the hand (palm up). Pronation is the same as medial rotation, resulting in a prone position of the hand (palm down).

Lower Arm Lateral Rotation (Supination)

This movement is important in such performances as the underhand pitch (Figure 6-10), the tennis backhand drive, and throwing of a curve ball. The supinator and biceps brachii muscles cause the movement.

Muscle	Description and actions
*Supinator (Figure 6-8)	This small muscle attaches proximally on the lateral epicondyle of the humerus and the radial ligament of the elbow. It extends downward to the posterior and lateral surfaces of the upper radius. It supinates the lower arm.

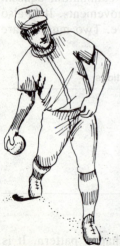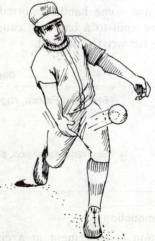

Figure 6-10 Lateral rotation of the arm, used to good advantage in the underarm pitch.

Muscle	Description and actions
*Biceps brachii (Figure 6-12)	This is a two-headed muscle. The proximal attachment of the long head is on the top of the scapula at the glenoid process. The short head attaches at the coracoid process of the scapula. The muscle extends down the anterior of the upper arm and attaches to the tuberosity of the radius just below the elbow. It crosses two joints, and it flexes the elbow and supinates (rotates laterally) the lower arm. The short head also assists in shoulder flexion horizontal flexion, and medial rotation, while the long head assists in shoulder flexion and abduction.

Lower Arm Medial Rotation (Pronation)

This movement is used extensively in handling balls, such as dribbling a basketball, certain arm-supported gymnastic movements, and wrestling. It is a stronger movement than lateral rotation, and it is caused by four muscles.

Muscle	Description and actions
*Pronator quadratus (Figure 6-5)	Attaches proximally to the lower fourth of the anterior of the ulna and extends across to its distal attachment on the lower fourth of the radius. It pronates the forearm.
*Pronator teres (Figure 6-6)	Attaches proximally to the medial epicondyle of the humerus and the coronoid process of the ulna, extends down the lateral side of the arm, and attaches onto the upper third of the radius. It pronates the lower arm and flexes the elbow.
Anconeus (Figure 6-9)	Proximal attachment is on the lateral epicondyle of the humerus. It extends diagonally around the arm to the posterior surface of the ulna and attaches at the olecranon process of the ulna. It pronates the forearm and extends the elbow.
Flexor carpi radialis (Figure 6-6)	See Wrist Flexion, page 82.

MUSCULAR ACTIONS OF THE ELBOW

The elbow joint is formed by the articulation of the ulna with the humerus. Because this joint is a hinge type, it is capable only of two kinds of movement—flexion and extension. Eight muscles contribute to flexion, and six contribute to extension. Of these fourteen muscles, nine are multijoint, some of which extend across the elbow and shoulder joints, while others cross over the elbow and wrist.

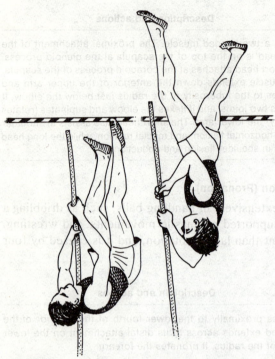

Figure 6-11 Elbow flexion, an important contributor in pole vaulting.

Elbow Flexion

Elbow flexion is one of the most powerful movements of the upper extremities and is used in a great variety of performances. Utilized frequently in pulling and lifting actions, elbow flexion is also a strong contributor to chinning, climbing, pole vaulting (Figure 6-11), several gymnastic movements, wrestling, football tackling, and curl lifts. In addition, it is the movement that must precede elbow extension, another frequently used movement. Eight muscles cause the elbow to flex.

Muscle	Description and actions
*Biceps brachii (Figure 6-12)	See Lower Arm Lateral Rotation, page 90.
Brachialis (Figure 6-12)	Attaches proximally to the lower half of the humerus, extends down the front of the arm, and attaches at the coronoid process of the ulna. It flexes the elbow.
*Brachio-radialis (Figure 6-6)	Proximal attachment is on the lateral surface of the lower third of the humerus. It extends downward and inserts at the base of the styloid process of the radius. It flexes the elbow.

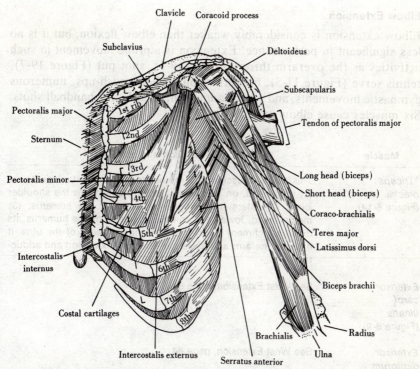

Figure 6-12 Deep muscles of the upper arm and chest. (*After C. M. Goss, Gray's Anatomy, 29th ed., Lea & Febiger, Philadelphia, 1973.*)

Muscle	Description and actions
Pronator teres (Figure 6-6)	See Lower Arm Medial Rotation, page 91.
Palmaris longus (Figure 6-6)	See Wrist Flexion, page 82.
Flexor carpi ulnaris (Figure 6-6)	See Wrist Flexion, page 82.
Flexor carpi radialis (Figure 6-6)	See Wrist Flexion, page 82.
Flexor digitorum sublimis (or superficialis) (Figure 6-6)	See Handgrip, page 80.

Elbow Extension

Elbow extension is considerably weaker than elbow flexion, but it is no less significant in performance. Extension is a prime movement in such activities as the overarm throw (Figure 19-3), shot put (Figure 19-7), tennis serve (Figure 11-5), basketball push shots, push-ups, numerous gymnastic movements, and some badminton, squash, and handball shots. Six muscles cause elbow extension.

Muscle	Description and actions
*Triceps brachii (Figure 6-14)	This unique muscle has three heads. Proximal attachments are (1) long head, on the scapula behind and below the shoulder joints; (2) lateral head, upper posterior of the humerus; (3) medial head, lower and middle posterior of the humerus. Its distal attachment is on the olecranon process of the ulna. It extends the arm and assists in shoulder extension and adduction.
Extensor carpi ulnaris (Figure 6-9)	See Wrist Extension, page 84.
Extensor digitorum communis (Figure 6-9)	See Wrist Extension, page 84.
Extensor carpi radialis brevis (Figure 6-9)	See Wrist Extension, page 84.
Extensor carpi radialis longus (Figure 6-9)	See Wrist Extension, page 84.
Anconeus (Figure 6-9)	See Lower Arm Medial Rotation, page 91.

MUSCULAR ACTIONS OF THE SHOULDER

The shoulder joint is formed by articulation of the humerus and scapula. It is one of the most versatile and frequently used joints in the body. A ball-and-socket joint, it allows seven different movements—flexion, extension, abduction, adduction, medial and lateral rotation, and circumduction. Twelve muscles, most of which are very powerful, cause movements in this joint. Each of the muscles contributes to more than one movement.

Shoulder Flexion

Flexion at the shoulder is movement of the arm forward and upward starting from the anatomical position. It is caused by four muscles, one of which (biceps) extends across both the elbow and shoulder joints. Shoulder flexion is very important in the common activities of walking and running and is a strong contributor to the underhand throw (Figures 6-10 and 19-1), pushing, striking, bowling, jumping, hurdling, some strokes in tennis, badminton, squash, and handball, and certain frequently used dance movements. Shoulder flexion may occur with the upper arm in the vertical position, as in the underarm pitch, in the horizontal position, as in the discus throw, and in an intermediate position, as in the sidearm throw (baseball). When flexion occurs in the horizontal plane, it is referred to as horizontal flexion. Muscles which cause shoulder flexion are listed below.

Muscle	Description and actions
*Deltoid (anterior) (Figure 6-13)	The deltoid muscle consists of three parts—anterior, middle, and posterior. The muscle attaches proximally on the anterior surface of the lateral third of the clavicle, the top of the acromion, and the outside edge of the spine of the scapula. It extends downward across the front, top, and back of the shoulder joint and attaches on the lateral side of the middle portion of the humerus. The anterior fibers cause shoulder flexion, abduction, and medial rotation. The middle fibers cause shoulder abduction. The posterior fibers cause shoulder extension, abduction, and lateral rotation.
*Pectoralis major (Figure 6-13)	The pectoralis major consists of two parts—the clavicular (upper) portion and the sternal (lower) portion. Its proximal attachment is on the anterior of the clavicle, the whole length of the sternum, and the cartilages of the first six ribs. The muscle lies horizontally, and the distal end attaches to the anterior of the humerus, about one-third of the way between the shoulder and elbow. The clavicular portion causes flexion, horizontal flexion, adduction, and medial rotation at the shoulder. The sternal portion causes shoulder adduction, horizontal flexion, medial rotation, and shoulder extension when the arm is in a flexed position, and flexion when the arm is hyperextended.
Biceps brachii (short head) (Figure 6-12)	See Lower Arm Lateral Rotation, page 90.

Muscle	Description and actions
Coraco-brachialis (Figure 6-12)	Attaches proximally onto the coracoid process of the scapula, extends diagonally downward, and attaches distally to the inner surface of the humerus about one-third of the way down the humerus. It contributes to flexion at the shoulder, especially when the arm is in the horizontal position, and adduction.

Shoulder Extension

Shoulder extension is movement of the arm downward and backward toward the anatomical position. Seven different muscles cause extension at the shoulder. One of these, the triceps, is a two-joint muscle. Shoulder extension is another very powerful movement and is important in such activities as chinning, climbing, pole vaulting, running, walking, rises in gymnastics, and opposite arm movements in the discus throw and shot put. Like flexion, shoulder extension may occur with the upper arm in a vertical, horizontal, or intermediate position. Shoulder extension beyond the anatomical position may occur and cause the arm to move to the rear

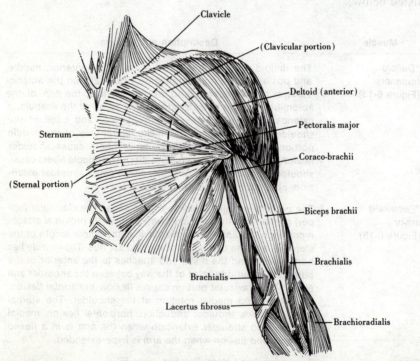

Figure 6-13 Superficial muscles of the upper arm and chest. (*After C. M. Goss, Gray's Anatomy, 29th ed., Lea & Febiger, Philadelphia, 1973.*)

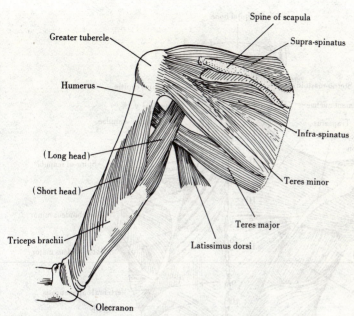

Figure 6-14 Triceps and deep muscles of the scapula. (*After C. M. Goss, Gray's Anatomy, 29th ed., Lea & Febiger, Philadelphia, 1973.*)

of the body, a movement known as hyperextension. Muscles causing shoulder extension are the following:

Muscle	Description and actions
*Latissimus dorsi (Figure 6-15)	Proximal attachment of this large flat muscle is on the spinous processes of the six lower thoracic and all of the lumbar vertebrae, the sacrum, the crest of the ilium, and the three lowest ribs. It extends diagonally up the back and attaches onto the upper anterior surface of the humerus. It extends, adducts, and medially rotates the arm at the shoulder.
*Teres major (Figure 6-14)	Proximal attachment is on the posterior surface of the lower scapula. It extends diagonally upward and attaches onto the anterior surface of the humerus. It causes extension, adduction, and medial rotation at the shoulder. Its actions are the same as the latissimus dorsi.
*Pectoralis major (sternal portion) (Figure 6-13)	See Shoulder Flexion, page 95.

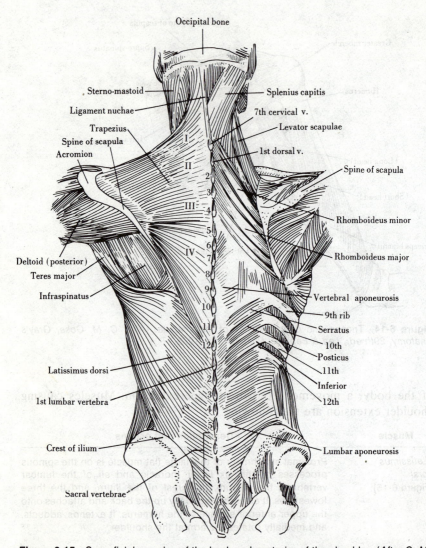

Figure 6-15 Superficial muscles of the back and posterior of the shoulder. (*After C. M. Goss, Gray's Anatomy, 29th ed., Lea & Febiger, Philadelphia, 1973.*)

Muscle	Description and actions
Deltoid (posterior) (Figure 6-15)	See Shoulder Flexion, page 95.
Triceps brachii	See Elbow Extension, page 94.

Muscle	Description and actions
(long head) (Figure 6-14)	
Infraspinatus (Figure 6-14)	Proximal attachment is on the infraspinous fossa of the scapula (posterior surface and lower portion). It extends diagonally upward and attaches onto the posterior surface of the humerus near the shoulder joint. It rotates the arm laterally and extends it in the horizontal position.
Teres minor (Figure 6-14)	Proximal attachment is on the lower posterior border of the scapula. It extends diagonally upward and attaches onto the posterior surface of the humerus near the shoulder joint. Its actions are the same as the infraspinatus muscle.

Shoulder Abduction

Shoulder abduction is movement of the arm outward and upward away from the body. This is probably the weakest movement of the shoulder joint. It is caused by the supraspinatus, biceps, and deltoid muscles. The pectoralis major (clavicular) also contributes to abduction above the horizontal position only. Although it is not considered a significant contributor in sports performances, this movement is used in elbow thrusting actions in football, soccer, and other body contact games, in basketball hook shots, and in various forms of modern dancing and ballet. Also, it is used with shoulder flexion in jumping actions and for maintaining balance as in the football punt, skiing, skating, and beam-walking.

Muscle	Description and actions
*Deltoid (Figures 6-13 and 6-15)	See Shoulder Flexion, page 95.
Supra- spinatus (Figure 6-14)	Attaches proximally to the supraspinous fossa of the scapula (upper posterior portion), lies horizontally, and attaches onto the greater tubercle (top) of the humerus. It abducts the arm at the shoulder, and may assist in outward rotation.
Biceps brachii (long head) (Figure 6-12)	See Lower Arm Lateral Rotation, page 90.

Shoulder Adduction

Shoulder adduction (Figure 6-16) is movement of the arm downward and inward toward the body. It is strong movement used often in arm-

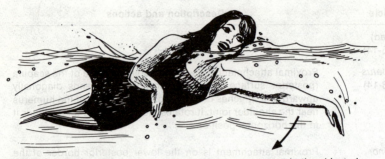

Figure 6-16 Shoulder adduction, a very strong movement in the sidestroke.

supported gymnastic skills, the swimming breaststroke, to some extent in the crawl stroke, and in numerous dance movements. Six muscles contribute to this movement.

Muscle	Description and actions
Latissimus dorsi (Figure 6-15)	See Shoulder Extension, page 96.
Pectoralis major (Figure 6-13)	See Shoulder Flexion, page 95.
Teres major (Figure 6-14)	See Shoulder Extension, page 96.
Triceps brachii (Figure 6-14)	See Elbow Extension, page 94.
Subscapularis (Figure 6-12)	Proximal attachment is on the anterior (front) side of the scapula, known as the subscapular fossa. It lies horizontally and attaches onto the lesser tubercle (top portion) of the humerus on the anterior surface. It medially rotates and adducts the arm at the shoulder.
Coracobrachialis (Figure 6-12)	See Shoulder Flexion, page 95.

Medial (Inward) Rotation at the Shoulder

This very significant movement is vital in the forehand tennis stroke; the overarm throw; certain shots in badminton, squash, and handball; rope climbing; and the crawl stroke, butterfly stroke, and breaststroke in swimming. Six muscles contribute to the movement. Care must be taken to be sure that humeral (shoulder) rotation is not confused with forearm rotation.

Muscle	Description and actions
*Teres major (Figure 6-14)	See Shoulder Extension, page 96.
*Pectoralis major (Figure 6-13)	See Shoulder Flexion, page 95.
*Latissimus dorsi (Figure 6-15)	See Shoulder Extension, page 96.
*Deltoid (anterior) (Figure 6-13)	See Shoulder Flexion, page 95.
Biceps brachii (short head) (Figure 6-12)	See Lower Arm Lateral Rotation, page 90.
Subscapularis (Figure 6-12)	See Shoulder Adduction, page 99.

Lateral (Outward) Rotation at the Shoulder

Examples of sports performances in which the upper arm is rotated laterally are the backhand tennis drive and the underhand pitch. The movement is caused by the coordinated actions of three muscles.

Muscle	Description and actions
*Infraspinatus (Figures 6-14 and 6-15)	See Shoulder Extension, page 96.
*Teres minor (Figure 6-14)	See Shoulder Extension, page 96.

Muscle	Description and actions
Deltoid (posterior) (Figure 6-15)	See Shoulder Flexion, page 95.
Supraspinatus (Figure 6-14)	See Shoulder Abduction, page 99.

Shoulder Circumduction

Circumduction at the shoulder is a circular, cone-shaped movement of the arm. Being a weak movement not frequently used, it results from the sequential combination of shoulder flexion, abduction, extension, and adduction.

MUSCULAR ACTIONS OF THE SHOULDER GIRDLE

The bone structure of the shoulder girdle consists of the scapula and clavicle. The shoulder girdle is capable of only a small amount of movement in any direction, but some of the movements have great significance in performance. The six movements performed by the shoulder girdle are elevation, depression, protraction (abduction), retraction (adduction), upward rotation, and downward rotation. Ten muscles work together in different combinations to cause these movements.

It is interesting to note the tremendous cooperation between the movements of the shoulder girdle and the upper arm. Whenever the humerus moves, the clavicle and scapula seem to follow, so that the glenoid cavity of the shoulder joint tends to point in the direction of the axis of the humerus. If the humerus is abducted, the scapula rotates upward. If the humerus is moved out front, as in flexion, the scapula abducts and tries to "turn the corner," following the curvature of the rib cage. Any movement of the humerus toward the rear, as in hyperextension, results in scapular adduction. It is important to note that the humerus does not drag the shoulder girdle along, but rather those muscles which move the shoulder girdle work cooperatively with the muscles causing the corresponding movement in the upper arm. It is also important not to interchange muscles affecting the shoulder joint and shoulder girdle. They are distinctly different muscles.

Shoulder-Girdle Elevation

Elevation of the shoulder girdle is important in lifting, vertical jumping where the arms and shoulders are thrust upward, and over-the-head reaching. Some specific performances in which the movement is significant are the tennis serve, the handstand, the shot put, pole vaulting (pushing action), basketball overhead shots and rebounding, the volley-ball spike and overhead push shots, and the high jump and long jump. Three muscles cause the shoulder girdle to elevate.

Muscle	Description and actions
*Levator scapulae (Figure 6-15)	Proximal attachment is on the transverse processes (side) of the four upper cervical vertebrae. It extends diagonally downward and attaches onto the upper and medial portion of the scapula. It elevates the shoulder girdle. It may also laterally flex the neck.
*Trapezius (I and II) (Figure 6-15)	This large fan-shaped muscle consists of four parts: I, II, III, and IV. The proximal attachment of the total muscle is on the base of the skull, ligaments of the neck, and the spinous processes down to and including the twelfth thoracic vertebra. It attaches onto the outer portion of the clavicle, the acromion process, and the upper surface of the scapular spine. Part I elevates the girdle; part II elevates, upward rotates, and retracts the girdle. Part III retracts the girdle, and part IV causes upward rotation, depression, and retraction.
Rhomboi-deus major (Figure 6-15)	Proximal attachment is on the spinous processes of the upper thoracic vertebrae. It extends diagonally downward and attaches to the lower half of the medial border of the scapula. It elevates and retracts the shoulder girdle and rotates the scapula downward.
Rhomboi-deus minor (Figure 6-15)	This muscle lies immediately above and parallel to the rhomboid major. Its proximal attachment is on the spinous processes of the last cervical and first thoracic vertebrae. The distal attachment is on the middle portion of the medial edge of the scapula. It elevates, and retracts the shoulder girdle and rotates the scapula downward.

Shoulder-Girdle Depression

Depression is the opposite movement from elevation. It is a very strong movement caused by three muscles. Specific performances in which it is a strong contributor are the pole vault (pulling action), chinning, climbing, swimming (pulling action), and numerous gymnastic activities such as the dip, iron cross (see Figure 20-5), giant swing, and parallel-bar movements. Three muscles cause this movement.

Muscle	Description and actions
*Pectoralis minor (Figure 6-17)	This muscle is underneath and entirely covered by the pectoralis major. Its proximal attachment is on the upper and outer surfaces of the third, fourth, and fifth ribs near their cartilages. It extends diagonally upward and attaches onto the coracoid

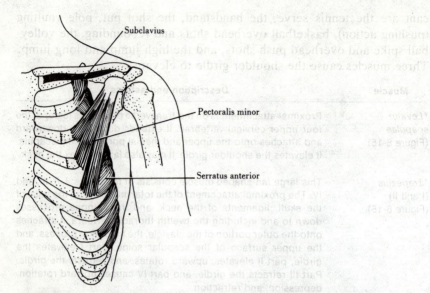

Figure 6-17 Serratus anterior, subclavius, and pectoralis minor muscles.

Muscle	Description and actions
	process of the scapula (anterior surface). It depresses the shoulder girdle and rotates the scapula downward and abducts it.
Subclavius (Figure 6-17)	Proximal attachment is on the anterior of the first rib and its cartilage. It extends upward and attaches along the middle underside of the clavicle. It depresses the shoulder girdle.
Trapezius IV (Figure 6-15)	See Shoulder-Girdle Elevation, page 102.

Shoulder-Girdle Protraction (Abduction)

Protraction occurs when the scapulae move outward from the spine, resulting in broadening of the shoulders. It is caused by the pectoralis minor and serratus anterior muscles. Protraction is important in performances such as baseball batting, the sidearm or overarm ball throw, the discus throw, the tennis forehand drive, and any performance in which reaching forward is involved.

Muscle	Description and actions
Pectoralis minor (Figure 6-17)	See Shoulder-Girdle Depression, page 103.

Muscle	Description and actions
*Serratus anterior (Figure 6-17)	Proximal attachment is on the upper outer surfaces of the first eight ribs. The fibers extend upward and backward and attach to the medial border of the anterior surface of the scapula. It protracts the shoulder girdle and rotates the scapula upward.

Shoulder-Girdle Retraction (Adduction)

Retraction is opposite from protraction, meaning the scapulae move toward the spine. This movement is short, but strong, and it is important in pull-ups, dips, climbing, and some gymnastic performances. Three muscles contribute to the movement.

Muscle	Description and actions
*Rhomboideus major (Figure 6-15)	See Shoulder-Girdle Elevation, page 102.
*Rhomboideus minor (Figure 6-15)	See Shoulder-Girdle Elevation, page 102.
*Trapezius (II and III) (Figure 6-15)	See Shoulder-Girdle Elevation, page 102.

Rotation of the Scapula Downward

Actually, when the anatomical position is assumed, the scapula is rotated downward to almost maximum; however, it may be purposely rotated slightly beyond that position. From the upward rotated position, the scapula may be rotated downward to the anatomical position. Three muscles cause this movement.

Muscle	Description and actions
*Pectoralis minor (Figure 6-17)	See Shoulder-Girdle Depression, page 103.
*Rhomboideus major (Figure 6-15)	See Shoulder-Girdle Elevation, page 102.
*Rhomboideus minor (Figure 6-15)	See Shoulder-Girdle Elevation, page 102.

Rotation of the Scapula Upward

Upward rotation of the scapula occurs when the scapula rotates around its own center in connection with rotation of the clavicle at the sternum through the frontal plane and on the clavicle's long axis through the sagittal plane, The lower point of the scapula moves away from the spine and the upper point moves upward and toward the spine. For example, upward rotation occurs when the arm is raised overhead. This movement is often accompanied by shoulder-girdle elevation. It is caused by two muscles.

---

*Serratus anterior (Figure 6-17)	See Shoulder-Girdle Protraction, page 104.
Trapezius (II and IV) (Figure 6-15)	See Shoulder-Girdle Elevation, page 102.

Since movements of the scapula are not easily observed, it is useful, and usually correct, to assume that scapular (shoulder-girdle) movements are closely related to movements of the upper arm at the shoulder joint. These relationships are usually as follows:

1 If the arm moves forward, the scapula abducts.
2 If the arm moves backward, the scapula adducts.
3 If the arm moves upward, the scapula experiences upward rotation.
4 If the arm moves downward, the scapula experiences downward rotation.

Usually shoulder-girdle elevation accompanies upward rotation, while shoulder-girdle depression usually accompanies downward rotation. However, these movements can be done independently of each other, as in the shoulder-shrug weight-training movement. Often abduction, upper rotation, and elevation go together as in purring the shot; adduction, downward rotation, and depression often go together as in the pull-up movement.

STUDENT LABORATORY EXPERIENCES

1. If a medcolator is available, electrically stimulate selected muscles of the upper extremity. For example, with one electrode held firmly in one hand, probe with the other electrode for the motor point of the flexors of the fingers (i.e., flexor digitorum superficialis, etc.)

2. If a cadaver laboratory is available, tag by number twenty-five muscles of the upper extremity and write the correct name of the tagged muscles.
3. Make tracings of Figure 6-1 and on the tracings place drawings of the muscles of the upper extremities which have been discussed in this chapter.
4. After carefully studying the muscular actions of the upper extremities and the following muscle-action table, make a duplicate table, leaving the action columns blank. Then practice filling in the table by memory. It will be helpful to visualize the joint, noting the location and the way in which the muscle crosses the joint, then judge whether or not the indicated action appears to be possible. Afterward, check your answers against the table given.

Muscle Action Table: Upper Extremities

| Muscle | Extension of fingers or thumb | Wrist | | | | | Lower arm | | Elbow | |
		Grip	Flexion	Extension	Abduction	Adduction	Medial rotation	Lateral rotation	Flexion	Extension
Flexor pollicis longus		X	X			X				
Adductor pollicis		X								
Abductor digiti quinti		X								
Abductor pollicis longus					X			X		
Flexor digitorum profundus		X	X							
Flexor pollicis brevis		X								
Flexor digitorum sublimis		X	X						X	
Flexor carpi ulnaris			X			X			X	
Flexor carpi radialis			X		X		X		X	
Palmaris longus			X						X	
Extensor carpi radialis brevis				X	X					X

Muscle Action Table: Upper Extremities

Muscle	Extension of fingers or thumb	Grip	Flexion	Extension	Abduction	Adduction	Medial rotation	Lateral rotation	Flexion	Extension
			Wrist				**Lower arm**		**Elbow**	
Extensor carpi radialis longus				X	X			X		X
Extensor carpi ulnaris				X		X				X
Extensor digiti quinti	X			X						X
Extensor digitorum communis	X		X							X
Extensor indicis				X						
Extensor pollicis longus	X			X				X		
Extensor pollicis brevis	X					X				
Supinator								X		
Pronator quadratus							X			
Anconeus							X			X
Pronator teres							X		X	
Brachialis									X	
Brachioradialis							X	X	X	
Biceps								X	X	
Triceps										X

Muscle Action Table: Upper Extremity

Muscle	Shoulder							
	Flexion	Extension	Abduction	Adduction	Medial rotation	Lateral rotation	Horizontal adduction	Horizontal abduction
Biceps (longhead)	X		X					
Biceps (shorthead)	X	X		X	X		X	
Coracobrachialis	X			X	X	X	X	
Deltoid (anterior)	X		X		X		X	
Deltoid (middle)			X					X
Deltoid (posterior)		X				X		X
Pectoralis major (clavicular)	X		X		X		X	
Pectoralis major (sternal)		X		X	X		X	
Latissimus dorsi		X		X	X			X
Infraspinatus		X						
Teres major		X		X	X			X
Teres minor		X				X		X
Triceps (long head)		X		X				
Supraspinatus			X			X		
Subscapularis	X		X	X	X		X	

Muscle Action Table: Upper Extremity

Muscle	Shoulder girdle					
	Elevation	Depression	Protraction	Retraction	Upward rotation	Downward rotation
Levator Scapulae	X					X
Trapezius I	X					
Trapezius II	X			X	X	
Trapezius III				X		
Trapezius IV		X		X	X	
Subclavius		X				
Serratus anterior			X		X	
Rhomboideus major	X			X		X
Rhomboideus minor	X			X		X
Pectoralis minor		X		X		X

Chapter 7

Muscular Actions of the Trunk and Neck

The trunk includes about one-half of the total body weight. The extremities attach to the trunk, which is the stable unit on which they move. The bone structure of the trunk includes: (1) all of the spinal column extending downward from the base of the neck (excluding only the cervical vertebrae), (2) bones of the rib cage, and (3) bones of the pelvic region (Figure 7-1). The bone structure of the neck consists of the cervical vertebrae and hyoid bone. In addition to causing a variety of movements, the muscles of the trunk often play the role of stabilizers, and many of them are among the postural (antigravity) muscles which must remain in partial contraction to hold the body erect.

This chapter covers only the large muscles of the trunk and neck, and those which contribute most to the particular movements discussed. Some of the smaller muscles in the spinal column and rib cage are not discussed because they are less significant in analysis of vigorous

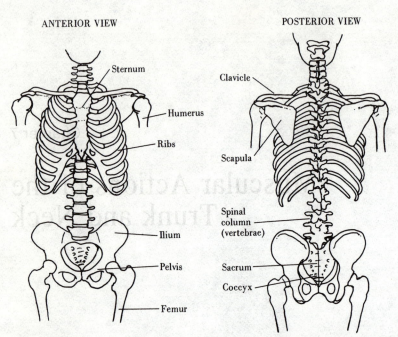

ANTERIOR VIEW   POSTERIOR VIEW

Figure 7-1 Anterior and posterior views of the bones of the trunk with portions of the upper and lower extremities attached.

body movements. The smaller muscles of the spine are illustrated in Figure 7-5.

MUSCULAR ACTIONS OF THE TRUNK

Excluding respiratory action and movement of the abdomen, all trunk actions involve movement in the spine (Figure 7-2). The structure of spinal vertebrae and the spongelike disks that separate them make possible a small amount of movement in any direction between each pair of vertebrae. When the movement between all vertebrae is combined, the result is extensive movement of the trunk. The trunk is capable of seven different movements: flexion, extension, lateral flexion to the right and left, rotation to the right and left, and circumduction.

The muscular system of the spine is very complex. It includes many small muscles which connect the individual vertebrae together and add support and stability to the spinal column. There are a few larger spinal muscles which are very significant in vigorous trunk movements. Added to these, the abdominal muscles and muscles of the pelvic region complete the muscular system of the trunk. All these muscles occur in pairs, designated either right or left. The effects are quite different depending on which side of the pair is active.

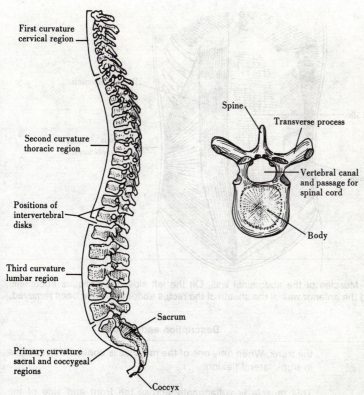

First curvature
cervical region

Spine

Transverse process

Second curvature
thoracic region

Vertebral canal
and passage for
spinal cord

Positions of
intervertebral
disks

Body

Third curvature
lumbar region

Sacrum

Primary curvature
sacral and coccygeal
regions

Coccyx

Figure 7-2   Side view of the spinal colum, and cross section of a vertebra.

Trunk Flexion (Forward Bend)

This movement occurs mostly in the lumbar (lower) region of the spine
and is used in almost all athletic performances. It is a prime contributor in
trampoline and diving maneuvers which involve the tuck and pike
positions, several gymnastic movements, the pole vault, javelin throw,
butterfly swimming stroke, overarm ball throw, and hurdling. Actually,
little range of motion is possible in trunk flexion, and it is often confused
with hip flexion. For example, in the sit-up exercise, only the curling
action is trunk flexion; most of the range of motion is due to hip flexion.
Following are descriptions of the trunk flexor muscles.

Muscle	Description and actions
*Rectus abdominis (Figure 7-3)	The two rectus abdominis muscles lie vertically up the front of the abdomen. Proximal attachment of each muscle is on the pubis bone and the ligaments covering the front of the pubis. The distal attachment is on the cartilages of the fifth, sixth, and seventh ribs. The muscle compresses the abdomen and flexes

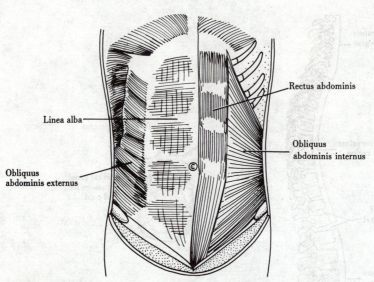

Figure 7-3 Muscles of the abdominal wall. On the left side, the obliquus abdominis externus and the anterior wall of the sheath of the rectus abdominis have been removed.

Muscle	Description and actions
	the trunk. When only one of the muscles is contracted, it assists in trunk lateral flexion.
*Obliquus abdominis externus (Figure 7-3)	This muscle lies diagonally across the front and side of the abdomen. Proximal attachment is on the eight lowest ribs. It extends diagonally downward and attaches onto the upper crest of the ilium, the pubis, and the linea alba. It compresses the abdomen and causes trunk flexion, lateral flexion to the same side, and rotation to the opposite side.
*Obliquus abdominis internus (Figure 7-3)	This muscle lies underneath the external oblique muscle, and the fibers of the two muscles run at right angles to each other. Proximal attachment is on the crest of the ilium. It extends diagonally upward and forward and attaches to the six lowest ribs and the linea alba. It compresses the abdomen and causes trunk flexion, lateral flexion, and rotation to the same side.
Psoas major (Figure 7-4)	See Hip Flexion, page 127.

*Throughout this chapter, this device indicates prime-mover muscle.

Trunk Extension (Straightening)

Like trunk flexion, this movement occurs mostly in the lumbar region of the spine. It is the most powerful movement of the trunk and is very

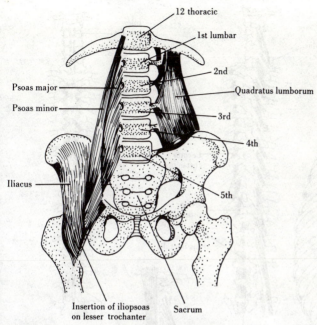

Figure 7-4 Muscles inside the pelvic region.

significant in athletics. Used in almost every kind of performance, trunk extension is of prime importance in several dance movements, the shot put, the butterfly stroke, the discus throw, lifting, wrestling, hurdling (final phase), and football blocking and tackling. In addition to the four muscles discussed below, several of the deep, small spinal muscles, especially the rotator muscles, contribute to extension. They are illustrated in Figure 7-5.

Muscle	Description and actions
*Semi-spinalis (thoracic) (Figure 7-5)	The muscle lies diagonally up the spine. The proximal attachment is on the transverse processes of the sixth to tenth thoracic vertebrae. It attaches distally to the spinous processes of the upper thoracic and lower cervical vertebrae. When the two muscles act together, they assist in extending the trunk. Separately, they assist in laterally flexing the trunk and rotate it to the opposite side.
*Erector spinae (sacrospinalis) (Figure 7-5)	This massive back muscle consists of three branches: the iliocostalis (lateral portion), longissimus (middle portion), and spinalis (medial portion). The muscle attaches proximally on the posterior surface of the sacrum, crest of the ilium, and spines of the lumbar and thoracic vertebrae. It extends up the back and

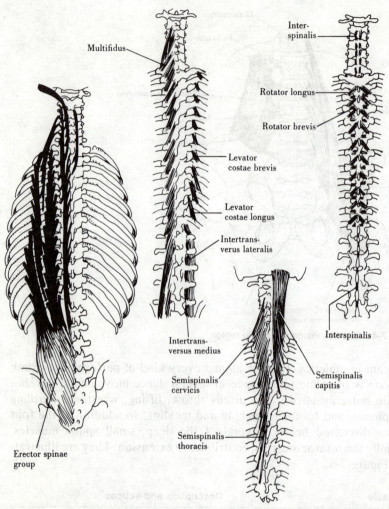

Figure 7-5 Back muscles which act on the spinal column. They contribute to trunk and neck extension, rotation, and lateral flexion.

Muscle	Description and actions
	attaches to the back portion of the ribs at several places, to the posterior of the thoracic and cervical vertebrae, and to the base of the skull. It extends, rotates, and laterally flexes the trunk and neck on the side of its location.
Quadratus lumborum (Figure 7-4)	This muscle lies up the side of the trunk between the ilium and the bottom of the rib cage. The proximal attachment is on the crest of the ilium and transverse processes of the four lowest

Muscle	Description and actions
	lumbar vertebrae. It extends upward and backward toward the spine and attaches to the upper two lumbar vertebrae and the last rib. It causes extension and lateral trunk flexion.
Multifidus (Figure 7-5)	This muscle (or group of muscles) lies down the side of the spine. The proximal attachment is on the posterior of the sacrum, the top of the iliac, and the transverse processes of the lumbar and thoracic vertebrae. The muscle extends diagonally upward and attaches to the spinous processes of the spine. Acting together, the two muscles extend the trunk and neck; singly, they cause trunk and neck rotation to the opposite side and lateral flexion.

Lateral Flexion of the Trunk (Sideward Bend)

The trunk may be flexed to either the right or the left by simultaneously contracting the trunk flexor and extensor muscles on the side where lateral flexion is desired. When beginning in a position of right lateral flexion, for example, a return to the upright position is a movement of left lateral flexion. Trunk lateral flexion is especially important in shot-putting, throwing, sideward lifts, and numerous gymnastic and dance movements. Practically all the trunk flexor and extensor muscles contribute to lateral flexion.

Muscle	Description and Actions
*Rectus abdominis (Figure 7-3)	See Trunk Flexion, page 113.
*Obliquus abdominis externus (Figure 7-3)	See Trunk Flexion, page 113.
*Obliquus abdominis internus (Figure 7-3)	See Trunk Flexion, page 113.
*Erector spinae (Figure 7-5)	See Trunk Extension, page 114.
*Quadratus lumborum (Figure 7-4)	See Trunk Extension, page 114.

Muscle	Description and actions
Semi-spinalis (thoracic) (Figure 7-5)	See Trunk Extension, page 114.
Multifidus (Figure 7-5)	See Trunk Extension, page 114.

Trunk Rotation

In addition to the deep rotator muscles of the spine (see rotator brevis in Figure 7-5), there are five larger muscles listed below which cause trunk rotation. They are of prime importance in the twisting actions in diving, trampoline, and dance. Trunk rotation is also used extensively in throwing and batting; golf, tennis, and badminton strokes; handball shots; the shot put (Figures 9-4 and 19-7); the discus throw (Figure 7-6); swimming; and other motor performances. The common term to describe trunk rotation is "turning the shoulders." *Right-handed* performers rotate *left* as they put the shot, hit a golf ball, or throw a baseball.

Muscle	Description and actions
*Obliquus abdominis externus (Figure 7-3)	It rotates the trunk to the opposite side. (*Same-side rotation* means that the trunk rotates to the side where the muscle is located. *Opposite-side rotation* means that when the muscle on the *left* contracts, it rotates the trunk to the *right*; and when the muscle on the *right* contracts, it rotates the trunk to the left.) See Trunk Flexion, page 110.
*Obliquus abdominis internus (Figure 7-3)	It rotates the trunk to the same side. See Trunk Flexion, page 113.
*Erector spinae (Figure 7-5)	It rotates the trunk to the same side. See Trunk Extension, page 114.
*Semi-spinalis (thoracic) (Figure 7-5)	It rotates the trunk to the opposite side. See Trunk Extension, page 114.
Multifidus (Figure 7-5)	It rotates the trunk to the opposite side. See Trunk Extension, page 114.

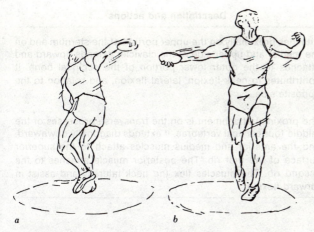

Figure 7-6   Trunk rotation is important in throwing a discus.

Trunk Circumduction

The trunk can circumduct, but this is not a frequently used movement. Trunk circumduction results from a sequential combination of flexion, lateral flexion, hyperextension, and lateral flexion to the other side.

MUSCULAR ACTIONS OF THE NECK

The bone structure of the neck consists of the upper seven (cervical) vertebrae of the spinal column. In addition to the smaller muscles of the spine, there are seven larger and more powerful muscles which cause movement in the neck. The neck is capable of extension (backward head tilt), flexion (forward head tilt), lateral flexion (sideward head tilt) to the right and left, rotation to the right and left, and circumduction. These are the same movements that occur in the trunk.

Neck Flexion

The neck is flexed by the coordinated actions of the three scalenus muscles and the sternocleidomastoid. Neck flexion, which is a much weaker movement than extension, is important in hurdling, diving and trampoline stunts where the pike and tuck positions are used, swimming, several dance movements, and "setting" the neck for contact in football and wrestling. The two muscles which cause neck flexion also contribute to forced inhalation because of the lifting effect they have on the upper portion of the rib cage.

Muscle	Description and actions
*Sterno-cleido-mastoid (Figure 7-7)	Attaches proximally on the upper portion of the sternum and on the medial and upper side of the clavicle; extends upward and attaches to the outer lower portion of the occipital bone. It contributes to neck flexion, lateral flexion, and rotation to the opposite side.
*Scalenus (anterior, medius, and posterior) (Figure 7-7)	The proximal attachment is on the transverse processes of the middle four cervical vertebrae. It extends diagonally downward, and the anterior and medius muscles attach to the superior surface of the first rib. The posterior muscle attaches to the second rib. The muscles flex the neck laterally and assist in forward flexion.

Neck Extension

Extension is the most powerful neck movement. It is caused by five large muscles, plus some of the smaller muscles which connect the vertebrae. Extensor muscles are used frequently in such performances as modern

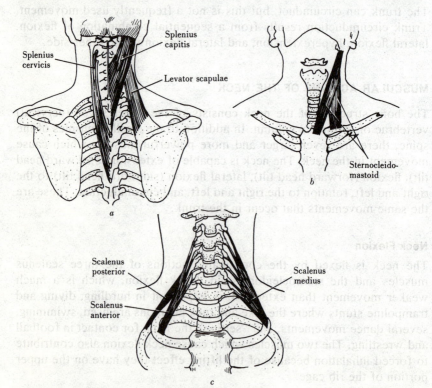

Figure 7-7 Major muscles of the neck.

dance and ballet, wrestling, some swimming strokes, especially the breaststroke and butterfly stroke, crouched football positions, and tumbling and gymnastic movements, especially those involving head-support positions.

Muscle	Description and actions
*Erector spinae (Figure 7-5)	See Trunk Extension, page 114.
*Semi-spinalis (capitis) (Figure 7-5)	Attaches proximally onto the articular and transverse processes of the lower four cervical and the upper six thoracic vertebrae. It extends diagonally upward and attaches to the base of the skull at the occipital bone. It contributes to extension, lateral flexion, and rotation of the neck.
*Semi-spinalis (cervicis) (Figure 7-5)	The proximal attachment is on the spinous processes of the lower cervical and upper thoracic vertebrae. It extends upward and attaches to the spinous processes of the upper cervical vertebrae. It contributes to extension, lateral flexion, and rotation of the neck to the opposite side.
*Splenius (capitis and cervicis) (Figure 7-7)	The proximal attachment is on the spinous processes of the seventh cervical and first three thoracic vertebrae. It extends upward and outward and attaches to the base of the skull on the occipital and temporal bones. It contributes to neck extension, lateral flexion, and rotation to the same side.
Multifidus (Figure 7-5)	See Trunk Extension, page 114.

Lateral Flexion of the Neck

Lateral flexion is caused by the following seven large muscles, plus smaller muscles which help connect the vertebrae together. Muscles on the right side cause lateral flexion to the right, while those on the left cause lateral flexion to the left. This movement is used frequently in such activities as modern dance and ballet, twisting and turning movements in diving and gymnastics, wrestling, and hard thrusting sideward and turning movements as in football blocking and tackling.

Muscle	Description and actions
*Splenius (capitis and cervicis) (Figure 7-7)	See Neck Extension, page 120.

Muscle	Description and actions
*Sterno- cleido- mastoid (Figure 7-7)	See Neck Flexion, page 119.
*Scalenus (anterior, medius, and posterior) (Figure 7-7)	See Neck Flexion, page 119.
*Semi- spinalis (cervicis and capitis (Figure 7-5)	See Neck Extension, page 120.
*Erector spinae (Figure 7-5)	See Trunk Extension, page 114.
Multifidus (upper portion) (Figure 7-5)	See Trunk Extension, page 114.
Levator scapulae (Figure 7-7)	See Shoulder-Girdle Elevation, page 102.

Neck Rotation

Five muscles on each side of the body contribute to neck rotation. Three of the muscles are opposite side rotators, meaning that when the left muscle contracts, the neck rotates to the right. Neck rotation is very important in total body twisting and turning movements, swimming (crawl stroke), all throwing activities, and the different forms of dance. This movement is used to some extent in almost all performances.

Muscle	Description and actions
*Sterno- cleido- mastoid (Figure 7-7)	It rotates the neck to the opposite side. See Neck Flexion, page 119.
*Semi- spinalis	It rotates the neck to the opposite side. See Neck Extension, page 119.

Muscle	Description and actions
(cervicis and capitis) (Figure 7-5)	
*Splenius (cervicis and capitis) (Figure 7-7)	It rotates the neck to the same side. See Neck Extension, page 120.
*Erector spinae (Figure 7-5)	It rotates the neck to the same side. See Trunk Extension, page 114.
Multifidus (upper portion) (Figure 7-5)	It rotates the neck to the opposite side. See Trunk Extension, page 114.

Neck Circumduction

This movement is not frequently used. As is the case with other body segments capable of this movement, circumduction in the neck results from the sequential combination of flexion, lateral flexion, and hyperextension.

MUSCLE ACTIONS IN RESPIRATION

Respiration results from muscle contractions. The process of inhaling is caused by the contraction of the costal and intercostal muscles which attach ribs to ribs. As these muscles contract, the ribs raise, and this causes expansion of the rib cage. At the same time the diaphragm muscle, which is a large flat muscle lying horizontally at the base of the rib cage, pulls downward as it contracts. These actions of the respiratory muscles result in enlargement of the chest cavity where the lungs lie. The expansion causes a lowering of the density of air (partial vacuum), which in turn causes lung expansion. This causes air to rush into the lungs (inhaling). When the diaphragm and intercostal muscles relax, the diaphragm muscle moves upward and the ribs lower. This reduces the space inside the chest cavity, forcing air out of the lungs (exhaling). The respiratory process goes on rhythmically at the rate of approximately sixteen times per minute in adults (at rest) without conscious control. The respiratory muscles are both voluntary and involuntary in the sense that they can be voluntarily controlled; but usually they function involuntarily.

Note It is interesting to note that the trunk or neck cannot experience a pure flexion, extension, or lateral flexion either right or left with the contraction of a single muscle because in all cases the muscles are located on or toward the corners of the trunk or neck and not directly in front, in back, or on either side. For example, if the trunk were to bend forward, abdominal muscles on both sides of the midline would have to contract. In trunk extension, muscles on both sides of the spine must contract. In order for the trunk to flex to the right, muscles on both the right front and right back must contract. Stated another way, if only a single muscle of the trunk or neck should contract, it would bend the body part diagonally in the direction of the muscle's location.

STUDENT LABORATORY EXPERIENCES

1. Trace Figure 7-1 and on the tracing place drawings of the muscles of the trunk and neck discussed in this chapter. Trace additional charts if needed.
2. After carefully studying the muscular actions of the neck and trunk in the text and in the following muscle-action table, duplicate the table, leaving the action columns blank. Then practice filling in the table by memory. It will be helpful to visualize the location of the muscles along the spine and neck to judge whether or not the indicated action appears to be possible. Afterward, check your answers against the table given.

Muscle Action Table: Trunk and Neck

Muscles*	Trunk				Neck			
	Flexion	Extension	Lateral flexion	Rotation	Flexion	Extension	Lateral flexion	Rotation
Rectus abdominis	X		X					
Obliquus externus	X		X	X				
Obliquus internus	X		X	X				
Psoás	X							
Semispinalis (thoracis)		X	X	X				
Semispinalis (capitis)						X	X	X
Semispinalis (cervicis)						X	X	X
Erector spinae		X	X	X		X	X	X
Quadratus lumborum		X	X					
Multifidus		X	X	X		X	X	X
Rotatores		X		X		X		X
Splenius (cervicis)						X	X	X
Splenius (capitis)						X	X	X
Sternocleidomasiod					X		X	X
Scalenus (anterior, medius, and posterior)					X		X	

*All muscles represent pairs, left and right.

Chapter 8

Muscular Actions of the Lower Extremities

This chapter includes the different movements that occur in the joints of the lower extremities, along with information about the muscles causing the movements. As in the two previous chapters, an illustration of each muscle is given.

The lower extremities include the feet and legs (Figure 8-1). It is the portion of the body which is used most extensively in locomotion, and in body support in an upright position. Because of these functions the lower extremities are very important in practically all motor performances.

MUSCULAR ACTIONS OF THE HIP

The joint at the hip is a ball-and-socket type, and is formed by the articulation between the femur and pelvis. It is capable of flexion, extension, abduction, adduction, rotation medially and laterally, and circumduction. It should be noted that the upper leg may be flexed and extended in either the vertical or horizontal position, or any position between the vertical and horizontal. Also, the leg may be hyperextended a

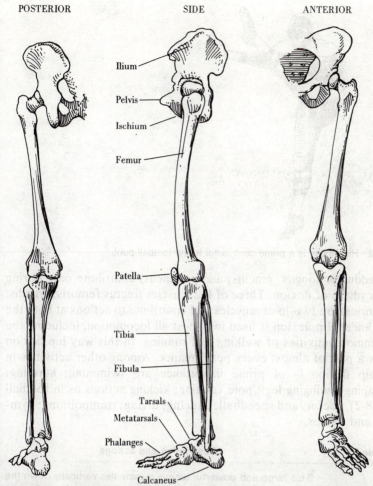

POSTERIOR SIDE ANTERIOR

Ilium

Pelvis

Ischium

Femur

Patella

Tibia

Fibula

Tarsals

Metatarsals

Phalanges

Calcaneus

Figure 8-1 Back, side, and front views of the skeletal structure of the lower extremity.

small amount, meaning that extension may continue beyond the vertical (anatomical) position. The twenty muscles surrounding the hip are some of the largest and most powerful muscles in the body. They contract in different combinations to cause the seven hip movements. Six of the twenty muscles also cross the knee joint, and contribute to movements in that joint.

Hip Flexion

Hip flexion is one of the strongest movements of the body, and it is caused by the contraction of ten muscles. Four of the muscles contribute all the way through the range of motion, while another four (adductor

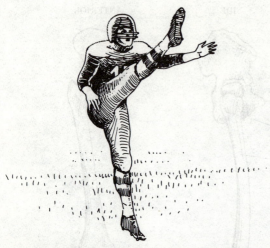

Figure 8-2 Hip flexion is a prime contributor in the football punt.

brevis, adductor longus, gracilis, and pectineus) contribute only during the early phase of flexion. Three of the muscles (rectus femoris, gracilis, and sartorius) are two-joint muscles and contribute to actions at both the hip and knee. Hip flexion is used in almost all locomotion, including the very common activities of walking and running. In this way hip flexion becomes a part of almost every performance. Among other activities in which hip flexion is of prime importance are swimming; hurdling; high-jumping (swinging leg); pole vaulting; kicking actions as in football (Figure 8-2), soccer, and speedball; dancing; diving; trampolining; gymnastics; and sit-ups.

Muscle	Description and actions
*Rectus femoris (Figure 8-3)	This large and powerful biceps muscle lies vertically down the front of the thigh. It attaches proximally by two tendons, one from the front and lower portion of the iliac spine, and the other just slightly higher on the iliac. Its distal attachment is on the upper patella. It flexes the hip and extends the knee.
*Pectineus (Figure 8-3)	The proximal attachment is on the lower surface of the pubis bone. It extends diagonally downward and attaches to the posterior surface about halfway down the femur. It adducts, flexes, and rotates the thigh laterally.
*Psoas major (Figures 8-3 and 7-4)	This strong muscle runs vertically through the inside of the pelvic region. The proximal attachment is on the bodies and transverse process of the last thoracic vertebra and all of the lumbar vertebrae. It extends downward and attaches to the inside of the head of the femur. It flexes and rotates the thigh laterally and assists in trunk flexion.

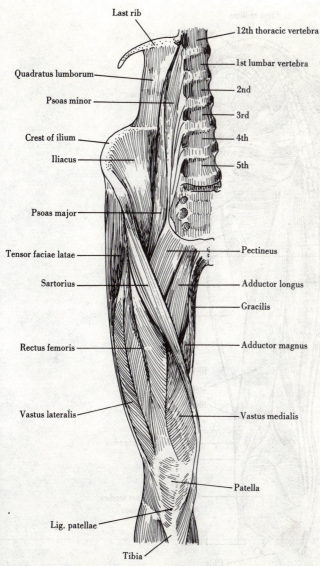

Figure 8-3 Muscles in the iliac region and the front of the thigh. (*After C. M. Goss, Gray's Anatomy, 29th ed., Lea & Febiger, Philadelphia, 1973.*)

Muscle	Description and actions
*Iliacus (Figures 8-3 and 7-4)	Attaches proximally on the interior surface of the iliac crest. It extends downward and joins the distal tendon of the psoas which attaches to the back of the upper portion of the femur on the lesser trochanter. It flexes the thigh and rotates it laterally.

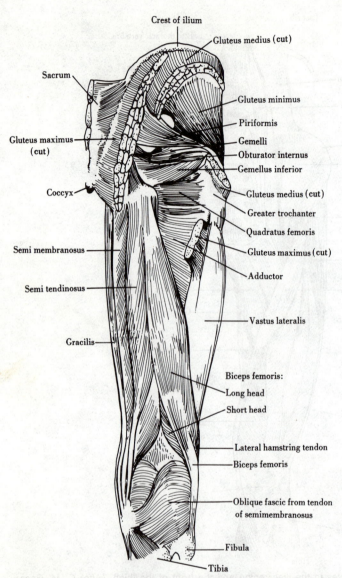

Figure 8-4 Muscles in the back of the hip and thigh. (*After C. M. Goss, Gray's Anatomy, 29th ed., Lea & Febiger, Philadelphia, 1973.*)

Muscle	Description and actions
Sartorius (Figure 8-3)	This slender two-joint muscle (the longest muscle in the body) attaches proximally on the anterior-superior spine of the ilium, and extends downward and inward to its distal attachment on the upper medial surface of the tibia. It flexes, abducts, and

Muscle	Description and actions

rotates the thigh laterally, and flexes and rotates the knee medially.

Adductor brevis (Figure 8-5)

The proximal attachment is on the front and lower surface of the pubis bone. It extends diagonally downward and attaches on the medial-posterior surface of the femur about one-third of the way between the hip and knee joints. It adducts, flexes, and rotates the thigh laterally.

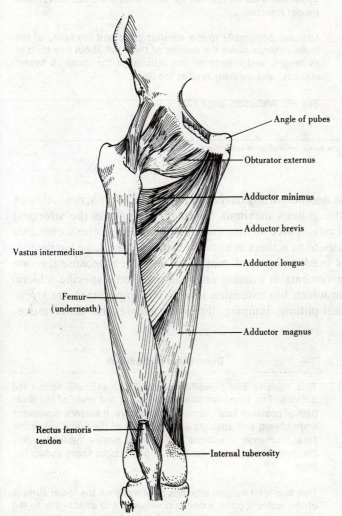

- Angle of pubes
- Obturator externus
- Adductor minimus
- Adductor brevis
- Vastus intermedius
- Adductor longus
- Femur (underneath)
- Adductor magnus
- Rectus femoris tendon
- Internal tuberosity

Figure 8-5 Muscles of the medial side of the thigh, and the vastus intermedius muscle.

Muscle	Description and actions
Adductor longus (Figure 8-5)	Attaches proximally on the front and lower surface of the pubis bone, extends diagonally downward and outward to its distal attachment on the medial surface of the femur about halfway between the hip and knee joints. It adducts, flexes, and rotates the thigh laterally.
Adductor magnus (Figure 8-5)	Attaches proximally to the lower portion of the pubis bone. It extends downward and outward to its distal attachment on the medial-posterior surface of the femur close to the knee joint. The upper fibers adduct and flex the thigh, while the lower fibers cause medial rotation.
Tensor fasciae latae (Figure 8-3)	Attaches proximally to the anterior crest and the spine of the ilium, extends down the outside of the thigh about one-third of its length, and inserts on the outside of the femur. It flexes, abducts, and medially rotates the thigh.
Gracilis (Figures 8-3 and 8-4)	See Hip Adduction, page 135.

*Throughout this chapter this device indicates prime-mover muscle.

Hip Extension

Hip extension is another strong movement. It is caused by six muscles, of which one is the gluteus maximus, often referred to as the strongest muscle in the body. Three of the muscles (hamstrings) cross over two joints and contribute to actions in both the hip and knee. Like hip flexion, hip extension is used in almost all motor performances, because it is one of the basic movements in running and walking. Some specific athletic performances in which hip extension is of prime importance are swimming, lifting, shot-putting, jumping, throwing, and several dance movements.

Muscle	Description and actions
Gluteus maximus (Figures 8-6 and 8-4)	This massive and powerful muscle lies diagonally across the buttock. The proximal attachment is on the crest of the ilium (lateral posterior face), sacrum, and coccyx. It extends downward and outward and attaches onto the back of the femur below the great trochanter. It extends and laterally rotates the thigh. Also, the lower fibers adduct the thigh and the upper fibers abduct the thigh.
Semimembranosus (Figure 8-4)	This two-joint muscle attaches proximally on the lower surface of the ischium bone, extends downward and attaches onto the medial epicondyle of the tibia. It extends and medially rotates the thigh, and flexes and medially rotates the knee.

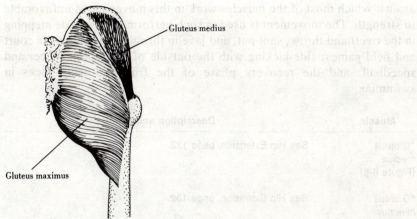

Figure 8-6 Gluteus maximus and gluteus medius muscles.

Muscle	Description and actions
*Biceps femoris (Figure 8-4)	This powerful, two-joint muscle lies vertically down the back of the thigh. Its long head attaches proximally to the lower portion of the ischium bone, and the short head attaches to the middle posterior surface of the femur. The distal end attaches onto the lateral side of the head of the fibula and the lateral condyle of the tibia. It flexes the knee and rotates it laterally. The long head also extends the hip.
*Semi-tendinosus (Figure 8-4)	The proximal attachment of this two-joint muscle is on the tuberosity of the ischium. It extends downward across the knee and attaches to the upper part of the medial surface of the tibia. It extends the thigh and rotates it medially. It also flexes and medially rotates the knee.
Gluteus medius (Figures 8-6 and 8-4)	Attaches proximally along the outside of the ilium near its crest, extends downward and attaches to the lateral surface of the great trochanter (top) of the femur. It is a strong abductor of the hip. Its posterior fibers also help with hip extension, which the anterior fibers assist in flexion and medial rotation.
Gluteus minimus (Figure 8-4)	The proximal attachment is on the middle part of the outer surface of the ilium. It extends downward and attaches to the front surface of the great trochanter (top) of the femur. The posterior fibers cause extension of the hip, while the anterior fibers cause medial rotation and flexion. The whole muscle causes hip abduction.

Hip Abduction

Abduction of the hip is a very weak movement and one not frequently used. It is caused by relatively small muscles, and the mechanical ratio against which most of the muscles work in this movement is unfavorable to strength. The movement is used in such performances as side-stepping in the overhand throw, shot put, and javelin throw; side-stepping in court and field games; side-kicking with the outside of the foot in soccer and speedball; and the recovery phase of the frog and whip kicks in swimming.

Muscle	Description and actions
*Gluteus medius (Figure 8-6)	See Hip Extension, page 132.
*Gluteus minimus (Figure 8-4)	See Hip Extension, page 132.
*Piriformis (Figures 8-4 and 8-7)	The proximal attachment is on the anterior surface of the sacrum. It passes in front of the pelvis and attaches onto the upper border of the great trochanter. It abducts the thigh and rotates it laterally.
Gemelli (Figures 8-7 and 8-4)	The proximal attachment is on the upper portion of the ischium bone. It lies horizontally and attaches to the medial surface of the great trochanter (top) of the femur. It rotates the thigh laterally and abducts it.
Sartorius (Figure 8-3)	See Hip Flexion, page 127.

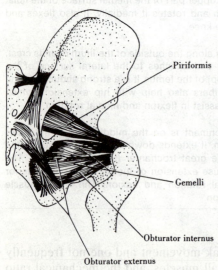

Piriformis

Gemelli

Obturator internus

Obturator externus

Figure 8-7 Interior muscles of the hip (deep lateral rotators).

Muscle	Description and actions
Tensor fasciae latae (Figure 8-3)	See Hip Flexion, page 127.
Gluteus maximus (upper fibers) (Figure 8-4 and 8-6)	See Hip Extension, page 132.

Hip Adduction

The six adductor muscles work against a much better mechanical ratio than the abductor muscles, and hip adduction is considerably stronger than abduction, but it is still a relatively weak movement. Adduction of the hip is used in such activities as side-stepping movements in various field and court games, side-kicking with the inside of the foot, and the frog and whip kicks in swimming.

Muscle	Description and actions
Adductor brevis (Figure 8-5)	See Hip Flexion, page 127.
Adductor longus (Figure 8-5)	See Hip Flexion, page 127.
Adductor magnus (Figure 8-5)	See Hip Flexion, page 127.
Gracilis (Figure 8-3 and 8-4)	It attaches proximally on the lower front portion of the pubis bone, and its distal attachment is on the medial surface of the tibia below the condyle. This muscle is very long. It runs the length of the upper leg on the medial surface. It adducts the leg at the hip, helps medially rotate the thigh, and flexes the knee.
Gluteus maximus (lower portion) (Figure 8-6)	See Hip Extension, page 132.
Pectineus (Figure 8-3)	See Hip Flexion, page 127.
Quadratus femoris (Figure 8-4)	It attaches proximally to the lateral margin of the ischial tuberosity; the distal attachment is at the quadrati tubercle. It is rectangularly shaped and adducts and laterally rotates the thigh.

Medial Rotation at the Hip

Medial hip rotation is a frequently used movement because it occurs in walking and running during the support phase of each stride. It is also used extensively in dodging and turning actions, the frog and whip kicks, batting, and golf and tennis strokes. It is a relatively strong movement in spite of the fact that most muscles contributing toward it do so as a secondary function. Five muscles contribute to medial rotation.

Muscle	Description and actions
*Gluteus medius (Figure 8-6)	See Hip Extension, page 132.
*Gluteus minimum (Figure 8-4)	See Hip Extension, page 132.
Gracilis (Figures 8-3 and 8-4)	See Hip Adduction, page 135.
Adductor magnus (lower fiber) (Figure 8-5)	See Hip Flexion, page 127.
Tensor fasciae latae (Figure 8-3)	See Hip Flexion, page 127.
Semi- tendinosus (Figure 8-4)	See Hip Extension, page 132.
Semimem- branosus (Figure 8-4)	See Hip Extension, page 132.

Lateral Rotation at the Hip

More muscles (seven prime movers and eight assistant movers) are required for lateral rotation at the hip than for almost any other movement. Yet it is not an extremely strong movement, because the muscles contribute to it as a secondary function, and the muscles work against a poor mechanical ratio. The movement occurs during the recovery phase (forward swing) of running and walking strides; it contributes to dodging and turning actions and certain swinging actions, as in tennis, golf, and baseball swings and in the final movement of the trail leg in high-jumping (roll). It is an essential movement of the pushing leg in the common side weight shift which turns the buckle (actually the pelvis) in the direction of the action.

Muscle	Description and actions
*Obturator externus (Figures 8-5 and 8-7)	Attaches proximally onto the obturator foramen on the inner wall of the pelvis. It lies horizontally, and attaches onto the femur just below the great trochanter. It rotates the thigh laterally.
*Obturator internus (Figure 8-7)	Attaches proximally to the inner surface of the wall of the pelvis on the obturator foramen. It lies horizontally and attaches to the greater trochanter of the femur. It rotates the thigh laterally.
*Gemelli (Figure 8-7)	See Hip Abduction, page 133.
Quadratus femoris (Figure 8-4)	See Hip Adduction, page 135.
*Gluteus maximus (Figure 8-6)	See Hip Extension, page 132.
Piriformis (Figures 8-4 and 8-7)	See Hip Abduction, page 133.
Sartorius (Figure 8-3)	See Hip Flexion, page 127.
Pectineus (Figure 8-3)	See Hip Flexion, page 127.
Adductor brevis (Figure 8-5)	See Hip Flexion, page 127.
Adductor longus (Figure 8-5)	See Hip Flexion, page 127.
Adductor magnus (Figure 8-5)	See Hip Flexion, page 127.
Gluteus medius and minimus (Figures 8-6 and 8-4)	See Hip Extension, page 132.

Muscle	Description and actions
Biceps femoris (long head) (Figure 8-4)	See Hip Extension, page 132.

Hip Circumduction

The hip joint is another one of the few joints capable of circumduction. As described earlier, circumduction is the sequential combination of flexion, abduction, extension, and adduction. It is not frequently used.

MUSCULAR ACTIONS OF THE KNEE

The articulation of the tibia and femur at the knee forms a joint which is usually considered capable of only two movements—flexion and extension. However, the lower leg can rotate slightly when the knee is in a flexed position. As the knee extends, the amount of possible rotation decreases, until when full extension is reached no rotation is possible. These rotating movements aid in changing direction during running, but otherwise they have little effect on performance.

Twelve muscles contribute to knee extension and flexion. Eight of these are two-joint muscles acting on either the hip or ankle joint in addition to the knee. Knee actions are relatively strong because the muscles causing them are mostly the large and powerful muscles of the upper leg.

Knee Flexion

Flexion of the knee is caused by the actions of eight muscles. Even though they work against a poor mechanical ratio, knee flexion is still a relatively strong movement. It is one of the important movements in walking and running (during the recovery phase of the stride). Therefore, it is one of our most frequently used movements. Also, it is used extensively in swimming, primarily during the preparatory phase of the various kicks. The knee flexors have a mechanical ratio of about 0.18.

Muscle	Description and actions
Biceps femoris (Figure 8-4)	See Hip Extension, page 132.
Semimembranosus (Figure 8-4)	See Hip Extension, page 132.

Muscle	Description and actions
*Semi-tendinosus (Figure 8-4)	See Hip Extension, page 132.
Gastrocnemius (Figure 8-8)	This large biceps muscle of the calf attaches proximally just above the knee on the medial and lateral condyles of the femur. It extends down the back of the lower leg and inserts onto the calcaneus bone by way of the Achilles tendon. It flexes the knee and plantar flexes the ankle.
Sartorius (Figure 8-3)	See Hip Flexion, page 127.

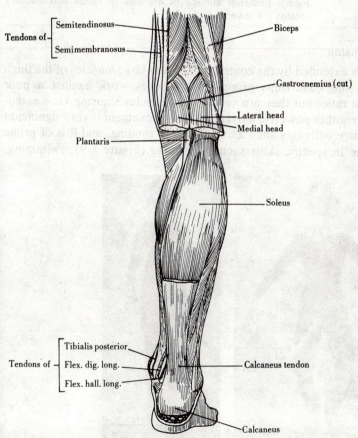

Semitendinosus
Tendons of
Semimembranosus
Biceps
Gastrocnemius (cut)
Lateral head
Medial head
Plantaris
Soleus
Tibialis posterior
Tendons of
Flex. dig. long.
Flex. hall. long.
Calcaneus tendon
Calcaneus

Figure 8-8 Superficial muscles of the back of the lower leg. (*After C. M. Goss, Gray's Anatomy, 29th ed., Lea & Febiger, Philadelphia, 1973.*)

Muscle	Description and actions
Gracilis (Figures 8-3 and 8-4)	See Hip Adduction, page 135.
Plantaris (Figure 8-8)	This two-joint muscle attaches proximally to the middle of the posterior surface of the femur just above the knee and extends down the back of the leg to its distal attachment on the upper surface of the calcaneus bone. It flexes the knee and plantar flexes the ankle.
Popliteus (Figure 8-10)	Attaches proximally to the lateral surface of the lateral condyle of the femur and extends diagonally downward across the posterior and upper part of the lower leg and attaches on the medial posterior surface of the tibia. It flexes and medially rotates the lower leg.

Knee Extension

The knee is extended by the contraction of four large muscles of the thigh known as the quadriceps group. The muscles work against a poor mechanical ratio, but they are very strong muscles, causing knee extension to be another powerful movement. This movement is very significant in locomotive activities such as walking and running, and it is of prime importance in specific skills such as jumping (Figure 8-9), swimming,

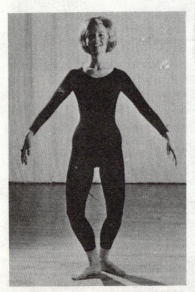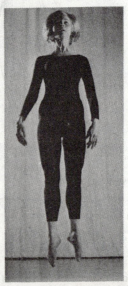

Figure 8-9 Hip, knee, and ankle extension are prime movements in a jump following a plie.

lifting, kicking, skiing, skating, and dodging. Also the knee extensors are principal postural muscles. The knee extensors have a mechanical ratio of about 0.37 compared to 0.26 for the flexors. This, plus four compared with three main muscles, explains why the extensors dominate when all units are simultaneously activated, as in the vertical jump. Also, the tension put on the hamstrings at the knee is effective in applying more force in the hip extension action.

Muscle	Description and actions
*Rectus femoris (Figure 8-3)	See Hip Flexion, page 127.
*Vastus intermedius (Figure 8-5)	This large muscle lies vertically along the front of the thigh, underneath the rectus femoris. Its proximal attachment is along the front of the femur, extending most of its length. The distal attachment is on the patella. It extends the knee.
*Vastus lateralis (Figure 8-3)	This muscle lies vertically alongside the vastus intermedius. Its proximal attachment is on the upper portion of the lateral surface of the femur. The distal attachment is on the top of the patella. It extends the knee.
*Vastus medialis (Figure 8-3)	This muscle lies along the medial side of the vastus intermedius. Its proximal attachment is on the medial surface of the upper portion of the femur. It extends downward and attaches to the top of the patella. It extends the knee.

Lower-Leg Rotation

When the knee is flexed, the lower leg may be slightly rotated medially and laterally. Because of the structure of the knee joint, these movements are not possible when the knee is fully extended. The movements are used in a few activities such as water and snow skiing. Following are the muscles which cause the lower leg to rotate when in a flexed position.

Medial rotation	Lateral rotation
*Semimembranosus	*Biceps femoris
*Semitendinosus	
Sartorius	
Popliteus	
Gracilis	

MUSCULAR ACTIONS OF THE ANKLE

The ankle joint is of the hinge type and is formed by the articulation of the talus bone with the tibia and fibula. Like other hinge joints, the ankle is

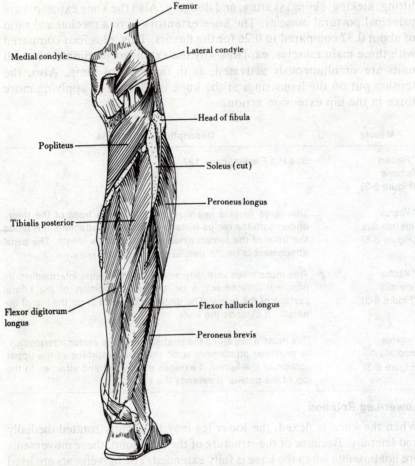

Femur

Lateral condyle

Medial condyle

Head of fibula

Popliteus

Soleus (cut)

Peroneus longus

Tibialis posterior

Flexor digitorum longus

Flexor hallucis longus

Peroneus brevis

Figure 8-10 Deep muscles of the back of the lower leg. (*After C. M. Goss, Gray's Anatomy, 29th ed., Lea & Febiger, Philadelphia, 1973.*)

capable of only two movements, flexion (dorsiflexion) and extension (plantar flexion). Dorsiflexion is a relatively weak movement, whereas plantar flexion is a very strong movement, and one which is highly significant.

Plantar Flexion (Extension)

Eight muscles contribute to plantar flexion, and seven of these are multijoint muscles. One (gastrocnemius) also crosses over the knee joint and contributes to knee flexion, and five other muscles extend into the foot and contribute to foot movements. Plantar flexion is a strong movement due to the favorable mechanical ratio of the calf muscles, which exceeds a two to one ratio in favor of force. This is also explained by the relatively small diameter of the calf compared with the thigh, which has about a four to one speed ratio, or a mechanical disadvantage of more than four to one. Therefore, the plantar flexors are so arranged as to be able to withstand the strong movements of the trunk and thigh which are often superimposed upon them. Plantar flexors make a significant contribution to walking and running. They are also significant in jumping, lifting, and throwing, actions which are used in a great number of physical performances.

Muscle	Description and actions
*Gastrocnemius (Figure 8-8)	See Knee Flexion, page 138.
*Soleus (Figure 8-8)	This large calf muscle lies underneath the gastrocnemius. Its proximal attachment is on the head of the fibula and medial border of the tibia. It extends down the back of the leg and attaches to the calcaneus bone, by way of the Achilles tendon. It causes plantar flexion.
Peroneus longus (Figures 8-10 and 8-11)	Proximal attachment is on the upper two-thirds of the lateral surface of the fibula and the upper tibia. It extends down the lateral side of the leg and attaches onto the first metatarsal and first cuneiform bones. It causes plantar flexion and eversion of the foot. It also helps to maintain the arch of the foot.
Peroneus brevis (Figure 8-11)	Attaches proximally onto the lateral surface of the lower two-thirds of the fibula, extends down the outside of the legs, and attaches at the fifth metatarsal bone. It causes plantar flexion and eversion of the foot.
Tibialis posterior (Figure 8-10)	This muscle lies vertically down the back of the lower leg, underneath the soleus and gastrocnemius. Its proximal attachment is on the upper posterior surface of the tibia and fibula. It passes diagonally downward across the inside of the ankle and attaches to the arch of the foot. It inverts the foot and assists in plantar flexion.
Flexor digitorum longus (Figures 8-10 and 8-13)	Proximal attachment is on the medial posterior surface of the tibia about one-fourth of the way down from the knee. It lies vertically down the inside of the lower leg and attaches to the last phalanges of the four outer toes by way of four tendons. It plantar flexes and inverts the foot and flexes the toes.

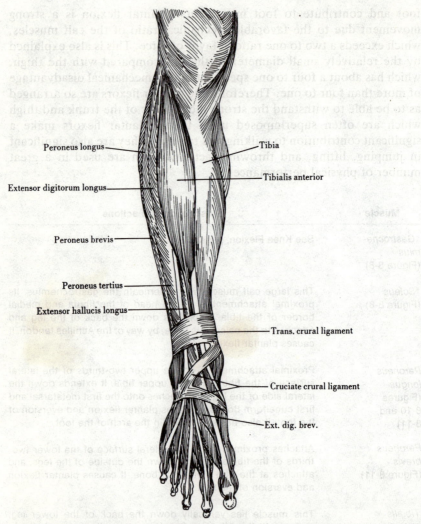

Peroneus longus

Extensor digitorum longus

Peroneus brevis

Peroneus tertius

Extensor hallucis longus

Tibia

Tibialis anterior

Trans. crural ligament

Cruciate crural ligament

Ext. dig. brev.

Figure 8-11 Muscles of the front of the lower leg. (*After C. M. Goss, Gray's Anatomy, 29th ed., Lea & Febiger, Philadelphia, 1973.*)

Muscle	Description and actions
Flexor hallucis longus (Figures 8-10 and 8-13)	Proximal attachment is on the distal two-thirds of the posterior surface of the fibula. It passes along the inside of the ankle and attaches to the base of the last phalanx of the big toe. It flexes the big toe and plantar flexes and inverts the foot.
Plantaris (Figure 8-8)	See Knee Flexion, page 138.

Dorsiflexion

Four muscles contribute to dorsiflexion, all of which are multijoint muscles extending across the ankle into the foot. This movement is relatively weak, but it is very important in swimming and in kicking. The dorsal flexors hold the foot in the desired position during kicking, and during walking and running they hold the swinging foot in position to clear the surface.

Muscle	Description and actions
*Peroneus tertius (Figure 8-11)	Proximal attachment is on the lower part of the fibula on the anterior lateral surface. It extends down the outside of the leg and attaches onto the fifth metartarsal bone. It flexes the ankle and everts the foot.
*Tibialis anterior (Figure 8-11	Proximal attachment is on the lateral and upper part of the tibia. It extends down the front of the leg and attaches at the metatarsal bone of the big toe. It flexes the ankle and inverts the foot.
*Extensor digitorum longus (Figure 8-11)	Attaches proximally to the lateral condyle of the tibia and upper anterior surface of the fibula. It extends down the outside of the leg and attaches onto the second and third phalanges of the four toes. It flexes the ankle, extends the toes, and everts the foot.
Extensor hallucis longus (Figure 8-11)	Attaches proximally to the anterior of the middle and lower fibula, extends down the anterior lateral side of the leg, and attaches to the big toe. It extends the big toe and flexes the foot.

MUSCULAR ACTIONS OF THE FOOT

The foot is a complex structure which is uniquely designed to play a major role in locomotion, balance, and cushioning of the force when landing. The foot includes several joints, and because of the actions of these joints it is able to invert, evert, plantar flex, dorsiflex, and circumduct. (Plantar flexion and dorsiflexion occur in the ankle joint and tarsal joint. The same muscles cause the movements in both joints.) The ankle joint also combines with the joints of the foot in circumduction. The toes may be flexed, extended, abducted, adducted, and circumducted.

There are twenty muscles contributing to foot movements which are worthy of mention here. Nine of the muscles extend from the lower leg, across the ankle joint, and attach to bones in the foot. The other eleven muscles are located totally in the foot. (See Figures 8-12, 8-13, and 8-14.)

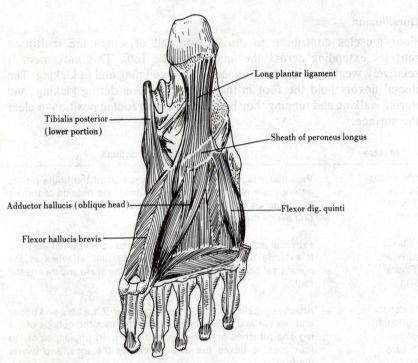

Long plantar ligament

Tibialis posterior
(lower portion)

Sheath of peroneus longus

Adductor hallucis (oblique head)

Flexor dig. quinti

Flexor hallucis brevis

Figure 8-12 Deep muscles of the bottom of the foot. (*After C. M. Goss, Gray's Anatomy, 29th ed., Lea & Febiger, Philadelphia. 1973.*)

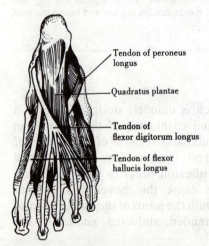

Tendon of peroneus longus

Quadratus plantae

Tendon of flexor digitorum longus

Tendon of flexor hallucis longus

Figure 8-13 Middle-layer muscles of the bottom of the foot. (*After Helen L. Dawson, Basic Human Anatomy, Appleton Century Crofts, New York, 1966.*)

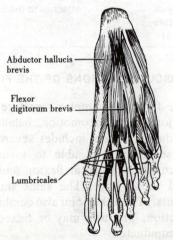

Abductor hallucis brevis

Flexor digitorum brevis

Lumbricales

Figure 8-14 Superficial muscles of the bottom of the foot. (*After Helen L. Dawson, Basic Human Anatomy, Appleton Century Crofts, New York, 1966.*)

Inversion of the Foot

Inversion is not a strong movement, but it is frequently used in sports. The invertor muscles are used in running and walking where zigzagging and dodging are involved, and in side-stepping and other performances where body weight is shifted in a lateral direction. Such movements are frequent in field and court games—tennis, badminton, baseball, soccer, football, skiing, etc. Four muscles are important contributors to foot inversion.

Muscle	Description and actions
*Tibialis anterior (Figure 8-11)	See Dorsiflexion, page 145.
*Tibialis posterior (Figure 8-10)	See Plantar Flexion, page 142.
*Flexor digitorum longus (Figures 8-10 and 8-13)	See Plantar Flexion, page 142.
*Flexor hallucis longus (Figures 8-10 and 8-13)	See Plantar Flexion, page 142.

Eversion of the Foot

Foot eversion is used with about the same frequency as inversion. As one foot is used in inversion, the other is generally used in eversion. Such is the case in dodging, side-stepping, and shifting the weight laterally from one foot to the other. For instance, if a field runner side-steps to the right the invertors of the left foot and the evertors of the right foot are important contributors. Also, the evertors and invertors of opposite feet work effectively together when the body weight is shifted laterally, as in a tennis stroke, golf swing, and batting, skiing, and throwing actions or when the body is "set" to resist lateral force. Four muscles evert the foot.

Muscle	Description and actions
*Peroneus brevis (Figure 8-11)	See Plantar Flexion, page 142.
*Peroneus longus (Figures 8-10 and 8-11)	See Plantar Flexion, page 142
*Peroneus tertius (Figure 8-11)	See Dorsiflexion, page 145.
Extensor digitorum longus (Figure 8-11)	See Dorsiflexion, page 145.

Toe Flexion

Toe flexion is one of the most important and frequently used movements. It is used extensively in locomotion, especially walking, running, and dancing. And it is of prime importance in all performances where the body is thrust, as in jumping (Figure 18-2). Seven different muscles are important contributors to toe flexion. In such instances the toes act in pushing against the surface. The flexion movement is a return to normal position from hyperrextension. The hyperextension occurs as a result of plantar flexor muscles lifting the heel.

Muscle	Description and actions
*Flexor dlgltorum longus (Figures 8-10 and 8-13)	See Plantar Flexion, page 142.
*Flexor hallucis longus (Figures 8-10 and 8-13)	See Plantar Flexion, page 142.
Flexor digitorum brevis (Figure 8-14)	Proximal attachment is on the medial process of the tuberosity of the calcaneus. It extends along the middle underside of the foot, and attaches to the phalanges of the second, third, and fourth toes. It flexes the toes.

Muscle	Description and actions
Flexor hallucis brevis (Figure 8-12)	Attaches proximally to the area known as the cuboid (under the arch of the foot) and extends diagonally to the lateral side of the foot. It attaches to the first phalanx of the big toe. It flexes the big toe.
Adductor hallucis (obliquus) (Figure 8-12)	Attaches proximally to the second, third, and fourth metatarsal bones and ligaments (approximately under the arch), extends along the medial side of the bottom of the foot, and attaches to the medial side of the first phalanx of the big toe. It adducts and flexes the big toe.
Lumbricalis (Figure 8-14)	Attaches proximally to the tendons of the flexor digitorum longus (about 1 inch behind the toes). It splits into four small muscles, which attach to the phalanges of the four outer toes. It extends the last phalanges of the toes, and flexes the first phalanges.
Quadratus plantae (Figure 8-13)	Attaches proximally to the anterior surface of the calcaneus, and extends to the arch of the foot, where it attaches to the tendon of the flexor digitorum longus. It flexes the toes.

The toes are also capable of extension, and a very limited amount of abduction, adduction, and circumduction. But these movements are not significant contributions to performance and so are not analyzed here.

STUDENT LABORATORY EXPERIENCES

1. If a medcolator is available, electrically stimulate selected muscles of the lower extremity. For example, hold one electrode in a hand and have a partner probe motor points of superficial muscles of the lower leg and foot. Notice the action and try to name the muscle responsible for the movement.
2. If a cadaver laboratory is available, tag twenty-five lower-extremity muscles by number and write the correct name of the tagged muscles.
3. On a tracing of Figure 8-1, place drawings of the muscles in the lower extremities.
4. After carefully studying the muscular actions of the lower extremities and the following muscle-action table, make duplicate tables, leaving the action columns blank. Then practice filling in the table by memory. It will be helpful to visualize the joint, noting the location and the way in which the muscles cross the joint, then judge whether or not the indicated action appears to be possible. Afterward, check your answers against the table given.

Muscle Action Table: Lower Extremities I

Muscle	Hip							
	Flexion	Extension	Abduction	Adduction	Medial rotation	Lateral rotation	Horiz. Adduction	Horiz. Abduction
Rectus femoris	X						X	
Pectineus	X			X		X	X	
Psoas major	X					X	X	
Iliacus	X					X	X	
Sartorius	X		X			X	X	
Adductor brevis	X			X		X	X	
Adductor longus	X			X		X	X	
Adductor magnus	X			X		X		
Gracilus	X			X	X		X	
Biceps femoris (long head)		X				X		
Semimembranosus		X			X			
Semitendinosus		X			X			
Gluteus maximus		PM	UF	LF		X		X
Gluteus medius	AF	PF	X		AF	PF		X
Gluteus minimus	AF	PF	X		AF	PF		X
Tensor fasciae latae	X		X		X		X	
Gemelli			X			X		X
Obturator externus						X		X
Obturator internus						X		X
Piriformis			X			X		X
Quadratus femoris						X		X

AF: anterior fibers: PF: posterior fibers: UF: upper fibers; LF: lower fibers.

Muscle Action Table: Lower Extremities II

Muscle	Knee and lower leg			
	Flexion	Extension	Medial rotation	Lateral rotation
Biceps femoris	X			X
Semimembranosus	X		X	
Semitendinosus	X		X	
Gastrocnemius	X			
Sartorius	X			X
Gracilis	X		X	
Plantaris	X			
Popliteus	X		X	
Rectus femoris		X		
Vastus intermedius		X		
Vastus medialis		X		
Vastus lateralis		X		

Muscle Action Table: Lower Extremities III

Muscle	Ankle and foot					
	Dorsiflexion	Plantar flexion	Inversion	Eversion	Toe extension	Toe flexion
Tibialis anterior	X		X			
Extensor digitorum longus	X			X	X	
Extensor hallucis longus	X		X		X	
Peroneus tertius	X			X		
Peroneus longus		X		X		
Peroneus brevis		X		X		
Gastrocnemius		X				
Soleus		X				
Plantaris		X				
Tibialis posterior		X	X			
Flexor digitorum longus		X	X			X
Flexor hallucis longus		X	X			X
Flexor digitorum brevis						X
Flexor hallucis brevis						X
Adductor hallucis						X
Lubricalis					X	X
Quadratus plantae						X

Chapter 9

Increasing the Effectiveness of Muscles

Presented in this chapter are important facts about muscular strength, endurance, power, speed of contraction, and tone that are pertinent to development and improvement of muscle use.

STRENGTH

Strength is the ability of the body or a segment of the body to apply force. People often have the impression that strength is simply the contractile force of a muscle or group of muscles. But strength involves a combination of three factors: (1) the combined contractile forces of the muscles causing the movement; (2) the ability to coordinate the agonist muscles with the antagonist, neutralizer, and stabilizer muscles; and (3) the mechanical ratios of the lever (bone) arrangements involved. The first factor depends on the maximum contractile force of each muscle agonistic to the movement. This force can be increased significantly through progressive resistance training. The second factor depends on the ability to coordinate the contractions of the individual muscles. This coordination can be improved by practicing the particular movements involved (develop skill in the movements). The third factor depends on the relative length of the resistance and effort arms of the levers. Sometimes this ratio can be altered advantageously by changing positions of certain body parts.

Strength is basic to motor performance, and it may be the most important single factor in performance. Because almost all vigorous performances depend on ability to apply great force against a resistance, increased strength will often contribute to better performance.

The contractile force of a muscle is directly related to the cross-sectional measurement of that muscle. As muscle strength increases, the cross section of the individual muscle fibers increases, resulting in a greater cross-sectional area of the total muscle. Theoretically, this measurement is proportionate to strength. However, this is not always true, because other factors are involved. For instance: (1) Two muscles having equal cross sections may differ in strength because of varying amounts of fatty tissue. Fat not only lacks ability to contract, but it also causes friction and interference with the shortening of muscle fibers. (2) The proportion of active fibers in different muscles influences strength. (3) The efficiency of contraction has an important influence on strength. Nevertheless, muscle size and strength are very closely related.

Conditions Influencing Strength Development

Several conditions influence the rate that strength develops and how long it is retained. Following are brief discussions of the more important facts which affect strength.

Strength May Be Increased by Training A muscle increases in strength when it contracts regularly against resistance greater than usual. If the rate of increase is to be rapid, the muscle must contract regularly against a heavy resistance, and the resistance must be increased as the muscle increases in strength. This is known as a *progressive resistance strength-building program*. Strength gains in certain muscles of over 100 percent in a week have been reported on rare occasions. But typically, strength gains of 5 percent weekly over several weeks are considered a fast rate of gain. Percent of gain is usually greater during the early part of training, especially if the muscles are weak in the beginning.

Not All Muscles Respond Equally When the same training program is used, the amount of strength development varies among different people. Within each individual, certain muscles respond better to strength stimuli than other muscles. When put on a strength-building program of equal intensity, some muscles may increase at 5 percent weekly, while others increase only 1 percent. This results partly because some muscles are in better condition at the beginning of training; ordinarily, those in poor condition increase more rapidly than those in good condition.

When Vigorous Muscle Use Ceases, Strength Decreases   Research results show that when a strength-building program ceases, the individual begins to lose strength almost immediately (seven to ten days). Strength developed at a slow rate lasts longer than strength developed rapidly. After strength training ceases, strength is lost at approximately one-third the rate it was gained. But a small amount of the gained strength remains indefinitely. If a segment of the body is completely immobilized, as when placed in a cast, strength decreases very rapidly (20 to 30 percent per week).

Strength Relates Closely to Age   Strength increases at a rather steady rate from birth to about age twenty-five, or twenty for women, at which time it levels off and then begins to decline at a gradual rate. At age sixty-five the typical person has approximately 70 percent of the prior peak strength remaining. Of course, the rate at which a person develops and loses strength is influenced by rate of maturation and the amount and kind of activity. As a result of training, a person can maintain near-maximum strength for several years beyond age twenty-five.

Contractile Force Varies with Muscle Length during Contraction   The contractile force of a muscle is greatest when the muscle is fully extended (at full extension, a muscle is about one-third longer than at rest). Force steadily diminishes as the muscle moves through contraction (shortens); when the muscle is fully contracted, its contractile force has been reduced to zero. This situation may be paralleled to a rubber band, which has its greatest tension when on stretch. It should be noted that contractile force does not reduce in the same proportion as the length of the muscle. During the early phase of contraction, force reduces much more slowly than muscle length; whereas during the late phase, force reduces proportionately faster than muscle length.

Strength Differs Slightly on the Two Sides of the Body   Even though right-handed people use the right side of the body considerable more than the left side (vice versa for left-handed people), the right side is only slightly stronger, and its musculature is only slightly larger than that of the left side. Physiologists generally attribute this to the cross-transfer theory, which means that training of one side of the body will influence the development of like muscles on the other side.

With Equal Training, Strength Develops More Slowly among Women than among Men   Research results on this topic are conflicting, but the available information indicates that after the age of approximately twelve years, females respond less readily to strength stimuli than males. When male sex hormones (testosterone) are injected into women during training, they develop strength at an increased rate. However, the reason men are stronger than women is not so much that they differ in response to strength stimuli, but that men are larger than women. Per cubic unit of muscle, women are nearly as strong as men.

Reserve Strength Becomes Available under Great Stress or Excitement   The reserve-strength theory is supported by observations of people who performed great feats of strength while under emotional stress or excitement and were unable to perform voluntarily the same feats after the emotional state had passed. This idea has little support from research, probably because the topic is difficult to treat experimentally. The excitement and stress cannot be provided under controlled conditions. Physiologists have explained reserve strength as a condition resulting from (1) increased secretion of adrenalin, causing the muscles to become more irritable, or (2) a stronger stimulus from the central nervous system and a reduction of inhibitions, causing more muscle fibers to respond.

Methods of Increasing Strength

To increase rapidly in strength, muscles must be contracted against heavy resistance, and the resistance must be increased as the muscles become stronger. In other words, the muscles are *overloaded,* meaning they are loaded beyond previous requirements, and *progressive resistance* is applied, meaning that as the muscles become stronger they are worked against resistance which is correspondingly greater.

There are several approaches to developing strength. In fact, any form of exercise which applies heavier than usual resistance will stimulate an increase in strength. Strength-building stimuli may be provided by:

1   Hard manual labor or vigorous athletic performance. (It is not possible to approach maximal strength by this method because of the absence of progressive resistance.)

2   Specific exercises against body weight, as in pull-ups or dips. (Additional weight must be added to body weight in order to get sustained gains in strength.)

3   Heavy resistance exercises against external movable resistance, such as weight-training equipment. (This method provides the greatest potential for gaining strength, because the resistance can be increased progressively, and muscle groups can be isolated and very heavy resistance imposed.)

4 Application of muscle tension (isometric contractions) against a fixed object or another body part. (This method has proven to be effective, but it has some pronounced limitations.)

The first three methods result in isotonic (dynamic) contractions, meaning the muscles change in length, and movement of body segments occurs. The fourth method results in isometric (static) contractions, where the muscles apply tension but do not shorten, and do not move the body segments.

Isotonic (Dynamic) Strength-Building Methods Before World War II, strength-building programs were used very little in athletic training. In fact, it was generally believed that "muscle-boundness" resulted from such programs. They were taboo to those seeking to improve performance. During World War II, therapists experienced success with heavy resistance exercises in the rehabilitation of hospital patients. Subsequently, additional research was done to determine the effectiveness of this kind of training for improving athletic performance. It was learned that increased strength was highly beneficial to athletic performance and that heavy resistance exercise was the most expedient method of increasing strength. Hence, weight training gained popularity among athletes and coaches.

Recently, another form of isotonic exercise, called *isokinetics*, is being advanced as a superior method for building strength. It affords the advantage of a variable resistance which allows the development of maximum tension by the performer throughout the full range of motion, while the fixed resistance of traditional isotonic exercise actually becomes a *reduced* resistance as the movement progresses (**62**).

Strength can be increased most rapidly by exercising against very heavy resistance for a few repetitions. After much study and experimentation, DeLorme and Watkins (**21**) declared that strength can be increased at the most rapid rate by employing heavy resistance for ten repetitions and three sets. They specifically recommended the following program to be executed every second day.

One set of 10 repetitions with 1/2 10 RMs
One set of 10 repetitions with 3/4 10 RMs
One set of 10 repetitions with 10 RMs

(RM means repetition maximum. Ten RMs is ten repetitions of an exercise using the maximum weight that can be lifted successively ten times.)

Recently, other investigators have produced evidence that fewer repetitions and heavier weight are more effective. For instance, Berger

(11) found that strength increases most when four to eight RMs are used with three sets. Other studies have added support to Berger's findings. Currently there is lack of agreement among experts about the exact program that is best for building strength, but the following points are well established and universally accepted:

1 Exercises must be selected to work the specific muscles in which strength is to be developed, because significant strength gains result only in exercised muscles.

2 Muscles should be contracted regularly (every second day; i.e., Monday, Wednesday, Friday) against *heavy* resistance.

3 Near-maximum weight for few repetitions (four to eight) should be used.

4 As strength increases, the weight must be progressively increased to provide continual overloading of the muscles (progressive resistance).

Suppose you want to design a strength-building program for a shot-putter, an athlete who requires great strength and speed. A typical procedure would be as follows:

1 Analyze the performance, and determine the contributing movements.

2 Select exercises which work the muscles that cause those movements.

3 Determine the maximum amount of weight that can be lifted for one repetition with each exercise, and use 70 to 80 percent of maximum weight.

4 Perform at least three sets of each exercise, doing as many repetitions as possible in each set. (If more than eight repetitions can be done, the weight is too light.) Some mature athletes prefer to do more sets (five to fifteen) with few repetitions (two or three) and very heavy weight (80 to 90 percent of 1 RM).

5 Rest 2 to 3 minutes between sets.

6 Do the workout on alternate days (Monday, Wednesday, Friday).

7 Increase the resistance as much as possible each week (progressive resistance, while staying within the selected range of four to eight repetitions).

Specific exercises for strengthening certain muscles can be obtained from weight-training charts and books. However, with knowledge of the actions of the major skeletal muscles, you should be able to design your own exercise program to suit your specific purpose. If in doubt, the exercise movement which most closely resembles the skill in which you are interested will probably be the correct choice. Be aware that the resistance must oppose the actions of the muscles you want to strengthen. (Figures 9-1 and 9-2 show isotonic exercise.)

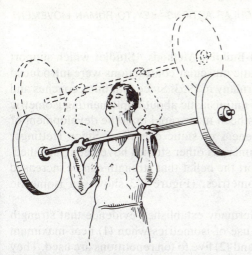

Figure 9-1 Two-arm press exercise (isotonic).

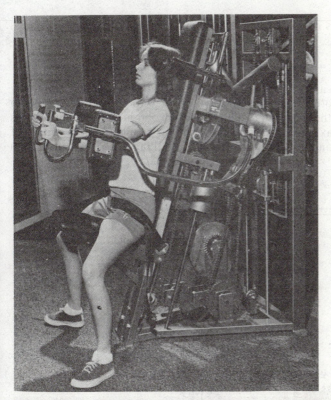

Figure 9-2 Nautilus equipment being used in muscle training. This sophisticated machinery is highly useful for the development of muscular strength, endurance, and power. Several different machines have been designed for developing different muscle groups.

Isometric (Static) Strength-Building Methods   Studies which support increasing strength through static muscular contractions were introduced by Hettinger and Muller of Germany in 1953. Since that time, coaches and athletes have been almost too enthusiastic about implementing isometric programs. Implementation has been more rapid than the development of knowledge about the effectiveness of static exercises. Since Hettinger and Muller's original study, numerous other studies have been published, most of which generally support the belief that strength can be increased at a rapid rate by use of isometrics. (Figure 9-3 shows an isometric exercise.)

Muller and Rohmert of Germany established evidence that strength will increase more rapidly by use of isometrics when (1) near-maximum muscle contractions are used and (2) five to ten repetitions are used. They also established the theory that strength will increase more evenly throughout the range of motion if the contractions are executed at various positions.

On the basis of presently available information, the following points are presented as guides for designing isometric strength-building programs:

1   Strength at a particular body position can be increased rapidly by using one or more maximum contractions of 8 to 10 seconds in length each day. Even though good results have been obtained with contractions of two-thirds maximum, it has been found that people are poor judges of how much tension they apply, so that the safe thing to do is use maximum tension.

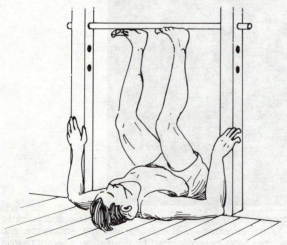

Figure 9-3   Two-leg press exercise (isometric).

2 If increased strength is desired throughout the full range, several (five to ten) contractions should be done at various positions. Where strength is needed only at the beginning of the motion, as in ballistic movements, the exercises should be designed accordingly.

3 If rapid development of strength is the primary concern, training should be done daily. However, if the objective is more long-range, training may be done on alternate days. Strength gained slowly tends to be more permanent.

4 One workout per day will produce as much strength as multiple workouts.

5 The best breathing technique is to take a deep breath at the beginning of the contraction, hold it for a few seconds, then exhale slowly during the latter part of the contraction. This technique protects the performer from fainting.

Comparison of Isometric and Isotonic Methods It has been found that static strength develops more rapidly by training statically, while dynamic strength develops more rapidly by training dynamically. Following are advantages of *isotonic training:*

1 There is a psychological advantage in isotonic exercises for some individuals, because they can see heavy work being done.

2 Isotonics cause more muscle hypertrophy. It is theorized that this is due to the increased capillarization which is stimulated much more by isotonics than by isometrics.

3 Isotonics causes strength to develop more uniformly throughout the range of motion.

4 More neuromuscular coordination results (smooth application of force) from isotonics, because the nerve-muscle innervation is much more complex than in isometrics.

5 Research indicates that even when strength gains from the two methods are equal, the strength from isotonics has more application to motor performance.

Advantages of *isometric training* are as follows:

1 It requires less time, less energy, less space, and very little equipment.

2 Isometrics can be used in many situations where isotonic programs are not feasible, such as in the home or the office.

Combining Isotonic and Isometric Exercises A limited amount of research supports the claim that strength can be gained at a rapid rate by combining isometrics and isotonics. This is done by contracting the muscles isometrically against a rope or cable arrangement for about 10 seconds, then reducing the resistance to allow a slow-motion isotonic contraction to occur. Several mechanical devices for use with this approach have been developed and sold commercially. With this method it is recommended that each exercise be repeated five to ten times daily.

Functional Overload A less effective and seldom-used method is functional overload. The activity itself is performed under resistive conditions. Weighted vests, ankle weights, and other weighted objects and implements have been used in the past. Throwing weighted baseballs and swinging weighted bats are still common practices. This method has the advantage of closely coordinating the strength gains into the movement patterns, but some experts think it reduces coordination and timing. Only mild strength gains result from this method, because typically the resistance is too little to provide a strong stimulus for strength. If too heavy a resistance is chosen, a falsification of the skill pattern may result using substitute muscle groups.

Physiological Changes with Strength

Several physiological changes consistently accompany increased strength. The more significant changes are:

1 Increased size of muscle fibers
2 Increased proportion of active fibers
3 Increased protein content
4 Increased fluid content
5 Increased capillarization (related to muscular endurance)
6 Increased connective tissue
7 Decreased fat within the muscle tissues
8 Changes in muscle chemistry
9 Decreased inhibitory control of muscles

The first six of these changes contribute to increased cross-sectional area of the muscle.

ENDURANCE

Endurance is defined as resistance to fatigue and quick recovery after fatigue. This definition may apply to the body as a whole, to a particular body system, or to a local area of the muscle system. For instance, we sometimes refer to total body endurance, circulorespiratory endurance, muscular endurance, or endurance of a particular part of the muscular system. But regardless of how many different names we give to endurance, the loss of it (fatigue) always has the same result—the muscles discontinue functioning effectively. They contract more slowly with less force, and predictability. The exact location of the fatigue which causes muscle failure is difficult to determine.

A high level of endurance implies that the person can maintain a given level of performance. When endurance gives way to fatigue as a result of muscular work, several elements important for good performance diminish: strength, timing, neuromuscular coordination, speed of movement, reaction time, and general alertness. Increased endurance postpones the onset of fatigue; therefore, endurance contributes to improved performance when fatigue is a limiting factor.

Conditions Influencing Endurance

Several factors influence endurance. Following are brief discussions of the more important factors.

Strength Contributes to Muscular Endurance   Suppose a person has a given amount of strength with which to move a particular amount of resistance through the range of motion one hundred times. If the strength were increased 50 percent, the person would be able to move the same resistance with greater ease; therefore, the movement could be repeated considerably more than one hundred times. Increased strength would result in increased muscular endurance.

The above statement refers to *absolute* endurance. In *relative* endurance, however, there are indications that strength hampers endurance. When the load (resistance) is a percentage of the maximum strength, those with less strength tend to endure longer. It is postulated that the strength element is partially factored out in this case and the shift is back to a more valid measure of true muscular endurance. Probably because of the hypertrophy of the muscle fibers associated with greater strength, the relative area of contact for the exchange of gases and nutrients between capillaries and muscle fibers is less with greater strength.

Neuromuscular Skill Influences Endurance   During performance, a certain amount of energy is wasted in unnecessary and uncoordinated movements. The skilled person wastes less energy than the unskilled. It has been found that an unskilled swimmer may use more than five times as much energy as a skilled person to swim the same distance. Similar but less dramatic comparisons could be made between skilled and unskilled performers in other activities.

Fatty Tissue Decreases Endurance   Fat lacks the ability to contract; therefore, it does not contribute to a person's performance. In fact, it hinders performance in three ways: (1) Fat within the muscle causes friction and contributes to inefficiency in muscle contractions; (2) fat within and surrounding the muscle adds dead weight, increasing resistance against the movement; (3) fatty tissue places an overload on the circulatory system. It is estimated that 1 pound of fat is equivalent to an increase in the vascular system of 1 mile.

Sustained Muscular Work Is Dependent upon the Circulatory and Respiratory Systems   For a muscle to continue to function, the individual muscle cells must receive nutrients and oxygen from the circulatory system, which also transports waste products from the muscles. The respiratory system supplies oxygen to the circulatory system and receives carbon dioxide and other waste from it. If the circulatory and cooperating systems do not keep the muscles adequately supplied with nutrients and oxygen and free of waste products, fatigue occurs.

Sustained Work Is Dependent upon the Nervous System   A muscle contracts only when it receives a stimulus, and the strength of its contraction is dependent partly upon the intensity of the stimulus. (An intense stimulus causes more motor units to respond, with each unit contracting to its maximum.) Therefore, under strenuous effort, if the nervous system does not continue to supply stimuli, the muscles will not continue to contract strongly. In such a case, the muscles appear to be fatigued, but the actual location of fatigue may be in the nervous system. Classic experiments with frogs reveal that in the connections between neurons (synapses) and between the neuron and the muscle fibers, fatigue occurs more readily than either in the nerve or in the muscle tissue itself.

Muscular Endurance Is Dependent upon Ability to Tolerate Acid Waste   The process of muscle contraction results in acid waste products, primarily lactic acid. Muscular activity is greatly hindered, and in fact it usually ends, when the lactate level in the blood is between 0.032 and 0.140 percent. Therefore, a person's endurance is strongly influenced by his ability to dispose of lactic acid and to tolerate a high level of this by-product. Tolerance increases as a result of forcing tissues to contend with high lactate levels in training, giving support to the contention that "the last repetition is most important." At this time highest lactate levels are present.

Endurance Is Related to Body Type, Sex, and Age   The following relationships exist: (1) On the average, mesomorphs (heavily muscled athletic type) and ectomorphs (slight body type) are more durable than endomorphs (obese type), with mesomorphs slightly more durable than ectomorphs. (However, there are exceptions to these rules.) (2) Up to the age of approximately thirteen, boys and girls possess about the same amount of endurance. After age thirteen, the durability of girls increases very little, while that of boys continues to increase to at least maturity, and sometimes considerably beyond that. Some men have been known to increase in endurance until they reach their middle thirties. (3) The relationship between age and endurance varies. Endurance increases with age up to a certain point, at which time endurance begins to decrease as age increases. Peak endurance potential occurs somewhat later than peak strength potential.

The Most Economical Pace Is an Even Rate over the Entire Distance In walking, running, swimming, and other locomotive activities, stopping, starting, accelerating, and decelerating are very costly in terms of energy. Therefore, the most economical approach is to distribute the available energy evenly over the entire distance. Theoretically, a 4-minute mile should consist of four 60-second quarter mile intervals; however, this is not feasible because the quarters are influenced by the start and finish of the race and by the necessity of gaining and holding position during the race. The idea of even pace also has strong application to long-duration games, such as basketball, soccer, tennis, or handball. Playing in "bursts" requires much additional energy. A comfortable rate of doing calisthenics results in more total repetitions than a rapid rate and even more than a slower rate.

Methods of Increasing Endurance

Because endurance is a factor in almost all vigorous performances, methods of increasing endurance are of prime concern. We have already talked of the need to apply the overload principle for the development of strength—that principle must also be applied if endurance is to be increased. Overload for muscle endurance simply means working the muscles beyond previous repetition levels under the appropriate resistance level.

Muscular Endurance

The most expedient method of increasing the *endurance of a particular muscle group* is to contract those muscles regularly against reasonably heavy resistance for near-maximum repetitions for three sets. Research results show that twenty to thirty RMs with three sets will increase endurance faster than 100 RMs with three sets. There is also evidence that ten RMs with three sets will increase endurance as fast as a greater number. Ten RMs will increase strength and endurance simultaneously, while twenty to thirty RMs will increase endurance but have little influence on strength and muscle size. Hence, if increased endurance and strength are desired, a strength-endurance building program is preferred (ten RMs for three sets). If increased endurance without increased strength and increased size is desired, then more RMs (twenty to thirty) with lighter weight should be employed.

Circulorespiratory Endurance

In *circulorespiratory endurance*, the main limiting factor is oxygen supply to the working tissues. The most effective method for increasing this form of endurance is interval training, which consists of a number of short bouts of vigorous exercise with a brief recovery period following each bout. Circulorespiratory endurance can also' be increased by long-duration continuous work, such as cross-country running or distance swimming.

Interval training for endurance makes very good sense from the physiological point of view because the prime objective of an endurance training program is to expose the person to the greatest work load before the onset of fatigue. This can be accomplished best through interval training. Research results (22) show that a work level which can be tolerated for an hour with the interval training technique will bring about exhaustion in 9 minutes when done continuously. Thus, the total work accomplished before fatigue is more than three times greater when interval training is used instead of continuous training. This greater output of work during a particular training session results in a stronger endurance stimulus.

The interval-training technique is used extensively for swimmers and distance runners and can be used successfully for total body conditioning of performers in activities such as wrestling, baseball, basketball, and various field sports. It has been found that interval training produces the best results when each exercise bout consists of approximately 3 to 5 minutes of vigorous work (running, swimming, or other forms of exercise), followed by light exercise or rest for 2 to 5 minutes. The work bout should be intense enough to maintain a heart rate of 90 percent of the maximum rate. (*Example:* Predicted maximum for a twenty-year-old is 200; ideal training level is 180 beats per minute.) DeVries (22) states that the rest interval is adequate when the resting heart rate returns to 120 beats per minute. (This figure undoubtedly varies for different individuals.) He also points out that training can be hampered by working the organism to total fatigue. The person should be able to recover from a workout within a few hours.

Interval training for swimmers or runners is the most effective for middle distances and relatively long distances (but not for extra-long distances). These events last from $1^{1}/_{2}$ to 15 minutes. Ideally the pace and the circulorespiratory endurance can be developed simultaneously. For example, a mile runner able to run a 4:20 time might follow this procedure in a given workout.

1   Under distance (less than the competitive event) of about one-fourth the total distance is selected.
2   The runner repeats quarter mile bouts slightly faster than the best pace for the total event (63 to 65 seconds each).
3   After about three bouts, interspersed with active rest periods, the heart rate should be approximately 180 at the completion of the bout.
4   The performer should be ready for the next work bout when the heart rate recovers to 120. After the pattern of recovery is established, time may be substituted for heart-rate monitoring.
5   The number of work bouts is determined by the condition of the performer and the rate of improvement that is desired. It is appropriate to start easily and increase gradually with subsequent workouts.

Endurance overload may result from interval training by adjusting the program in any of the following ways:

1   Gradually increase the intensity of the work in each bout by increasing speed or duration.
2   Shorten the interval between work bouts.
3   Increase the number of work bouts in a particular training session.

MUSCULAR POWER

Muscular power is a combination of speed and strength. It is the ability to apply force at a rapid rate. Power is typically demonstrated in projecting the body (as in the long jump) or an object (such as putting the shot, Figure 9-4) through space, wherein the muscles must apply strong force at a rapid rate to give the body or object the momentum necessary to carry it the desired distance. When expressed by formulas,

$$\text{Power} = \text{force} \times \text{velocity} \quad \text{or} \quad \text{Power} = \frac{\text{work}}{\text{time}}$$

It is possible for a person to be extremely strong and still not be extremely powerful; also, a person may be able to move with great speed against a very light resistance but lack the strength to move rapidly against heavier resistance. One who possesses great strength combined with great speed of movement, however, is powerful.

Muscular power is very important to vigorous performances because it determines how hard a person can hit, how far a person can throw, how

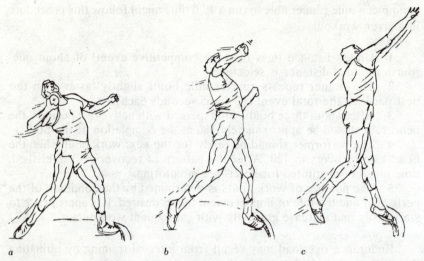

a   *b*   *c*

Figure 9-4 Shot-putting is primarily a power event, because success is dependent primarily upon the correct combination of strength and speed of contraction (assuming correct technique).

high a person can jump, and, to some extent, how fast a person can run or swim. All explosive maximum efforts depend directly upon power.

Power can be increased by increasing strength without sacrificing speed, by increasing speed of movement without sacrificing strength, or by increasing both speed and strength. The usual approach to increasing power is to increase strength (force). However, speed can also be increased a limited amount as a result of training. Both speed and force can be stressed by applying strong force through rapid (explosive) motion in exercising.

SPEED OF CONTRACTION

In different species the rate of contraction of muscle tissue varies greatly, and generally, the smaller the species, the faster its muscles contract. (However, there are exceptions to this rule.) In addition, among individual members within a particular species, muscle tissue varies a limited amount in its rate of contraction. And within an individual, different muscles contract at different rates of speed. In the human being, for instance, postural muscles (which are red) are relatively slow contractors, while most of the other motor muscles (which are pale) contract rapidly. In addition, there is a relationship between the size of different muscles and their speed of contraction; the smaller muscles tend to contract faster than the larger ones. However, there are also many exceptions to these rules.

Research completed since 1975 has used a muscle-stain technique of quick-frozen muscle biopsies from human subjects. Fiber typing has shown that each muscle is composed of slow-twitch (ST) fibers and fast-twitch (FT) fibers in varying ratios. For example, in normal subjects the soleus muscle is about 88 percent ST fibers and 12 percent FT fibers, while the triceps is about 33 percent ST fibers and 67 percent FT fibers; however, there is great variability in these ratios. The mechanical advantage of the soleus is 2.6 to 1, which favors a force ratio or strong effect against the resistance, while the triceps has a mechanical ratio of 0.1 to 1, which favors a speed ratio in its effect on the resistance. This suggests that the muscle-fiber-type ratio is related to mechanical ratio.

A study by Bangerter (2), reported in the June 1982 southwest district AAHPERD research section, showed a curvilinear correlation of 0.933 when using fiber ratios of nine selected skeletal muscles and the mechanical ratio of the respective levers these muscles move. Structure and function would appear to hold to an expected relationship.

The relative speed of contraction of different muscles varies greatly among individuals. For example, person A may have faster leg actions while person B has faster arm actions. Moreover, person A's arm extensor muscles may contract relatively fast while the arm flexors contract relatively slowly. In other words, speed varies with the individual body movement. A person may be a slow runner but have very fast arm and finger movements.

If all else is equal, a longer muscle will produce proportionately greater speed than a shorter one. Assume that muscle A and muscle B contract at the same rate of speed per linear centimeter of muscle and that muscle A is five times as long as muscle B. Muscle A will fully contract in the same time period as muscle B, thus moving the distal attachment of A five times as far in the same time interval.

Increasing Speed of Contraction

A muscle almost always contracts against some resistance, even if the resistance is only the weight of the body segment being moved. Because of this, strength can influence the rate of contraction. If all else remains equal, as a muscle becomes stronger, the resistance has less retarding effect on speed of contraction. As the amount of resistance against which one performs becomes greater, strength has a greater influence on speed of contraction; where resistance is very light, strength is a relatively insignificant factor in speed of contraction.

Increased coordination of muscles (skill) can increase the speed of specific movements. As the mover muscles become better coordinated, they can cooperatively overcome the external resistance with greater speed. When muscles are well coordinated, one contractile force arrives at the peak velocity of the previous force; consequently, the second force is more effective (Newton's law of inertia). Also, as the agonists and antagonists become better coordinated, the antagonists furnish less resistance to the contractile efforts of the agonists (reciprocal inhibition is improved). If increased speed is desired in a particular performance, the skills should be practiced at rates equal to or exceeding those used in performance.

A. V. Hill (**39**) claims that speed of contraction can be increased by approximately 20 percent by raising body temperature 2°C. The magnitude of this claim lacks sufficient evidence, but it is well established that increased body temperature does increase rate of contraction to some degree. Apparently such increase is due to decreased viscosity of the muscles when body temperature is raised. Raising body temperature a measurable amount requires much work, which is one argument in favor of warm-up in preparation for explosive-type performances. The major problems with warm-up are to prepare the correct muscles (selective activities) and to exercise an amount which is adequate, yet not fatiguing. Another factor is to time the warm-up properly, so its effects are maximum.

The efficiency of muscle contraction can be increased by training, which may result in increased contractile speed. For example, if fatty tissue within a muscle is eliminated or if viscosity is reduced, then friction is reduced. This results in greater efficiency and a faster contraction. If flexibility of antagonist muscles is inadequate, an increase in flexibility will cause those muscles to furnish less resistance to the movement, resulting in greater speed. Also, reducing neural inhibitions as a result of training will allow the performer to call voluntarily upon greater numbers of available motor units. The more motor units involved, the greater the strength and the more quickly the resistance can be overcome.

Influence of Speed on Muscular Power

When the mechanical ratio (leverage) of a body movement remains constant, the speed of movement is directly proportionate to the speed of contraction of the mover muscles. If the rate of contraction were increased by 5 percent, the speed of movement would increase by the same percentage. In turn, the increased speed of movement would contribute to increased power ($P = F \times V$). If other factors remain constant, power will increase in proportion to speed of movement.

Influence of Speed on Energy Cost

The energy cost of a muscle contraction varies with the cube of the speed of contraction. For example, if muscle X contracts twice as fast as muscle Y, the energy cost of muscle X is eight times as great as that of muscle Y. Whereas if muscle X contracts three times as fast as muscle Y, the energy cost of muscle X is twenty-seven times as great as that of muscle Y. This factor has great significance because it explains why maximum efforts produce fatigue so rapidly. In determining one's pace in endurance activities, energy cost is the prime consideration. This explains why spurts of speed and unnecessary rapid movements are undesirable in endurance events.

FLEXIBILITY

Flexibility is a condition of muscle and connective tissue which contributes to range of motion (Figure 9-5). It is a characteristic that can be improved on an immediate or long-term basis. For *immediate improvement* flexibility can be increased a limited amount by doing preparatory stretching exercises. Before warm-up, antagonist muscles relax slowly and incompletely when the agonists contract, and thus retard free movement and accurate coordination. Warm-up exercises cause the antagonists to relax more completely, and the movements become

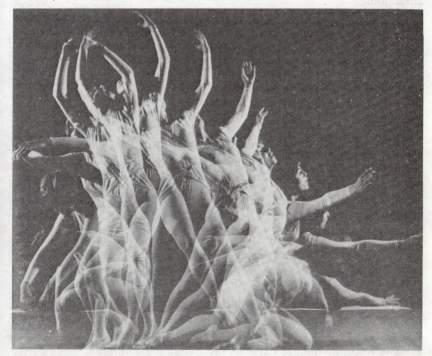

Figure 9-5 Flexibility is often very important in creative dance. This photograph also illustrates the fact that in some performances visual impression is more important than strength or endurance.

smoother and better coordinated. Improved flexibility on a *long-term* basis can be accomplished by performing flexibility (stretching) exercises on a regular basis.

Two forms of exercises have been used to stretch muscles and connective tissues: *ballistic* (bobbing) and *slow stretch*. Flexibility can be increased effectively with either method, but the slow-stretch method is recommended because it has these advantages:

1   There is less danger of exceeding the limits of extensibility of the tissues, which would cause injury and soreness.
2   It does not activate the stretch reflex
3   It provides the opportunity to relax the antagonist muscles consciously and allow them to s-t-r-e-t-c-h.

Slow-stretch exercises can be done either passively (muscles are consciously relaxed while another person moves the body segment) or actively (movement is caused by muscle contraction). Passive exercises are useful in therapy but are less desirable than active exercises in athletic conditioning.

The following is the recommended procedure for improving flexibility. Go through the movement slowly until the muscles and connective tissues stretch far enough to experience the "stretch pain." Hold the position for 8 to 10 seconds while consciously relaxing the antagonist muscles, thus allowing them to stretch as freely as possible. Repeat this procedure five or six times for each movement in which greater flexibility is desired. The best results are accomplished when stretching is done daily.

Changes in flexibility brought about by stretching exercises persist for several weeks after exercising is discontinued. A sizable percentage of the increased flexibility will be retained for as long as 10 to 12 weeks.

MUSCLE TONE

Muscle tone is a condition which gives firmness and proper shape to muscles. It relates to the state of conditioning; that is, a well-conditioned muscle possesses good tone while a poorly conditioned muscle is poorly toned.

Traditionally, muscle tone has been defined as "a constant state of contraction of part of the muscle fibers." Supposedly, this constant contraction results from a steady flow of impulses from the nervous system. Recent evidence expands the traditional definition.

As a result of electromyographic study, Basmajian (8) found that both a *passive* and an *active* component compose muscle tone. The passive component consists of constant electricity in muscles and connective tissues plus turgor, which is the pressure of body fluids tending to distend their surrounding tissues. Always present in muscles, this passive component varies in amount depending upon muscle condition. The active component consists of contraction of certain muscle fibers which are stimulated by the stretch reflex. This dependence on the stretch reflex makes the active component rely upon body posture for its existence. The reflex causes nervous stimulation of certain muscle fibers which contributes to muscle firmness.

Effects of Exercise on Tone

Devries (22) reported results of one limited study which indicated that increased strength did not change muscle tone. However, practical experience and observation strongly support the idea that one of the benefits of exercise is increased muscle tone. Increased strength and muscle endurance resulting from exercise are generally accompanied by firmness and proper shape, the most obvious qualities of tone. Lack of exercise produces the opposite results. The loss of strength, endurance, and tone is especially noticeable when a body segment is totally immobilized, as when cast for a fracture. It must be concluded that muscular strength and endurance-building exercises do increase tone. The relationship between tone and other muscular characteristics such as speed, efficiency, and flexibility is not established. But highly toned muscles seem to have a degree of tension already available; so they should be better prepared to act.

EFFECTS OF WARM-UP

Several studies have produced evidence that cooling of the muscles below normal temperature causes a loss of contractile time and reduces excitability of the muscles. Supposedly warming of the muscles will reverse these effects. A.V. Hill (38) found that increasing the temperature of the muscle improved both contractile force and contractile speed. DeVries (22) reasoned that warm-up which results in increased temperature of the blood and muscles should improve the performance because (1) muscles would contract and relax faster, (2) muscles would contract with greater efficiency because of lower viscosity, (3) hemoglobin would give up more oxygen and also dissociate more rapidly, (4) myoglobin would show effects similar to those of hemoglobin, (5) metabolic processes would increase, and (6) resistance of the vascular bed would decrease.

In a thorough review on the research of warm-up the authors found that about half the reports support the idea that warm-up is beneficial while the other half support the claim that warm-up has no effect on performance. None of the reports indicated negative effects of warm-up. The advocates of warm-up consider it important on the basis of the following claims:

1 Warm-up increases the rate and force of muscular contraction.
2 Warm-up related to that particular activity improves the necessary coordinations.
3 Warm-up helps to prevent injury.
4 In endurance activities warm-up brings on second wind more readily.

Unfortunately some of these claims are not well substantiated by research; this does not indicate that they are untrue, however, because there is also no evidence against them.

Most coaches seem to believe that warm-up is valuable and want their athletes to continue using warm-up until further evidence is accumulated. The authors firmly agree with this position, but it must be recognized that indiscriminate warm-up may waste energy and result in limited effects on the essential muscles. The warm-up should be specific to the activity being performed and should be increased in intensity as the performer becomes better conditioned. The timing of the warm-up in relation to performance must be correct; otherwise the beneficial effects may be reduced or eliminated. The following are some important guides:

1 Warm-up should be intense enough to increase body temperature and cause perspiration but not so intense that it causes fatigue.
2 Warm-up should include some stretching and loosening exercises along with some total body work.
3 Warm-up should include movements that are common in the performance at hand.
4 The warm-up should begin to taper off 10 to 15 minutes before the performance and end at least 5 minutes before performance except for light stretching. This will allow recovery from any temporary fatigue without losing the effects of the warm-up.
5 Warm-ups should *avoid* muscular strength or endurance-building activities and should not be limited to one body area.

Regarding the effect of warm-up on injury, several experts claim that failure to warm up may relate to tearing of muscle fibers. Frequently a pulled muscle occurs in a relaxed fiber, one that is antagonistic to the contracting fibers. This happens because the opposing (relaxed) fibers do

Regarding acceleration, it must be realized that in body movements muscle contractions provide the force, and more forceful contractions expend more energy. The energy cost of a muscle contraction varies with the cube of the speed of contraction. If muscle X contracts twice as fast as muscle Y, its energy cost is eight times as great as that of muscle Y. If muscle X contracts three times as fast as muscle Y, its energy cost is twenty-seven times as great as that of muscle Y. This fact has much application in determining the rate at which a performer should accelerate. It especially has great application in endurance activities.

Maximum Acceleration and Efficiency of Motion

Principle: To achieve maximum acceleration, all available forces should be applied sequentially with proper timing and as directly as possible in the intended line of motion, and body actions extraneous to the desired movement should be reduced to a minimum, because they waste energy and interfere with productive movements.

Example A: A swimmer performing the crawl stroke should attempt to increase the forces which propel the body in the desired direction and decrease all other actions, such as lifting the body upward or weaving it from side to side. *Example B*: Watching the head of a runner or hurdler from the side reveals whether or not the forces are properly directed forward rather than upward. In either case, the objective is to move forward, and excessive up-and-down head motion indicates misdirected force.

In some cases maximum acceleration (and thus maximum speed) is not the prime objective of the performance. Acceleration may be sacrificed for quickness of release, such as some throws in baseball other than pitching, or it may be sacrificed for greater accuracy, as in basketball shooting. In these cases, usually fewer joint actions, and thus fewer forces, are used.

Effects of the Body's Radius on Rotational (Angular) Speed

Principle: When a body rotates, lengthening of the radius slows the rotation, whereas shortening of the radius increases the rotation, because the resistance against the rotating force becomes proportionately less effective when the radius is shortened.

Example A (Figure 12-4): In springboard diving, the rate of rotation (and thus the number of turns) is increased as the tuck is tightened, causing the body's radius of rotation to shorten. A pike position produces a slower rotation, and a lay-out position allows a still slower rotation. *Example B*: A skater or dancer may increase the speed of spin by bringing the arms close to the body, or may decrease the speed by reaching outward. *Example C*: Pole vaulting involves several rotational

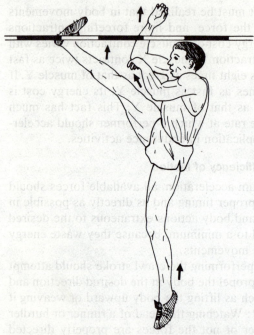

Figure 12-3 The high-jumper swings the arms and the free leg vigorously, using them to pull the total body upward. This is transfer of momentum from swinging body parts.

PRINCIPLES RELATED TO THE LAW OF ACCELERATION

Application of the following principles results in acceleration or conservation of velocity and momentum.

Acceleration Is Proportional to Force

Principal: Acceleration is proportional to the force causing it, providing the mass is held constant, meaning that if the force is doubled, the rate of acceleration is also doubled, etc. [except for effects of air or water resistance which vary with the theoretical square law (Chapter 13)].

Example A: A sprinter increases acceleration by increasing the force that he or she applies backward and downward against the running surface. If the runner were able to increase the force by 25 percent, the rate of acceleration would be increased by 25 percent (less the effects of air resistance). Furthermore, if the runner could reduce the mass and keep the force constant, acceleration would increase. *Example B*: A swimmer can increase acceleration proportionate to the increase in force that is applied against the water with the stroke and kick.

not yield to the pull suddenly placed on them by the rapidly contracting muscles. Morehouse and Miller (57) support this idea by stating that muscles most frequently torn because of inadequate warm-up are those antagonistic to the strong contracting muscles. These cold antagonistic muscles relax slowly and incompletely when agonists contract and thus retard free movement and hinder accurate coordination. Morehouse and Rasch (58) state, "The danger of injury is lessened when an athlete is thoroughly warmed-up, which increases the speed with which he is able to react." They imply that this increased reaction helps to prevent injury.

Sometimes, especially during sprints, the muscle pull occurs after full stride has been achieved and repeated several times (at about 75 meters in the 100, for example). In this case it is illogical to assume that the muscle was not adequately warmed or stretched. The cause could be a skill error resulting from an attempt to accelerate, especially when the performer perceives himself losing, or losing his advantage. If neural impulses get out of sync, muscle groups that are alternately relaxing and contracting (quads and hamstrings) may, at a given instant, *co*contract. This momentarily takes the flexibility (slack) out of the muscle that should be antagonistic at the moment (almost invariably the hamstrings), forcing something to "give." Muscle fibers of the hamstrings or the tendon attachments tear, resulting in a "muscle pull."

By increasing *strength, endurance, power,* or *speed of contraction* of the muscles, one's ability to perform can frequently be improved. In fact, such increases are often the best approach to improving performance. Teachers, coaches, and athletes should not overlook these possibilities for improving performance. Increasing *flexibility* of the muscles antagonistic to the primary movements in a performance may help to forestall fatigue and avoid injury.

IMPORTANT CONCEPTS

1 When body systems are stressed (overloads imposed) on a regular basis, they tend to respond by the improvement of function (*law of use*).

2 *Progressive training* implies that overload increments of greater intensities are gradually imposed, resulting in continuous steplike improvements.

3 Regardless of which fitness component is being improved, two general outcomes can be predicted:

    a Initial gains are larger than later gains; and as one approaches capacity, gains that appear inconsequential may be the difference between success and failure.

    b Day-to-day variations in ability to perform, and plateaus of nonimprovement, lasting months in some instances, should be expected.

4 Near maximal contractions regularly imposed appear to be the most rapid means of developing *muscular strength*. The *heavy resistance* needed fatigues the exercised muscles rapidly, thus limiting the number of contractions.

5 Stronger individuals have an advantage in the demonstration of muscular endurance when using submaximal resistance of an absolute nature (*absolute muscular endurance*; all performers use the same resistance). In *relative muscular endurance* (resistance varies in proportion to the performer's strength) greater strength is not an advantage; in fact it is a slight disadvantage.

6 True *muscular endurance* is most effectively developed with maximum repetitions under the appropriate resistance load. If the use of the muscular endurance is to be primarily in submaximal tasks, it may be desirable to add more resistance and gain a greater strength component (concept 5), but unfortunately at the expense of true endurance.

7 *Circulorespiratory endurance* is best achieved through interval training of sufficient intensity (based on speed and duration of the work bout) to elevate the heart rate to 80 to 90 percent of maximum. Within this intensity range, an increase in the number of work bouts in each training session is advantageous.

8 Explosive kinds of performance rely upon *power* as the prime ingredient. Power can be developed by strength or speed training as long as the other component is not sacrificed. Both components may be developed in rapid, resisted exercises, where either component can be emphasized based on the selected resistance.

9 *Speed* or quickness of a movement or series of movements may be enhanced by repeatedly attempting to duplicate them as rapidly and as often as possible. At times it may be better to communicate "higher," "farther," or "harder" rather than "faster" to the performer. Such emphasis naturally achieves rapid movements of the body parts, while the latter emphasis may disturb timing and coordination.

10 *Muscle tone* may be achieved through muscular-strength or muscular-endurance development, and its apparent contribution to function relates to the muscle's readiness to respond.

11 Although *warm-up* has undoubtedly been abused on occasion, resulting in deterioration of performance, no substantial evidence to contradict the value of correct warm-up has been presented. Empirical evidence plus logical support seems to justify the retention of well-planned warm-up to precede performance.

12 The particular exercise selected *does not* determine the effect produced in terms of fitness. The result is dependent upon how several *factors* of the exercise situation are varied. In particular:

    a Amount of resistance
    b Speed of repetition

     c Number of repetitions
     d Number of sets
     e Appropriate selection of muscle or movement or both

STUDENT LABORATORY EXPERIENCES

Select a specific skill which requires a large amount of strength, endurance, or speed. Describe in detail how to best increase muscle effectiveness to cause improvement of that skill. Give specific exercises and procedures to be followed. Do not include any exercise or procedure that you cannot justify.

Chapter 10

Muscular Analysis of a Skill

This chapter is a model for a student to follow in doing a muscle analysis. The project involves selecting a performance such as a track and field event, swimming stroke, or gymnastic skill and writing a muscular analysis of the performance similar to the one illustrated here. The purpose of performing a muscular analysis of a skill is to help the analyst:

1 Become fully aware of the specific body actions involved in the performance

2 Become better informed of all the muscles involved in different roles and develop a greater insight into the complexity of the coordination patterns

3 Identify the specific muscles and muscle groups used, so that muscle-strength and endurance-building programs may be designed to benefit those muscles

4 Identify the muscles in which flexibility is needed

The analysis should consist of three major phases. *First,* describe the objectives and nature of the performance, that is, what the performer is attempting to accomplish and exactly how the skill should be done. *Second*, determine the specific body actions that are part of the performance and identify their sequence. *Third*, identify the muscles which contribute to each action and indicate each muscle's role in the performance. Following is an example of a muscle analysis of a specific skill. (*Note*: It should be recognized that a more exact analysis of muscle involvement would result from the use of electromyographic equipment. But such equipment is rarely available to teachers and college students.)

Muscle Analysis of Hurdling

In hurdling (high hurdles), the objective of the performer is to clear the hurdle as quickly as possible and come off the hurdle in good running position to sprint rapidly to the next hurdle. Three running strides are taken between hurdles, and the hurdle is cleared on the fourth stride. The barrier is not taken in three strides and a jump, but rather in four running strides, the last of which is longer and accentuated in action. The hurdler should leave the ground approximately 2 meters in front of the hurdle and land about 1 meter behind it.

The pattern of specific body actions in hurdling (Figure 10-1) is complex. In clearing the barrier, the forward leg, led by the knee, should be driven forward and upward to clear the hurdle. At the same time, the upper portion of the body is thrust forward and downward to meet the upward-driven leg. The arm opposite the lead leg is extended forward, and the chest is dipped toward the knee of the lead leg. These movements are coordinated with the upward-forward drive from the push-off leg.

As the lead leg clears the hurdle, it is driven downward. The upper body should still be well forward to aid in the downward drive of the leg. As the leg is driven downward, the upper body becomes more erect. At this time the trail leg is whipped forward into the next running stride.

To clear the hurdle as quickly as possible, the runner's body weight is

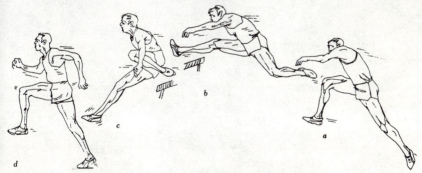

Figure 10-1 Sequence drawings of body actions in running the high hurdles.

thrust *forward*, much the same as a high-jumper's weight is thrust *upward*. This forward thrust of weight tends to pull the runner over the hurdle and to the ground in a minimum length of time.

In working for perfection in hurdling action, the athlete should keep these points in mind: (1) clear the hurdle in the shortest possible time and with as little vertical height as possible, (2) let the hurdle interfere as little as possible with running rhythm, and (3) maintain as near-perfect balance as possible and come off the hurdle into a good sprint position.

On the muscle-analysis chart that follows are (1) the more important specific body movements that occur in hurdling and (2) indentification of the muscles which are involved in each of the movements and the specific role that each muscle plays in the movement. It is not practical to identify all body movements and all muscles that contribute to hurdling; therefore, only those actions and muscles which make major contributions to hurdling are identified.

In order to conserve space, only a portion of the analysis of muscle function is presented here. The portion is sufficient to provide a model for students to follow.

Specific movements	Agonist muscles (mover)	Main stabilizing actions	Antagonist muscles (must be relaxed to allow movement)	Main neutralizing actions
Movements into the hurdle				
Hip flexion of lead leg (approximately 100°)	Adductor brevis Adductor longus Gracilis Rectus femoris Pectineus Psoas major Sartorius Iliacus (The gracilis and sartorius are probably only partially used in hip flexion in this case, because they also flex the knee. In this case knee extension occurs simultaneous to hip flexion.)	The obliquus abdominis externus and internus and rectus abdominis muscles contract to stabilize the pelvic region on which the leg moves.	Gluteus maximus Biceps femoris Semimembranosus Semitendinosus	The adductor brevis, adductor longus, pectineus, and gracilis muscles all adduct the thigh as they flex it. The sartorius abducts and flexes the thigh, tending to neutralize the adduction of the other four muscles. Probably other hip abductors contract slightly to assist the sartorius. The adductor brevis and longus and the pectineus also laterally rotate the thigh. This is a necessary movement in hurdling; therefore, it is not neutralized.
Knee extension of lead leg (100°)	Rectus femoris Vastus medialis Vastus intermedius Vastus lateralis	In this case the hip flexor muscles are the main stabilizers. While they are contracting to flex the hip, they also give the upper leg the stability it needs so the knee can extend. Several other muscles which control movements of the upper leg contribute to its stability in this case, but the hip flexors are by far the greatest contributors.	Biceps femoris Semimembranosus Plantaris Popliteus Semitendinosus Gastrocnemius	No neutralizing actions occur in knee extension.

181

Specific movements	Agonist muscles (mover)	Main stabilizing actions	Antagonist muscles (must be relaxed to allow movement)	Main neutralizing actions
Movements into the hurdle (continued)				
Trunk forward flexion (50°) and rotation toward lead leg (25°)	Rectus abdominis Obliquus externus Obliquus internus Psoas (These muscles all appear in pairs, and when both members of each pair contract, trunk flexion occurs. In order for the desired trunk rotation to occur simultaneously with flexion, one member of each pair of muscles contracts with greater force than the other member. See trunk rotation in Chapter 7 for details. Also, the deep spinal rotator muscles are probably active in this case.)	Ordinarily the hip and leg extensors contract to stabilize the legs and pelvis to provide a base on which the trunk can flex. But, in this case, hip flexion and knee extension occur simultaneously with trunk flexion. The weight of the leg and trunk pulled toward each other provides most of the stability necessary for their movement.	Erector spinae Quadratus lumborum Multifidus The small and deep posterior muscles of the spine	The opposite members of each pair of active muscles neutralize each other's tendencies to flex the trunk laterally.

Note: If the analysis of muscle function were to be completed using this same format, the following additional movements would appear in the left-hand column with corresponding information in the other columns—*Moving into the hurdle (continued)*: shoulder flexion of the opposite arm (90°), elbow extension of the opposite arm (90°). *Pushing off with the leg*: hip extension of push-off leg (20°), knee extension of push-off leg (20°), plantar flexion of push-off foot (40°), toe flexion of push-off foot (25°). *Clearing the hurdle*: hip abduction of trail leg (80°), horizontal flexion of trail leg (90°), knee flexion of trail leg (100°). *Coming off of the hurdle*: hip extension of lead leg (100°), trunk extension (30°), shoulder extension of lead arm (100°). Some additional movements are involved in hurdling that are less significant than those identified above, and they are not included in this sample analysis.

APPLICATION OF MECHANICAL LAWS AND PRINCIPLES

Part Three

Application of Mechanical Laws and Principles

Part Three deals with important principles derived from the fields of physics, particularly mechanics, which influence performance. As these chapters are studied, the reader will become more aware of how modern techniques of performance evolved from basic scientific laws and principles. The simplified statements of the laws and principles, along with the many practical examples, make the content easy to understand and apply. The content of this part forms the basis for mechanical analysis of performance.

Chapter 11 explains the use of simple machines in human motion, with the emphasis on use of levers and leverage. Chapter 12 deals with the principles of motion, which are derived from Newton's three basic laws of motion. In Chapter 13 important factors relative to force are identified and discussed. Chapter 14 covers the important principles governing projections; Chapter 15 deals with balance, stability, and posture; and Chapter 16 is an example of the practical application of the content of the preceding five chapters. After studying Part Three, readers should be well prepared to analyze performances from the mechanical point of view. This will assist them greatly in becoming better teachers and performers.

A review of basic material useful in mechanical analysis of motion now follows. This will enable the student to solve problems and perform the laboratory experiences suggested in the subsequent chapters.

Displacement, velocity, and force may be represented by vectors, that is, arrows indicating direction and magnitude. To find a resultant from a number of vectors the graphic polygon method of solution is recommended as the most simple. For example, consider the following four vectors based on compass points representing displacement.

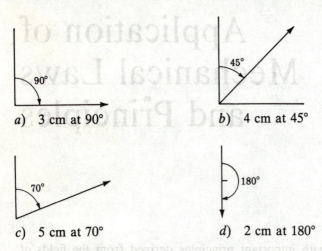

a)   3 cm at 90°   *b*)   4 cm at 45°

c)   5 cm at 70°   *d*)   2 cm at 180°

To sum them and find the resultant, the arrows may be drawn as represented below, with *R* representing the summed displacement.

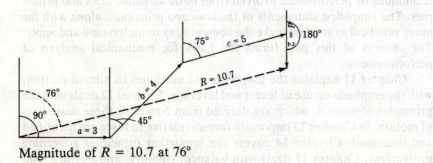

Magnitude of *R* = 10.7 at 76°

An example using triangulation could be made of an athlete performing the long jump. Suppose the horizontal running velocity is 9 meters per second and the vertical velocity imparted at takeoff is 3 meters per second; the resultant velocity is the graphic sum of the velocities, or

$$R = \sqrt{(9)^2 + (3)^2} = \sqrt{90} = 9.4868 \text{ meters per second}$$

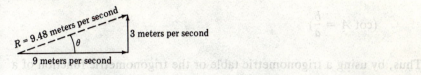

In this instance, the angle of projection (θ) is defined by the following trigonometric relationship. The $\sin \theta = \dfrac{\text{opposite side}}{\text{hypotenuse}}$ or $\dfrac{3 \text{ m/s}}{9.4868 \text{ m/s}} = 0.3162$ (which is the arc sine). Therefore $\theta = 18.43°$ with the horizontal. The same answer is achieved by a second trigonometric relationship as follows. The $\tan \theta = \dfrac{\text{opposite side}}{\text{adjacent side}}$ or $\dfrac{3 \text{ m/s}}{9 \text{ m/s}} = 0.333$ (which is the arc tangent). Therefore $\theta = 18.43°$ with the horizontal. Each trigonometric relationship seeks and achieves the same answer. (To test these values see the trigonometric table or use a pocket calculator.)

Because problems involving triangular configurations will be encountered in many situations, pertinent trigonometric functions and their definitions are given here. Notice the following statements about a right triangle.

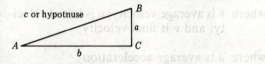

In the given right triangle ABC

1 The sine of an angle $= \dfrac{\text{length of side opposite that angle}}{\text{length of hypotenuse}}$

  ($\sin A = \dfrac{a}{c}$)

2 The cosine of an angle $= \dfrac{\text{length of side adjacent to that angle}}{\text{length of hypotenuse}}$

  ($\cos A = \dfrac{b}{c}$)

3 The tangent of an angle $= \dfrac{\text{length of side opposite that angle}}{\text{length of side adjacent to that angle}}$

  ($\tan A = \dfrac{a}{b}$)

4　The cotangent of an angle = $\dfrac{\text{length of side adjacent to that angle}}{\text{length of side opposite that angle}}$

$(\cot A = \dfrac{b}{a})$

Thus, by using a trigonometric table or the trigonometric function of a pocket calculator, if two parts are known about the right triangle, we may solve for any of the other parts. There are, of course, six parts: three angles (A, B, C) and three sides (a, b, c). If the A or B is known, the other is arrived at by simply subtracting the known angle from 90°. C always is equal to 90°, and the sum of the three angles in any triangle is equal to 180°. in dealing with force or velocity vectors, the same system is used.

In presenting the material that follows it is assumed that college students can handle basic algebraic expressions. The following formulas are commonly used when dealing with linear kinematics, angular kinematics, kinetics, kinematics and kinetics, and force and equilibrium.

A　Linear Kinematics (Linear Motion)

1　$v = \dfrac{d}{t}$　　　　where v is velocity; d is displacement or distance; and t is time

2　$\bar{v} = \dfrac{u + v}{2}$　　　where $\bar{v}$ is average velocity; u is initial velocity; and v is final velocity

3　$\bar{a} = \dfrac{v - u}{t}$　　　where $\bar{a}$ is average acceleration

4　$v = u + at$　　　where v is final velocity when acceleration is uniform (derived from $a = \dfrac{v - u}{2}$)

5　$s = ut + \frac{1}{2}at^2$　　where s is vertical distance traveled when acceleration is constant, as in the case of gravity (gravity constant $g = 9.8$ m/s² or 32.2 ft/s²)

6　$s = \frac{1}{2}gt^2$　　　when　initial velocity is zero (0)

In dealing with projectiles, freely falling bodies, and gravity we use the following.

7　$v_y^2 = u_y^2 + 2gs$　　where v_y is vertical takeoff velocity; u_y is initial vertical velocity at top of flight

8 $v_y^2 = 2gs$ when initial velocity is zero (0)

If the angle of takeoff and landing (θ) is other than vertical (90°), then the following projectile formulas, as derived from the above, apply.

9 $t = \dfrac{u \sin \theta}{g}$ where t is time required for an object to reach its highest point

or

10 $t = \sqrt{2s/g}$ where t is time to fall from highest point

11 $T = \dfrac{2u \sin \theta}{g}$ where T is time object is in flight

12 $s = \dfrac{(u \sin \theta)^2}{2g}$ where s is vertical height the object attains

13 $R = \dfrac{u^2 \sin 2\theta}{g}$ where R is horizontal distance the object covers from takeoff to landing at the same level as takeoff

14 $R = \dfrac{u^2 \sin \theta \cos \theta + u \cos \theta \sqrt{(u \sin \theta)^2 + 2gh}}{g}$

where R is range of a projectile when height of takeoff is different from height of landing; h is height difference between takeoff and landing

15 $v_x = v_\theta \cos \theta$ where v_x is horizontal velocity; v_θ is velocity in the direction of projection

16 $v_y = v_\theta \sin \theta$ where v_y is vertical velocity

17 $v_x = v_y \tan \theta$

18 $v_y = v_x \tan \theta$

19 $v_\theta = v_x/\cos \theta = v_y/\sin \theta = \sqrt{v_x^2 + v_y^2}$

B Angular Kinematics (Angular Motion)

20 $\omega = \dfrac{\theta}{t}$ where ω (omega) is angular velocity

21 $\bar{\alpha} = \dfrac{\omega_f - \omega_i}{t}$ where $\bar{\alpha}$ (alpha) is average angular acceleration

22 (a) $v_T = \omega r$ where v_T is tangential velocity (linear, curvi-
       (b) $\omega_1 r_1 = \omega_2 r_2$ linear, or circular velocity at a point on the radius); r is radius

23 $\quad v_T = \dfrac{\omega r}{57.3} \qquad$ converts ω from degrees to radians, hence to linear units

24 $\quad C = 2\pi r \qquad$ where C is circumference of circle and π is 22/7 or 3.1416; therefore, 1 radian equals length of the radius on the circumference

25 $\quad$ 1 rev = 360°

26 $\quad$ 360° = 6.28 radians

27 $\quad$ 1 radian = 57.3°

C Kinetics (Force)

28 $\quad Wt = mg \qquad$ where Wt is weight; m is mass; g is gravity

and

29 $\quad m = \dfrac{Wt}{g}$

30 $\quad T = Fr \qquad$ where T is torque; F is force applied perpendicular to the radius (usually expressed in meter-newtons)

When forces act perpendicular (at 90°) to the radius of rotation

31 $\quad F \times FA = \qquad$ where F is force; FA is length of force arm; R
$\quad\quad R \times RA \qquad$ is resistance; RA is length of resistance arm

If forces act at other than 90° to the arms

32 $\quad F \times FMA = \qquad$ where MA is moment arm for force or resist-
$\quad\quad R \times RMA \qquad$ ance (this must be calculated using trigonometry)

33 $\quad M.A. = \dfrac{R}{F} \qquad$ where $M.A.$ is mechanical advantage

and

34 $\quad M.A. = \dfrac{FA}{RA}$

35 $W = Fd$ where W is work; F is force; d is distance (usually expressed in meter-newtons or foot-pounds)

36 $P = \dfrac{W}{t}$ where P is power, the rate at which work is accomplished

or $P = \dfrac{Fd}{t}$

37 $P.E. = mgh =$
$Wt \times h$
where $P.E.$ is potential energy; m is mass; g is gravity; h is height of center of gravity of mass above ground level; also mg equals Wt, since m is $\dfrac{Wt}{g}$

38 $P.E. = K.E.$ where $K.E.$ is kinetic energy

As long as a body moves it has kinetic energy in proportion to its mass and velocity. Thus

39 $K.E. = \frac{1}{2}mv^2$

Because of the principle of conservation of momentum

40 $W = K.E. = Fd$ or work done is equal to kinetic energy acquired

Therefore,

41 $Fd = \frac{1}{2}mv^2$

D Kinematics and Kinetics (Motion and Force)

Newton's Laws of Motion Newton's second law, the law of acceleration, states that the force developed is in proportion to the product of the mass and acceleration of an object. Mass is usually expressed in kilograms and acceleration in meters per second squared (m/s²). Force is expressed in newtons.

42 $F = ma$ where F is force; m is mass; a is acceleration

From that equation we derive the impulse equation; if we set $a = \dfrac{v - u}{t}$, then $F = \dfrac{m(v - u)}{t}$ and

43 $Ft = mv - mu$

44 Impulse = Ft or,   impulse is the product of force and the time over which the force acts

45 $M = mv$ where M is momentum; m is mass; v is velocity

Newton's third law of motion, or reaction and conservation of momentum in a system, states that the momentum lost by a striking object is gained by the object which is struck, or

46 $M_1v_1 - M_1u_1 = M_2v_2 - M_2u_2$

Rotational Equivalents Newton's first principle, the law of inertia, is expressed by the formula which says that the moment of inertia about an axis is the sum of the mass of particles multiplied by the square of the distance of each particle from the axis. It expresses the force required to start or stop motion and is written.

47 $I = mr^2$

48 $A.M. = I\omega$ where $A.M.$ is angular momentum; I is inertia; ω is angular velocity ($\omega = v_T/r$)

and

49 $A.M. = mrv_T$ where m is object's mass; r is radius of rotation at object's center of gravity; v_T is tangential velocity at that point (derived from $A.M. = mr^2[v_T/r] = mrv_T$)

The centripetal force (Fc) is center-seeking and is equal in magnitude and opposite in direction to the centrifugal, or center-fleeing force. This is the force required to hold an object in a curved path and is expressed in the formula

50 $Fc = \dfrac{mv_t^2}{r}$ where m is object's mass; v_t^2 is object's tangential velocity squared; r is radius measured from object's center of rotation to center of gravity

Forces Modifying Motion The coefficient of friction (μ) is the quotient of the force of pull (P) needed to overcome the friction caused by weight of the object holding the two surfaces together. The value is usually less than 1. It is expressed as

51 $\mu = \dfrac{P}{Wt}$

The coefficient of friction is the arc tangent and determines the amount of lean possible by a player or

52 $\tan \theta = \dfrac{P}{Wt} = \mu$ where θ is an angle of lean with the vertical

53 $\epsilon = \sqrt{\dfrac{h_b}{h_d}}$ where ϵ is coefficient of elasticity or resolution of an object; h_b is height of bounce; h_d is height of drop

The neutral coefficient of restitution of two moving objects can be determined by a formual based on the conservation of momentum.

54 $\epsilon = \dfrac{v_2 - v_1}{u_1 - u_2}$

E Force and Equilibrium

The formula for determining the location of the center of gravity of an individual in a lying position on a reaction board used with a weighing scale is expressed as

55 $X = \dfrac{Fl}{Wt}$ where X is distance above soles of the feet; F is scale reading of partial weight of subject and board minus scale reading of partial weight of board; l is length of reaction board between knife-edges; and Wt is weight of subject

56 $\%h = \dfrac{X}{h} \times 100$ is the location of center of gravity (as measured from soles of feet) where h is total height of individual

The problems in the subsequent chapters will refer to the above formulas by number as a help to their respective solutions. While it is recommended that problems associated with student laboratory experiences be solved using the metric units system (the international requirement), a list of useful conversion factors follows for the convenience of students accustomed to dealing with English customary units, so that by using conversions they may have a better quantitative "feel" for human performance paramenters.

Conversion factors included allow for change from metric units to English units or vice versa. Metric system interconversions have not been given, as they are always expressed in terms of powers of 10. The following prefixes indicate the most commonly used factors.

micro	0.000001	10^{-6}
milli	0.001	10^{-3}
centi	0.01	10^{-2}
kilo	1,000	10^{3}
mega	1,000,000	10^{6}

	To change from	To	Multiply b or to revers divide by
Acceleration	Meters per second^2	Feet per second^2	3.28
	Meters per second^2	Miles per hour per second	2.237
Angle	Radians	Degrees	57.296
	Radians	Revolutions	0.159
	Revolutions	Degrees	360
	Revolutions	Radians	6.28 or
Distance	Meters	Feet	3.28
	Meters	Yards	1.094
	Kilometers	Miles	0.621
	Centimeters	Inches	0.3937
Energy	Meter-newtons (joules)	Foot-pounds	0.738
	Joules	Kilocalories	0.0002:
	Foot-pounds	Joules (meter-newtons)	1.356
Force	Newtons	Pounds	0.225
Impulse	Newton-seconds	Pound-seconds	0.225
Mass	Kilograms	Slugs	0.0685
Moment of	Kilogram-meters^2	Slug-feet^2	0.738
inertia	Kilogram-meters^2	Pound-feet^2	23.7
	Slug-feet^2	Pound-feet^2	32.174
Momentum	Kilogram-meters per second	Slug per feet per second	0.225
	Kilogram-meters per second	Pound-feet per second	7.227
	Slug-feet per second	Pound-feet per second	32.174
Power	Kilocalories per second	Watts	4186
	Kilocalories per second	Horsepower	0.0015(
	Kilocalories	Foot-pounds per second	0.858
	Horsepower	Foot-pounds per second	550.
	Horsepower	Watts	745.2
	Foot-pounds per second	Watts	1.356
Pressure	Kilograms per centimeter^2	Pounds per inch^2	14.22
	Kilograms per meter^2	Pounds per inch^2	0.0014
	Newtons per centimeter^2	Pounds per inch^2	0.0145
	Dynes per centimeter^2	Pounds per inch^2	1.45
Torque	Meter-newtons	Pound-feet	0.737
Velocity	Meters per second	Feet per second	3.28
	Kilometers per hour	Miles per hour	0.621
	Miles per hour	Feet per second	1.467
	Meters per second	Miles per hour	2.237

Chapter 11

Levers and
Other Simple Machines

There are six kinds of simple machines; the more complex machines are combinations of these simple machines. The six simple machines are the lever, the pulley, the wheel and axle, the inclined plane, the wedge, and the screw. The first three of these are found in the human body, with the lever being by far the most prevalent.

LEVERAGE

In mechanics a lever is defined as a rigid bar which revolves around a fixed point known as an axis (A), with a force (F) to move it, and a resistance (R) to be overcome by it. (The force is sometimes referred to as the effort, the axis as the fulcrum, and the resistance as the weight.) Levers are useful for various purposes depending upon the kind of lever and the mechanical ratio it provides.

Classes of Levers

There are three kinds (classes) of levers, determined by the relative arrangement of the axis (A), the point of force (F), and the point of

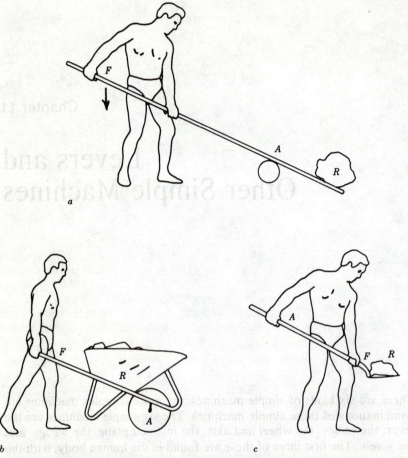

Figure 11-1 Practical examples of the three different classes of leverage. (a) First-class leverage. (b) Second-class leverage. (c) Third-class leverage.

resistance (R). A first-class lever has the arrangement F-A-R; a second-class lever has the arrangement F-R-A; a third-class lever has the arrangement of A-F-R. The outside components may be switched, for only the middle component determines the class of lever. Figure 11-1 shows examples of the three kinds of levers used in practical situations.

Inasmuch as practically all movements of the body involve levers, the following points will help to understand human movement better.

1 In the body a bone or a combination of bones composes a rigid bar known as a lever.
2 The axis passes through a joint, and is the point around which the lever moves.

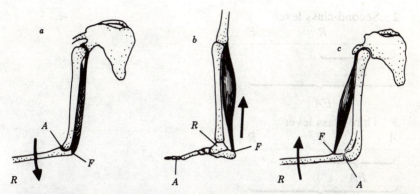

Figure 11-2 The three classes of leverage used in human movement. (a) Triceps muscle causes first-class leverage as it extends the elbow. (b) Gastrocnemius muscle causes second-class leverage as it plantar flexes (extends) the foot. (c) Biceps muscle causes third-class leverage as it flexes the elbow.

3 The application of force is at the attachment of one or more muscles producing the force, and the force is caused by the contractions of the muscles.

4 The point of resistance is the center of gravity of the body segment being moved, plus the center of gravity of any external weight or resistance. (The resistance may be either the weight of the body segment alone, weight of the segment plus external weight, or the application of an external force as in working against an opponent.)

Figure 11-2 shows examples of how the three classes of levers are used in human movement. It is interesting to know that in every kind of movement at every joint one of the three classes of levers is involved.

Lever Arms

Every lever, regardless of its kind, has two separate arms known as the force arm FA and the resistance arm RA. The force arm is the perpendicular distance from the axis A to the line of force F (or line of pull), while the resistance arm is the perpendicular distance from the axis A to the resistance R. The exact ratio between the force arm and resistance arm varies with each class of lever, and with different levers of the same class. This can be readily understood by examining the following drawings. Further, the ratio changes as the lever moves through its range of motion, because the line of pull changes.

1   First-class lever

$$\underbrace{F \qquad\qquad A}_{FA} \quad \underbrace{\qquad R}_{RA}$$

2 Second-class lever

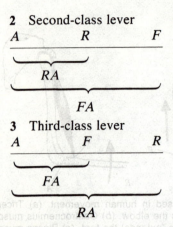

3 Third-class lever

Figure 11-2 The three classes of leverage used in human movement. (a) Triceps muscle causes first-class leverage as it extends the elbow. (b) Gastrocnemius muscle causes second-class leverage as it plantar flexes (extends) the foot. (c) Biceps muscle

In a *first-class* lever either arm (*FA* or *RA*) may be longer than the other, depending on the location of the lever's axis; in *second-class* levers the *FA* is always the longer, and in *third-class* levers the *RA* is always the longer.

Mechanical Ratio

The ratio that exists between the two arms of the lever determines the mechanical ratio of the lever. For example, if the two arms were the same length, as in a perfectly balanced teeter-totter, the mechanical ratio would be one to one and there would be no mechanical advantage. If the *force arm* were five times as long as the resistance arm, the mechanical ratio would be one to five in favor of *force*. Conversely, if the *resistance arm* were five times as long as the force arm, the mechanical ratio would be one to five in favor of *resistance*.

It is conceivable that in the human body the exact mechanical ratio is different in every movement at every joint. Further, it is known that the ratio varies at different points through the range of motion. Therefore, it can be correctly stated that even though the mechanical ratio might appear to be a constant in any particular joint, it is actually a variable. Further, in some cases the mechanical ratio can be purposely adjusted by changing the point of resistance or by shortening the lever. In some sports, such as gymnastics and wrestling, knowing how to adjust the leverage to your advantage is a very important part of the technique.

Force versus Speed

Whenever the force arm *FA* of a lever is longer than its resistance arm *RA*, the mechanical advantage favors the application of force at the sacrifice of speed, and the lever is called a *force lever*. Conversely, when the resistance arm *RA* is longer than the force arm *FA*, the lever favors

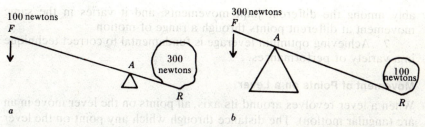

Figure 11-3 Influences on mechanical ratio of different relative lengths of force arm and resistance arm. In (a), the force arm is three times as long as the resistance arm, while in (b), the resistance arm is three times as long as the force arm.

speed and range of motion at the sacrifice of force, and is called a *speed lever*.

Figure 11-3 involves two first-class levers. In the lever on the left the *FA* is three times as long as the *RA*. This lever has a mechanical ratio of one to three in favor of force, meaning that 100 newtons of force would balance 300 newtons of resistance. The lever on the right has an *RA* three times as long as the *FA*. This lever has a mechanical ratio of one to three in favor of *speed*, meaning that it would take 300 newtons of force to balance 100 newtons of resistance; but if the point of force were moved 1 meter, the point of resistance would move 3 meters in the same amount of time, and therefore would move three times as fast. This is why it is called a speed lever.

The following statements will help understanding of the application of *speed levers* and *force levers* as they apply to human movement.

1   First-class levers may produce either kind of advantage depending on the relative position of *A*. If the *A* is closer to the *F* than it is to the *R*, the *FA* will be shorter than the *RA*, and the lever will favor *speed*. Conversely, if the *A* is closer to the *R*, the *RA* will be shorter than the *FA*, and the lever will favor *force*. It is interesting to note that the first-class levers in the human body have their axes *A* close to the point of force *F* and are therefore speed levers.

2   In a second-class lever the *RA* is always shorter than the *FA*, and there is no way that this can be untrue in a second-class lever. Therefore, second-class levers are always *force* levers.

3   In a third-class lever the *FA* is always shorter than the *RA*, and there is no way that the opposite can be true in a third-class lever. Therefore, third-class levers are always *speed* levers.

4   Most of the levers in the human body are either first-class or third-class, with third-class levers being the most prevalent.

5   Most of the levers in the human body are *speed levers*, meaning that the force arms are shorter than the resistance arms.

6   The exact mechanical ratio (amount of leverage) varies considerably among the different joint movements, and it varies in the same movement at different points through a range of motion.

7   Achieving optimum leverage is fundamental to correct technique in a variety of performances.

Movement of Points on a Lever

When a lever revolves around its axis, all points on the lever move in an arc (angular motion). The distance through which any point on the lever moves is directly proportional to its distance from the axis. For example, in Figure 11-4:

1   Point y is twice as far from the axis as point x, and z is three times as far as x. If point x moves a distance of 3 centimeters, point y will move 6 centimeters, and z will move 9 centimeters.

2   Points x, y, and z move through their arcs of 3, 6, and 9 centimeters, respectively, in the same amount of time. This illustrates that a point which is farther from the axis not only moves a proportionately greater distance but also moves with proportionately greater speed.

Sports Implements as Levers

When an implement such as a baseball bat, a golf club, or a tennis racket is held in the hand, it becomes a lever. In some cases the implement can be viewed as a separate lever, and in other cases it is an extension of a body lever. An implement which extends beyond the hands moves faster than the hands themselves, and the farther the implement extends the greater is its velocity (refer to Figure 11-4). This means that in the golf swing, the head of a longer club will move faster than the head of a shorter club, if the angular velocity is the same. Further, it means that a point on a bat 50 centimeters from the grip will move faster than a point 35 centimeters from the grip. This would lead one to believe that a baseball should be struck near the end of the bat where the velocity of the bat is the greatest. This is true as far as velocity is concerned, but another factor must be considered. If the ball is struck at a distance from the center of weight of the bat, the force of the ball will tend to rotate the

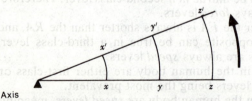

Axis

Figure 11-4   The length of a lever influences the linear speed and distance it will travel when the angular speed and distance are constant. Point y moves twice as fast and twice as far as x. Point z moves three times as far and three times as fast as x.

bat, and part of the force of the bat will be dissipated. In order to make the most solid contact, the center of gravity of the bat should meet the center of gravity of the ball. Since the idea of maximum velocity of the bat and solid striking force are not in complete harmony, a compromise between the two will produce the best results. That is, the ball will travel the farthest if it is struck solidly by the bat at a point slightly beyond the center of gravity of the bat. At this point on the bat, velocity is relatively high and the impact is close to the center of weight of the bat.

In connection with this same idea, full extension at the joints as opposed to partial extension will lengthen the total lever or combination of levers, and will thereby produce more speed at a particular point along the lever. This means that if angular velocity at the joints remains constant, then during a service stroke in tennis (Figure 11-5) the racket head will be moving faster if the arm is fully extended at the moment of contact with the ball. Strengthening of the muscles producing the angular motion ensures no loss in angular velocity as the lever is lengthened.

Obviously in the use of sports implements it is important to analyze the effects that each implement has on leverage, and utilize the implement in the manner that will produce optimum results.

Practical Application

Nothing can be done in the human body to change the length of force arms, but much can be done to change resistance arms, and thus the

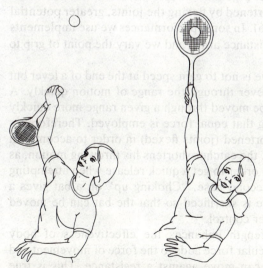

Figure 11-5 The tennis serve demonstrates a long resistance arm to gain speed at the end of the lever. The tennis racket adds length to the moving lever, causing the racket face to move considerably faster than the hand.

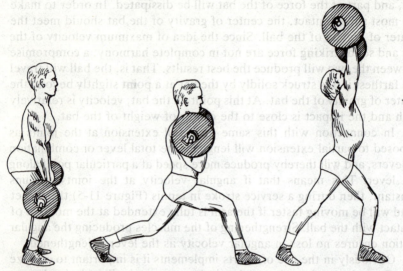

Figure 11-6 Lifting maximum weight demonstrates the need for a short resistance arm (weight is kept close to the body) so that maximum force may be applied against the resistance.

proportionate length of the two. Variations occur by extending or flexing the acting joints, thus increasing or decreasing the length of the lever. As levers are lengthened, greater potential for *speed* occurs at the end of the lever. When the lever is shortened by flexing the joints, greater potential for *force* occurs (Figure 11-6). In some performances we use implements to increase the length of resistance arms, and we vary the point of grip to suit our purpose.

Sometimes the objective is not to gain speed at the end of a lever but rather to move the whole lever through the range of motion quickly. A shorter resistance arm can be moved through a given range more quickly than a longer one, assuming that equal force is employed. Therefore, in some cases the lever is shortened (joints flexed) in order to accomplish the act better. For example, the catcher shortens his throwing motion, as compared with a pitcher, in order to get a quick release when attempting to throw out a runner at second base. "Choking up" on a bat gives a similar effect; striking force is sacrificed so that the bat can be moved more quickly and with better control.

Building additional strength enhances the effectiveness of body levers, because greater muscular force adds to the force of movement and to the speed at which we can move against a resistance. This is true regardless of the class of lever or the amount of leverage.

WHEEL AND AXLE

The wheel and axle consists of a wheel-type device attached to the axle about which it revolves. The revolving action may result either from force applied to the wheel, as in steering an automobile, or from the axle, as in the case of the driving force of the automobile. The larger the diameter of the wheel the greater is the magnification of the rotary movement. The turning effect of the wheel is the product of the force and the radius.

The wheel and axle is similar to the lever, because the radius of the wheel corresponds to the force arm of a lever. This is easier to understand if you visualize the wheel as consisting of a single spoke as in the case of a pencil sharpener.

When the force is applied to the wheel in order to turn the axle, the mechanical advantage favors force; so it would correspond to a *force* lever. Conversely, when the force is applied to the axle in order to turn the wheel, the leverage favors speed. It is interesting that in pedaling a bicycle both kinds of leverage are involved, because when the rider applies force to the pedals (wheel), this turns the axle which connects the two pedals. The chain then conveys the force to the rear axle, which turns the rear wheel.

Most of the wheel and axle arrangements in the human body are designed to gain speed at the expense of force. However, both kinds of leverage are represented. The most clear-cut examples occur in the trunk. Figure 11-7 shows a cross section of the trunk representing a wheel and axle where the force of the oblique abdominal muscles is applied to the

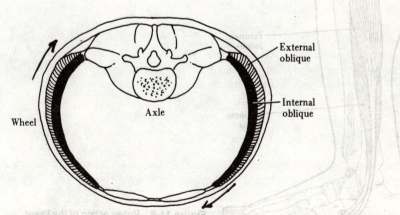

Figure 11-7 Wheel and axle action of the trunk. The external and internal oblique muscles contract to cause rotation of the trunk (wheel) around the spine (axle).

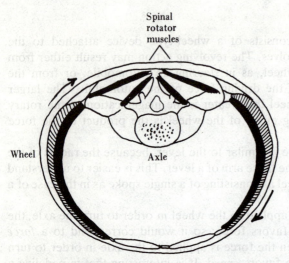

Figure 11-8 Axle and wheel action of the spine. The spinal rotator muscles contract, applying force to the spine (axle), thus causing the wheel to turn.

wheel. The axle is represented by the spinal column around which the wheel rotates.

Figure 11-8 shows an opposite situation where the rotator muscles of the spine apply force to the axle (spinal column), resulting in the turning

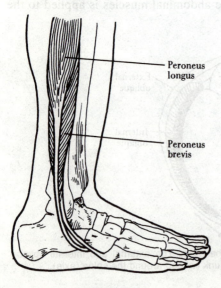

Figure 11-9 Pulley action of the lower tendons of the peroneus longus and peroneus brevis muscles.

of the wheel (trunk). Another example of force applied to the wheel is the muscles which attach to the base of the skull to rotate the head (wheel) on the top vertebrae of the spine.

PULLEY

A pulley is thought of as a wheel-type device with a rope running over it. Even though there are no pulleys of this kind in the human body, there are actions that resemble pulley movements. Pulleys in the body are represented by tendons which wrap over portions of bones and thus change the direction of pull. Possibly the best example is the lower tendon of the peroneus longus muscle which wraps around a protruding portion of the lower end of the fibula (Figure 11-9). The tendon of the peroneus brevis follows a path almost parallel to that of the peroneus longus. In much the same manner, the tendons of the flexor hallucis longus, flexor digitorium longus, and tibialis posterior wrap around the bone structure of the inside of the ankle. An example in another portion of the body is the lower attachment of the sartorius where the tendon wraps around the inside of the condyles of the knee joint. The adductor magnus and the gracilis muscles have lower tendons which lie parallel to the tendon of the sartorius. The lower tendon of the rectus femoris muscle also illustrates a pulley arrangement when the knee is bent.

All the pulleys in the human body are simple pulleys, which means that no mechanical advantage is either gained or lost.

BODY PLANES AND MOVEMENT PLANES

There are three reference planes of the body, and each plane is perpendicular to each of the other two. Likewise, there are three planes of motion corresponding (parallel) to the planes of the body. The planes are as follows (see Figure 11-10):

1 The *sagittal plane* is represented by an imaginary vertical plate passing through the body dividing it into right and left portions (also known as the *anterior-posterior* or *median* plane). The arm and leg actions in walking are examples of movement in this plane (parallel to it). Other examples are the arm actions in the underarm pitch and in bowling, and forward and backward rotary actions of the body.

2 The *frontal plane* is represented by an imaginary vertical plate passing through the body, dividing it into front and back portions (it is also known as the *lateral* or *coronal* plane). Examples of movement in this plane are the arm actions during the elementary backstroke and the arm actions associated with the iron cross in gymnastics.

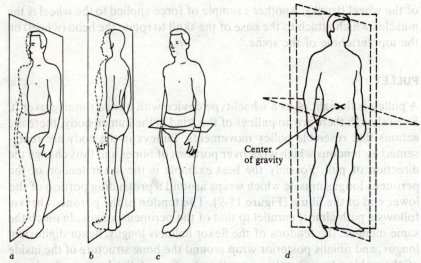

Center
of gravity

a   b   c   d

Figure 11-10 The three primary (cardinal) planes of the body. (*a*) Sagittal. (*b*) Frontal. (*c*) Transverse. The center of gravity is at the point of intersection of three planes (*d*).

3 The *transverse plane* is represented by an imaginary horizontal plate passing through the midsection of the body and dividing it into upper and lower portions. Movement in this plane is represented by twisting actions of the body or by the action of the throwing arm in the discus throw.

The position of each plane that divides the body into equal halves is known as the *cardinal plane.* The point at which the three cardinal planes intersect represents the exact center of the body and is therefore the body's center of gravity.

IMPORTANT CONCEPTS

1 All motor movements of the body involve the use of simple machines, with the lever being by far the most frequently used machine in the body. But the pulley and the wheel and axle are used a limited amount.

2 There are three kinds of levers, known as *first-*, *second-*, and *third*-class. In the *first*-class lever, the axis is between the force and the resistance. In the *second*-class lever, the resistance is between the axis and the force. In the *third*-class lever, the force is between the axis and the resistance.

3 Third-class levers are the most prevalent in the human body. There are several first-class levers and very few second-class levers in the body.

4 Each lever has a *force arm* which is the perpendicular distance from the line of force to the axis, and a *resistance arm* which is the perpendicular distance from the resistance to the axis. The ratio between the two arms is the mechanical ratio of the lever. The mechanical ratio can be changed by adjusting the relative length of the two arms.

5   From the practical point of view a body lever can be lengthened by adding to the body part an implement such as a golf club, tennis racket, or baseball bat.

6   In the use of a lever or any other simple machine, either *speed* or the ability to apply *force* can be gained by sacrificing the other. In other terms, in order to gain one advantage, the other is always sacrificed in the same amount.

7   In the wheel and axle arrangement, the ability to apply *force* is gained when the wheel is turned in order to apply force with the axle. Conversely *speed* is gained when the axle is turned, causing the extremity of the wheel to move much faster than the axle. Both speed and force arrangements exist in the human body.

8   The pulleys that exist in the human body are simple pulleys which only change the direction of pull and do not change the mechanical ratio.

9   The correct application of machines (mechanics) in the human body is fundamental to correct technique of motor performances.

Chapter 12

Motion

Athletic performances require the performer to move himself or herself, and sometimes to impart motion to an external object; therefore, motion is basic to athletic performance. It is impossible for a movement to occur unless a force produces it. The forces most often used in athletics are those produced by muscular contractions in combination with the ever-present force of gravity.

There are two kinds of motion: *rotary* and *translatory*. Rotary (or angular) motion does not transport an object from place to place; it is simply a turning of the object about an axis, or fulcrum. Appropriate synonyms for rotary motion are spinning, twisting, and turning. In rotary motion any point on the object describes the arc of a circle, with the axis of the movement being at the center of that circle. Translatory motion, on the other hand, is movement over a distance from one point to another. *Linear* translatory motion takes place when the path of movement is a straight line; *curvilinear* translatory motion occurs when a curved pathway is followed. Curvilinear motion is distinguished from rotary motion in that while curvilinear motion may be in a perfectly circular path, the axis of rotation is not within the mass of the moving object. An object often experiences both rotary and translatory motion simultaneously, as does the earth when it spins about its axis (rotary) and follows a curvilinear (translatory) path around the sun. During walking, the body experiences translatory motion while the arms and legs experience rotary (angular) motion about the active joints. An object often experiences linear and curvilinear motion (both translatory) successively. For example, when an object is hurled through space, it starts its flight in a linear path but soon changes to a curved path as a result of the forces of air resistance and gravity. When a baseball pitcher throws a curve ball, the motion of the ball appears to be linear, but almost immediately after release, the ball follows a curvilinear path (rotation continues). The curvilinear path is governed by the direction and amount of the spin, which usually causes a left or right movement, and the force of gravity, which causes a downward movement. The curved path the ball travels is dependent upon the combined magnitudes of the linear and rotary forces applied to the ball.

TRANSLATORY MOTION

Following are facts which contribute to understanding the role of linear motion in human performance. Curvilinear motion is discussed further in Chapter 13.

   1   An object will move in a straight line when:
      a   The object is freely movable, and the force is applied on center. As the force is applied at a point farther from the center of gravity, the object will rotate around its center of gravity at a faster speed.
      b   Regardless of where the force is applied, the object is free to move only in a linear path. Example: a sliding door or window.
   2   The human body experiences linear motion when it is pushed or pulled by an outside force or glides over a smooth surface. Examples: skiing (straight) or sliding down a slide.
   3   In many instances, the body experiences linear motion due to rotary motion of some of its segments. Examples: swimming, walking, running (Figure 12-1), and vertical jumping.
   4   In some instances a distal segment may experience linear motion due to rotary motion of the proximal segments. Examples: the hand in fencing and the foot in pushing, as in the vertical jump.

ROTARY (ANGULAR) MOTION

Following are important facts about rotary motion:

   1   An object will rotate under the following conditions:
      a   If the object is freely movable, and the force is applied

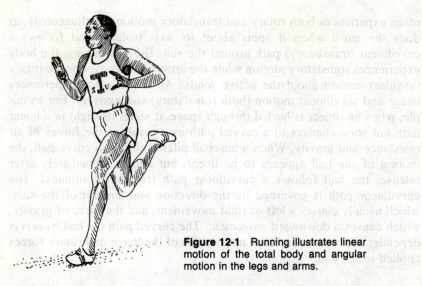

Figure 12-1 Running illustrates linear motion of the total body and angular motion in the legs and arms.

off-center. As the force is applied at a point farther from the center of gravity, the object will rotate around its center of gravity at a faster speed.

   b If force is applied to any part of the object, and it is free to move only in a rotary path. Examples: swinging door, arm moving around the shoulder joint, and leg moving around the hip joint.

  2 The human body as a whole experiences rotary motion under the following conditions:

   a When it is unsupported and revolves around its center of gravity. Examples: diving stunts (Figure 12-2), trampoline stunts, tumbling stunts, and certain gymnastic movements. Examples: cartwheel and handspring (both rotary and translatory); giant swing (only rotary).

  3 Individual body segments experience angular movement by causing the segment to revolve around an axis which passes through the joint. Examples: arm rotates around the shoulder joint, lower leg rotates around the knee joint. Rotary motion may also occur around an axis which passes through the length of a segment. Examples: inward or outward rotation of the upper arm at the shoulder, pronation or supination of the forearm.

  Note The terms *angular motion* and *rotary motion* are interchangeable. *Angular* is the term usually used when the moving part has a point of contact at one end and rotates around that point, such as the movement of a body limb around a joint. *Rotary* is the term usually used for rotational movements of freely moving bodies that are unattached.

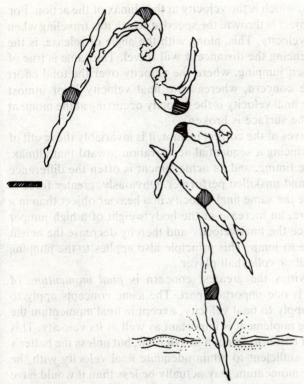

Figure 12-2 The forward one-and-one-half somersault illustrates rotary motion of the total body as it moves through a curvilinear path of flight.

VELOCITY AND MOMENTUM

The distance an object travels in a given direction in a period of time represents its velocity. Usually an expressed velocity represents the average speed of movement and does not take into account the velocity for any portion of the total distance. However, it is important to be aware that velocity of an object is seldom constant. Therefore, one must, at different times, think in terms of average velocity, maximum velocity, and final velocity. Increase in velocity is referred to as *acceleration*. The opposite of acceleration is *deceleration*. Acceleration may be uniform or varying, but, as with velocity, acceleration is seldom constant.

When the mass of a moving object is combined with its velocity, the object is said to have *momentum*. Momentum is the product of velocity and mass. Therefore, an increase of either velocity or mass will cause a proportionate increase in momentum.

In explosive athletic events, one of the real concerns is the *final velocity* of the object, which is the velocity at the climax of the action. For instance, when an object is thrown, the speed at which it is traveling when released is its final velocity. This, along with the angle of release, is the primary factor influencing the distance it will travel. The same is true of the human body when jumping, where the velocity over the total effort (average) is of little concern, whereas the final velocity is of utmost concern. In this case final velocity is the velocity occurring at the moment when contact with the surface is broken.

If velocity climaxes at the correct instant, it is invariably the result of muscular forces producing a sequential acceleration toward that climax. This calls for precise timing, and its achievement is often the difference between the skilled and unskilled performer. Obviously, greater force is necessary to produce the same final velocity in a heavier object than in a lighter one. Therefore, an increase in the body weight of a high-jumper could seriously reduce the final velocity and thereby decrease the height the performer is able to jump. This principle also applies to the jumping ability of a basketball or volleyball player.

In striking activities the greatest concern is *final momentum*, of which final velocity is one important part. The same concepts apply to final momentum as apply to final velocity, except in final momentum the weight of the striking implement is important as well as its velocity. This may cause a baseball batter to select a heavier bat, but unless the batter's muscular forces are sufficient to attain adequate final velocity with the heavier bat, the final momentum may actually be less than it would have been with a lighter bat. If a football player can develop greater momentum with his moving body, he can strike a more forceful blow, which may mean that he should gain weight to be more effective. However, unless he can attain the same velocity at impact that he had before the weight gain, his momentum may be either unchanged or less.

BASIC LAWS OF MOTION

Many teaching hints and coaching tips related to skill are derived from a number of principles of motion. These principles, in turn, are derived from just three basic laws of motion developed by Isaac Newton (1642–1727). If the teaching technique cannot be traced back to a basic Newtonian law, assuming the technique has to do with motion, its soundness should be viewed with serious doubt. It is important to understand that some performance techniques may have evolved from performers who have been successful *in spite of* the use of unsound techniques. Furthermore, at times performers are convinced they do something in a certain way when actually it is done quite differently. For example, few divers are aware that most twisting movements are initiated while they are still in contact with the board.

At times, one law must be violated in order to observe another. One law may produce effects of such magnitude that the effects of the other are made inconsequential. Following are Newton's three laws of motion:

Law of inertia   A body at rest tends to remain at rest, whereas a body in motion tends to continue in motion with consistent speed and in the same direction unless acted upon by an outside force.

In effect, the first law refers to *resistance to any change* relating to motion. It takes force to begin motion, to retard motion, to accelerate an object, to change its direction, or to stop its motion. The greater the change is to be in the existing condition of motion, the more force will be needed to produce the change. Resistance to change of motion is called *inertia*. In terms of application, the law means that if an object is at rest (stationary), it will remain at rest unless some force puts it into motion. Conversely, if an object is in motion, it will continue in the same direction and at the same speed unless changed by the forces of gravity, friction, air resistance, or other forces.

Law of acceleration   The velocity of a body is changed only when acted upon by an additional force. The produced acceleration (or deceleration) is proportional to and in the same direction of the force.

This means that if the propelling or driving force of the body or an object is doubled, the rate of acceleration will double, and if the driving force is tripled, the acceleration will increase proportionately.

It also means that if a resisting force is applied directly opposite the movement of an object, then (1) it will decelerate the object and finally stop it, if the force is weak but continuous (air resistance or water resistance); (2) it will stop the object if the magnitude of the resistance is equal to the momentum of the object; or (3) it will reverse the direction of the object if the magnitude is greater than that of the object. If a force is applied to a moving body at an angle (neither directly with nor against the path of motion), the resulting change in both velocity and direction of the body depends upon the magnitude and the angle of that force (determined by a parallelogram of forces).

Law of counterforce   The production of any force will create another force which will be opposite and equal to the first force.

In the vertical jump, for example, the resistance of the earth makes the thrust possible. The muscular force that is directed downward against the earth is insufficient to overcome the inertia of the earth, and the counterforce of the earth pushing back is effective in propelling the performer.

Another example of counterforce is in swimming, where the hands are directed backward against the water and the water produces the counterforce necessary to propel the body. It is the *counterforce* which makes it possible for the performer to move.

When the body is unsupported (suspended in space), as during the long jump, the action of one of its parts will provide a counteraction of another part but will not alter the flight path of the body's center of gravity because the air does not provide sufficient resistance to generate a significant counterforce, as does a solid (earth) or a liquid (water). Skydiving and ski jumping are exceptions to the rule that air resistance is insufficient to change the flight path of a mass as great as the human body. The great speeds achieved in these instances pile up air molecules in sufficient quantity to cause a significant effect. Similarly, an arm extending from the window of an automobile traveling at 30 kilometers per hour feels little if any effective air resistance, but at 100 kilometers per hour the difference is evident.

PRINCIPLES RELATED TO THE LAW OF INERTIA

Derived from basic laws, principles of performance are generalized statements which govern the techniques of performance. It is difficult to separate principles of motion from those of force, but for convenience, the attempt is made here, despite some overlaps. If the following principles are observed, the law of inertia will not be violated, and performance will be aided rather than hindered.

Combining Translatory and Rotary Motions

Principle: Successful performance often calls for effectively combining translatory and rotary motions.

Example A: The discus throw results from a combination of movements. The performer moves the total body linearly from the back to the front of the circle, and in doing so overcomes the inertia of the discus to motion in that direction. The performer rotates the total body with ever-increasing velocity in progressing forward. Then, near the end of the total body rotary movement, the discus is thrown by means of upper-body rotation and rotary actions of the throwing arm. These three kinds of motion, if performed correctly with proper sequence and timing, will produce maximum final velocity of the discus in the desired direction at release. *Example B*: A long-jumper or high-jumper uses both the translatory motion of the approach and angular motion of the body segments at the takeoff. The approach overcomes the inertia to forward progress while the vertical thrust overcomes the inertia to vertical progress. The relative emphasis on each kind of motion depends upon the objective of the jump (vertical or horizontal). *Example C*: Shift of body weight is a movement common to many activities, especially throwing and striking actions. It is commonly referred to as "getting your body into the act." This means transferring the body weight from one foot to the other in the direction of the action and is another example of linear motion of the total body combined with rotary motion of the body segments. Batting a baseball, performing a stroke, and throwing an object are all examples in which the weight shift is valuable. *Example D*: A dancer doing a leap turn experiences translatory motion (curvilinear) during the leap, and at the same time experiences rotary motion of the total body as it turns in space. At the same time certain separate body segments experience angular motion around their joints. Similar examples could be stated for diving and gymnastic tumbling activities.

Continuity of Motion

Principle: When performing activities in which two or more consecutive motions contribute to movement in the same direction, there should usually be no pause between the motions. The accomplishment of the first motion represents the overcoming of a certain amount of inertia. Any hesitation before the next motion will result in loss of some or all of the advantage gained by the previous motion.

Example A: When a pole-vaulter pulls the body upward, then reverses and pushes farther upward, there should be no pause between the pull and the push (except as influenced by the reaction of the pole). Both motions contribute to movement in the same direction. *Example B*: During the kip, the gymnast pulls the body upward and then pushes farther upward. Again there should be no pause between the pull and the push. *Example C*: Less muscular force is required to do a backward roll if the tumbler starts from a standing position and allows the force of gravity to begin the movement, thereby overcoming some of the resistance to backward rotary motion. This is accomplished by moving backward and downward to a sitting position. If the tumbler stops in the sitting position, nothing is gained. The next movement must continue immediately after the previous one. *Example D*: If the shot-putter hesitates between the movement across the ring and the final thrust, the value of the former movement is lost. This principle also applies to swimming, running, kicking, throwing, and other basic motor skills.

Effects of Momentum

Principle: Momentum is the product of mass and velocity; therefore, if either of these components is increased, the object possesses proportionately greater momentum, and the greater the momentum of an object, the greater resistance (inertia) it will present to a change in direction or velocity. Further if the motion of the object becomes a force (as it contacts another object), the force will be equal to the momentum.

Example A: As a football player moves with greater momentum, he becomes less susceptible to forces which attempt to alter his speed and direction. Therefore, weight is advantageous if it does not reduce speed. To completely stop the player's momentum, a body possessing equal or greater momentum must hit him head on. If that body has less weight, it can develop greater momentum only by attaining greater speed. If the contact is made from any direction other than straight on, the result will depend on the principle of multiple forces (discussed in Chapter 13). *Example B*: The basketball player who wishes to change direction of movement quickly will find the change more difficult with greater momentum. The change will also be more difficult as the degree of change in direction increases. Change of direction requires that a retarding force and a redirecting force be applied, and these forces, which overcome momentum, must be increased as momentum is increased. *Example C*: The selection of a heavier baseball bat, or any striking implement, provides opportunity for developing greater momentum, but only if sufficient muscular force is available so that the speed of the swing is not decreased. More momentum can be produced with a longer implement, because if angular velocity is the same, the end of a longer implement will move faster than a shorter implement. (A more thorough explanation of this point was offered in Chapter 11).

Transfer of Momentum

Principle: Momentum developed in a body segment may be transferred to the total body, and the longer and heavier the body segment is, and the greater its speed, the greater will be its contribution to total body momentum.

Example A (Figure 12-3): In jumping, the swinging action of the arms and the free leg transfers momentum to the rest of the body. If the swinging leg or arm is straight, thereby causing its center of weight to be farther from the axis of rotation, it contributes more to momentum, if angular speed of the swinging limb is held constant. (While this example may seem to illustrate a transfer of momentum, it is really a case of conservation of angular momentum.) *Example B*: In the track start, the forward driving actions of the arms contribute momentum to the total body.

Note Any movements of body parts after contact has been broken with the surface, such as swinging the arms or "running in the air" by the long-jumper, will not change the flight of the body as a whole.

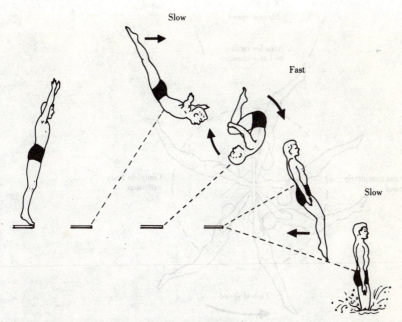

Slow

Fast

Slow

Figure 12-4 When a performer who is rotating moves from the lay-out to the tuck position, the rate of rotation increases. In a tight tuck the performer will rotate about twice as fast as in a lay-out position. This principle is also apparent in turning movements in ice skating, dance, and gymnastics.

movements. The two primary ones are the pole rotating about the box and the total body rotating about the handgrip. By lowering the grip on the pole, the speed of the pole rotating about the box is increased, but the height to which the body is raised is decreased. By pulling the body toward the grip at the correct time, the rate of body rotation about the grip is increased, and the momentum resulting from the early phase of the swing is conserved.

Conservation of Momentum in Swinging Movements

Principle: To build or to conserve momentum in any swinging movement, the radius of rotation should be shortened on the upswing and lengthened on the downswing, because this maximizes the effects of gravity when moving with it and minimizes gravity's effects when moving against it.

Example A (Figure 12-5): In doing a giant swing on a high bar (or other circling movements), the performer shortens the radius of rotation during the upswing to reduce the effects of gravity and lengthens the radius on the downswing to enable gravity to exert maximum effects. Shortening during the upswing is achieved by depressing the shoulder girdle and flexing slightly at the hips (within the limits that good form will

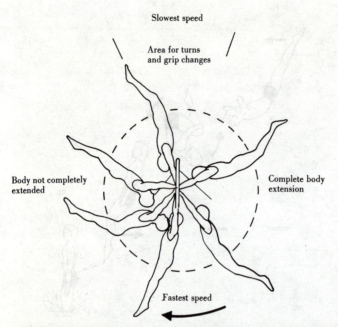

Slowest speed

Area for turns
and grip changes

Body not completely
extended

Complete body
extension

Fastest speed

Figure 12-5 When the body performs swinging movements, its center of gravity is moved away from the grip on the downswing and toward the grip on the upswing. Radius of the circle is greater on the right side than on the left side.

allow). Opposite movements cause lengthening during the downswing. *Example B*: In the pole vault, the vaulter swings on the pole, with the handgrip serving as the center of rotation. The body is extended away from the grip during the initial phase of the swing, then pulled toward the grip during the middle and latter phases, thus conserving the momentum that has been gained to carry the body forward and upward. If the vaulter shortens the radius from the box to the grip, speed will be gained, usually at the expense of height. If this radius is lengthened, height is gained at the expense of speed (and distance). With the fiber-glass pole, the vaulter usually wants to delay the forward momentum in order to allow time for the energy stored in the bend of the pole (the same as that energy stored in a diving board) to be returned at just the right time. Holding the body behind the pole (seated hang position) and delaying the swing accomplishes the desired effects. *Example C*: On either a child's swing, the flying rings, or a trapeze, the technique of swinging remains essentially the same. Performers move their weight away from the point of rotation on the downswing and pull toward the point of rotation on the upswing.

Movements while Unsupported

Principle: When the body is unsupported, movements of body segments may cause the body to rotate about its center of gravity, but its flight path will be unaffected. Such movements are useful in controlling rotation and balance, and they are especially useful in preparation for landing. While the body is unsupported, if a segment moves on one side of an axis of rotation, it causes movement of an equal magnitude on the opposite side of that axis (Newton's third law of motion).

Example A: In the straddle-roll high-jumping technique the sequence of moving the body parts over the bar may determine the success of the jump provided that the center of gravity is projected high enough to clear the bar. The problem is usually that the trailing leg does not clear the bar. In order to get the trail leg over the bar, the jumper should thrust the lead arm backward and upward, because this causes a countertwist of the trunk which will lift the trail leg. The countertwist can be demonstrated by having an athlete stand on a turntable (this simulates being free in the air) and instructing him to rotate his arms and shoulders in one direction. The hips and legs automatically rotate in the opposite direction (counterrotate). *Example B*: When hurdling, the arm opposite the lead leg must be thrust forward and slightly toward the lead leg to enable the performer to keep balance in a straight forward direction. If this is not done, the body tends to rotate away from the lead leg, and the performer does not land in the direction of the run. Furthermore, the trunk should be well flexed forward, because as the lead leg is snapped down to make early contact with the surface after clearing the hurdle, the upper body tends to straighten. If too much straightening occurs, the runner loses the forward lean, which is necessary for driving toward the next hurdle.

In many common activites, such as running, the countermoves of body segments in maintaining balance are automatic, and although the performer is unaware of them, they are essential to the performance. This principle applies at least partially to bodies in water as well as in air. However, bodies in water do not follow this principle entirely. The movement of a part does result in the displacement of the center of gravity, because water provides more resistance than air against body movements.

Twisting Movements

No new principles are stated here, but it is useful to emphasize principles which have already been discussed and which have special application to twisting actions.

Example A: Twisting movements are based largely upon the principle of conservation of angular momentum. Usually a body segment is "thrown" in a given direction while the body is still in contact with the supporting surface. The body then follows by twisting in the same direction in which the segment was thrown *Example B*: If the body segment is thrown after the body is airborne, the effects will follow the principle of counterrotation of unsupported bodies. This means that a movement of a segment will cause a countermovement of another segment or segments. For example, if the right arm is thrown forward in a horizontal plane in front of the chest (motion to the left), the remainder of the body will counterrotate to the right (toward that arm). The longer and heavier the body segment is which initiates the twisting movement, the greater will be the resulting counterrotation (all other factors being equal). *Example C*: The principle governing the effects of the body's radius on rotational speed applies here, meaning that the shorter the radius, all else being equal, the faster will be the rotation (or twisting action). For example, a diver who wants to twist rapidly should keep the legs together and the arms tucked in tight to the chest. By extending the arms sideward-out-ward from the body, the diver will slow down the twisting action considerably.

PRINCIPLES RELATED TO THE LAW OF COUNTERFORCE

The following principles depend upon the performers's applying muscular forces against a surface or object:

Surface Variation and Counterforce

Principle: When a force is applied to a stable surface, a counterforce is returned to the body from which the force came. The less stable the surface, the less will be the counterforce.

Example A: When running or jumping, the surface pushes back with force equal to the application of force, thus propelling the body. If the surface "gives," as in the case of sand, much of the counterforce is dissipated, thus limiting the amount of force that can be applied, and the performer receives less propulsion. *Example B*: If the surface is slippery or if footwear is inadequate to cause proper friction, the results are the same as those described in example A. *Example C*: Water offers less resistance than a solid surface; therefore, the propulsive force returned to the body is less in water than on a solid surface.

Direction of the Counterforce

Principle: The direction of the counterforce is directly opposite that of the applied force, and the applied force is the most effective when it is perpendicular to the supporting surface, because then slippage or "give" is minimized.

Example A: To achieve maximum height in jumping, the force must be applied directly downward, meaning that to get best results, the center of weight must be above the takeoff point. *Example B*: If a person runs or jumps while assuming too wide a stance, forces are poorly directed, resulting in inefficient movements, and some surface slipping may result. *Example C*: In water the body moves directly opposite to the applied force. If the force is downward, the counterforce propels the body upward: if the force is backward, the body moves forward. Only those forces which propel the body forward should be emphasized. *Example D*: Track starting blocks change the angle of the supporting surface, so that the surface is more perpendicular to the desired direction of propulsion. For this reason the performer should be sure to get the right amount of the foot on the block.

Counterforces in Striking Activities

Principle: The amount of force a striking implement imparts to an object depends on the combined momentum of the implement and the object at the moment of impact. Any give in the implement or the object at impact reduces the propulsive force (unless the implement or object is highly elastic, in which case propulsive force may be increased).

Example A: If the implement is held in the hands, the grip must be firm at impact to reduce or eliminate give at the grip. All clubs, bats, paddles, and rackets used in sports should be gripped in this manner if the objective is to impart maximum force. *Example B*: If an object is struck by a body segment (foot in kicking, fist in boxing, hand in volleyball and handball, etc.), then all joints not actively moving should be firm in their positions in order to reduce give.

Temporarily Stored Counterforce

Principle: If a surface or implement used in a performance has elasticity (ability to respond from disfigurement), an applied force which produces bend or compression will represent an amount of stored energy, and the stored energy increases the propulsive force over what it would be if elasticity were not present. The amount of energy depends upon the amount of disfigurement of the object, combined with its ability to spring back to its original shape.

Example A: When contacting the bed of a trampoline, the legs should be stiff in order to depress the bed a maximum amount, thus causing it to respond with greater force. In fact, the technique used to dissipate the force provided by the bed is to flex the supporting joints at the moment of contact. In the compressed position the trampoline bed possesses stored counterforce which is released as the bed resumes its normal position. *Example B (Figure 12-6):* After the vaulting pole (fiber glass) has been inserted in the planting box, the amount it will bend depends upon the final momentum the vaulter develops against the pole as a result of the approach and takeoff. Excessive give in the arms and shoulders of the

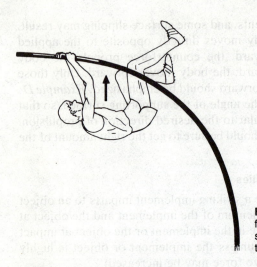

Figure 12-6 The excessive bend of a fiber-glass vaulting pole represents stored energy which becomes available to the vaulter when the pole responds.

vaulter cushions the amount of force transferred to the pole. The more limber the pole, the less force required to bend it, but also the less propulsive energy produced by it as it springs back to its original shape. Other examples of stored energy can be observed when the diving board is depressed or when the golf club is swung forcefully, causing the shaft to bend during the early phase and to straighten during the middle phase of the swing.

Surface Contact while Applying Forces to External Objects

Principle: In throwing, pushing, pulling, and striking activities one or both feet should be kept in firm contact with the supporting surface until the force providing motion is complete. Otherwise maximum force is reduced. However, it must be recognized that when applying force to objects, greater momentum may be gained by developing maximum total body momentum (with a running approach) in the desired direction. In order to maintain this momentum, it may be impossible to comply with the "firm contact principle"; however, even then the principle holds true to some extent and cannot be ignored. The influence of the firm contact principle increases as the external object becomes heavier.

Example A: If a football lineman removes his feet from the ground before his maximum momentum is complete, the force of his block or tackle will be reduced. *Example B*: If a shot-putter breaks contact between the feet and the ground before the main force—providing movements are complete—the force will be reduced. The same is true for a baseball batter and golf driver.

IMPORTANT CONCEPTS

1 There are three basic laws of motion known as Newton's laws, and the principles of motion are derived from the three laws.

2 There are two basic forms of motion, *translatory* and *rotary* (angular). Translatory means the object is transported from one point to another, while rotary means the object rotates around an axis within itself. Translatory motion can be further divided into linear (straight-line) and curvilinear (curved-line).

3 *Velocity* is frequently of great importance. In some performances *maximum velocity* is of paramount importance, while in other cases the *average velocity* is more important. *Acceleration, deceleration,* and *pace* are factors influencing velocity.

4 *Final velocity* is of utmost importance in activities of projecting the body or an object, because it is the speed of movement at the climax of the performance (when contact is broken). When all else remains constant, increased final velocity results in increased projectile speed and increased distance.

5 *Momentum,* which is the combination of velocity and mass, is of fundamental importance in activities where impetus or striking force is needed. By increasing either velocity or mass, momentum is increased a proportionate amount.

6 *Final momentum* is of utmost importance in imparting a force to a body or object. It is the amount of momentum at the moment of impact, and it becomes the striking force.

7 The correct application of principles of motion is fundamental to correct technique. However, in some instances one principle will have to be violated or not fully applied in order to enhance the application of another principle which might be more important to the performance.

Note Numerous other important concepts are stated in the chapter in the form of principles, and there is no need to restate them here.

STUDENT LABORATORY EXPERIENCES

The best conceptual benefit will come to the student from solving the following problems:

1 How many meters would a runner go in a straight line if he or she were to run for 4 seconds at a velocity of 7.5 meters per second? How far would that runner go in the same situation on a curved track? (See formula **1**.) Name the two types of motion in the problem. *LINEAR + ANGULAR*

2 A sprinter runs the 100-meter dash in 12 seconds. (*a*) What is the runner's average velocity? (*b*) If acceleration is constant for the first 20 meters and velocity constant at 10 meters per second for the last 80 meters, what is this sprinter's acceleration? (*c*) Average velocity for the first 20 meters? (See formulas **1**, **2**, **3**.)

A 4.15 n/s   B

3 It takes a dancer 0.5 second to do a complete turn. (*a*) What is the angular velocity (ω) in revolutions? (*b*) In radians? (*c*) In degrees? (See formulas **20, 24, 25, 26, 26, 27**.)

4 What is the tangential velocity (v_T) of a golf-club head if its radius—shoulder to head of club—is 1.4 meters and it moves through the last 22° before impact in 0.015 seconds? (See formulas **22, 22**.)

5 If the angular velocity (ω) of a gymnast doing a giant swing is $\omega_1 = 180°$/second at the horizontal on the downswing and $\omega_2 = 380°$/second at the bottom of the swing, what is the average angular acceleration ($\bar\alpha$) if the swing takes 0.35 seconds? (See formula **21**.)

6 The radius of rotation of a skater who is spinning is 0.9 meter. The angular velocity is 2π radians/second. The skater then reduces the radius of rotation to 0.33 meters. (*a*) What is the new angular velocity (ω) in radians? (*b*) In revolutions? (*c*) In degrees? (See formula **22**.)

7 A 7.7-kilogram shot is dropped from a height (s) of 6 meters. (*a*) With what velocity (v_y) does it hit the ground? (*b*) What is its momentum at the instant it is dropped? (*c*) What is its final momentum at impact? (See formulas **8, 45**.)

3 A 1/4 RPS 1REV   4

B 6 2°

C 360°

7

1 M = 7.7 X

A =

Chapter 13

Force

Force is described as push or pull, but it is more precisely defined as the product of the *mass* and *acceleration* of an object. The motion of a body never truly becomes a force unless it contacts another body or object. Usually one body exerts force, and the other receives it, but in some cases both bodies exert force against each other. A force is not effective in producing motion unless it is of sufficient magnitude to overcome the inertia of the body receiving the force.

Principles have been formulated which apply to all activities in which the development of force is desired. Although most of the principles are based on the *assumption* that the objective is to produce maximum force, one must be aware that such a result is not always desired. The golf putt, football pass, toss to initiate a baseball double play, and baseball bunt are examples in which less than maximum force is desired. Principles of force are logically grouped under the following headings: (1) general principles, (2) self-produced and other positive forces, (3) environmental forces, and (4) force dissipation.

225

GENERAL PRINCIPLES OF FORCE

In striking activities, *final momentum* is the most important factor in producing striking force. *Final velocity* is the prime factor in jumping and throwing, and *average velocity* is the prime consideration in locomotive activities where the objective is to cover a distance in the shortest time. Any human motion arises from the cooperation of muscular and gravitational forces acting on the body in a state of either motion or rest. If the body already possesses momentum in the correct direction before force is applied, the force will be more effective.

Total Force

Principle: A total force (or velocity) is the sum of the forces (or velocities) of each body segment contributing to the act, if the forces are applied in a single direction and in the proper sequence with correct timing.

Example A: At the moment of release, a ball which is thrown is traveling at a velocity approximately equal to the sum of the velocities of all the body movements contributing at the time of release. *Example B*: At the moment of release, the discus is traveling at a velocity approximately equal to the sum of the velocities of all the contributing forces. This includes the linear movement across the ring, the rotary movement of the total body (spin), and the angular movements of the different body segments contributing to the throwing action. *Example C*: In *any* explosive performance, the next force in sequence contributing to velocity should be applied at the peak of the previous force. To accomplish this, maximum coordination of specific movements is required. If the second force is applied too late, momentum from the first force is lost; if the second force is applied too soon, superimposing the force reduces the possible total effect of the two forces.

Constant Application of Force

Principle: Application of force should be constant and as even as possible so that maximum force is used to overcome the resistance of gravity and air or water, and minimum force is used to overcome inertia.

Example A: When pushing a car, less force is required to keep the car in motion at a constant rate than to increase the velocity of the car. The cost of running a car is more economical (less energy required) when driven at a constant speed as opposed to varying speeds. Frequent starting and stopping expends additional energy. *Example B*: A distance runner or swimmer moves more efficiently and economically when traveling at a constant speed and with smooth application of force, in which case a minimum amount of energy is used to overcome inertia.

Direction of Force Application

Principle: In general, all forces should be applied as directly as possible in line with the intended motion. Forces applied in other directions either retard motion in the desired direction or result in wasted energy.

Example A: A swimmer or runner should reduce to a minimum all forces which do not directly contribute to forward progress. Unproductive muscular contractions are characteristic of unskilled performers. *Example B*: A runner who points the toes outward ("duck-footed") with each stride cannot direct his or her forces straight ahead. Only part of the lever (foot) is used, and certain muscles that would otherwise contribute are ineffective; thus the force of the push is reduced. *Example C*: When the pole-vaulter makes the final push from the pole, it is necessary for the pole to be close to the body, with the center of the body weight generally above the hands. Otherwise, the pushing force will add momentum toward the horizontal rather than the vertical direction.

Distance of Force Application

Principle: If a constant force is applied to a body, the body develops greater velocity as the distance over which the force is applied increases.

Example A: In the shot put if the performer begins with the back instead of the side toward the direction of the put, the advantage of another quarter of a turn over which to apply force is gained. Still another quarter of a turn enable one professional shot-putter (Brian Oldfield) to outdistance all others. The same idea applies to the discus throw. *Example B*: Most throwing (Figure 13-1) and striking events (performed right-handed) should end with the striding foot slightly to the left of the intended line of flight. This slightly "open" stance at the completion of the action permits a greater distance over which to apply the force. Also

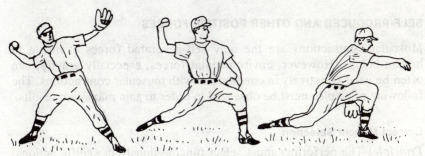

Figure 13-1 The baseball pitch illustrates the application of force over a long range of motion, thus allowing more time to increase the velocity. (*Clarence Robison, Clayne Jensen, Sherald James, and Willard Hirschi, Modern Techniques of Track and Field, Lea & Febiger, Philadelphia, 1974.*)

in throwing, the greater the range of motion of each contributing body segment, the greater the velocity resulting from that segment.

Multiple Forces

Principle: When two or more forces act upon a body, or two or more forces act upon each other, the resulting movement is determined by the direction and magnitude of the acting forces. If two forces act in the same general direction, the direction of the resulting force is somewhere between the two, and the magnitude of the resulting force is more than either, but not as much as the total, of the two contributing forces. The magnitude and direction of the resulting force can be determined exactly by constructing a parallelogram of forces.

Example A: The *gather* in the high jump or long jump means to "ready" the body just at takeoff to apply a vertical force with the least possible loss of horizontal momentum, which has already developed in the approach. The resulting magnitude and direction of flight are dependent upon the relative contributions of both the horizontal and vertical forces. *Example B*: If two football opponents make contact, each will change direction and speed, depending upon the momentum of each at the time of contact and the angle at which they collide. If they collide exactly head on with equal momentum, both players will totally lose their momentum. If they collide at an angle (not head on), they both maintain part of their momentum, but it will be transferred to a new direction. *Example C*: A high-jumper applies force to the surface with the push-off leg, adds force in the vertical direction with the swinging leg, and adds more force with the arm swing. All these contributing forces are in the same general, but not the exact, direction. Therefore, the total vertical force is less than the sum of all contributing forces.

SELF-PRODUCED AND OTHER POSITIVE FORCES

Muscular contractions are the only self-generated forces available to human beings. However, environmental forces, especially gravity, can often be used effectively in conjunction with muscular contractions. The following principles must be observed in order to gain maximum results.

Correct Muscle Selection

Principle: The performer must select (unconsciously in skillful actions) the muscles which are most effective for the task at hand. In a maximum effort the stronger the muscles and the more muscles that are brought into the action, the greater will be the force, and the less likely that muscle strain will occur.

Example A: When lifting heavy objects, the muscles of the legs provide greater strength than the extensor muscles of the back; therefore, lifting with the legs is more effective and much less hazardous. However, heavy lifts require the combined use of both the legs and the back. *Example B*: In boxing, the force of a left hook is greatest when it is initiated from hip and torso rotations, whereas the force is minimal when developed only from shoulder and arm actions. The same can be said of throwing or striking an object with arm action only as opposed to total body action (involvement of more and stronger muscles).

Stability and the Loss of Effective Force

Principle: Certain muscles must be "set" in performance of certain skills, especially those skills which involve heavy resistance. Also, a firm base of support, which contributes to stability of the body and its parts, helps to reduce loss of force.

Example A: The thrusting (putting) action against a shot is most effective if all joints not used in the development of force are stabilized, and contact of the back foot with the surface is firm. The follow-through or reversal occurs after the propelling forces have contributed all they can to the final velocity of the shot. *Example B*: Striking forces are more effective if all joints are either stabilized or moving in the direction of the action at the time of contact, and the feet are in firm contact with the surface.

Effect of the Angle of Force Application

Principle: In angular movements of body segments, the maximum effect on force occurs when the limb is at right angles to the direction in which the object is moved. The same applies to the angle of muscle pull (see example C).

Example A (Figure 13-2): A swimmer using the crawl stroke is most effective in the application of force when the hand and arm are directly

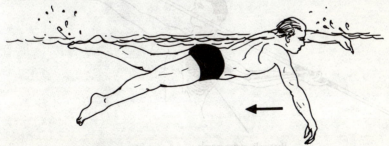

Figure 13-2 A swimmer can apply the greatest amount of effective force when the arm is at right angles to the direction of movement and the body.

below the shoulder—in other words, when the limb is at right angles to the direction of body movements. In this position the application of force has its greatest effect. *Example B*: In batting a baseball, the position of the greatest effective force occurs when the bat is in front of the body. At this point the bat is approximately at right angles to the flight of the ball. Force applied to the ball at any other angle is less effective. *Example C*: In movement of the elbow joint, the force applied by the elbow flexor muscles has its greatest effect when the elbow forms a right angle (90°). Consequently the difficult phases of a pull-up occur when the arm positions deviate farthest from the right angle (either straight or greatly bent), never at the midpoint of the movement.

Initial Muscular Tension

Principle: The force of muscular contraction may be increased by increasing the initial tension of the muscle (putting the muscle on stretch). The nearer a muscle is to complete contraction, the less force it can apply. It is not possible to adhere completely to both this principle and the previous one (effect of the angle of force application) at the same time. A compromise is necessary.

Example A: Drawing the arm backward in preparation to pitch a ball or to thrust a javelin (Figure 13-3) places the mover muscles on stretch, thereby increasing their initial contractile force. *Example B*: Although the legs are bent initially in preparation for a vertical jump, an additional slight dip prior to extension provides increased stretch of the extensor muscles and adds to the force of their contraction. *Example C*: Backward lean of the trunk prior to kicking places the rectus femoris muscle on stretch, enabling it (and other muscles) to extend the knee with greater force. (See section on stretch reflex, Chapter 4, for additional information about this principle.)

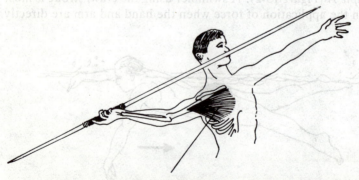

Pectoralis major muscle

Figure 13-3 The powerful pectoralis major muscle is on stretch in preparation for the thrust of the javelin. Numerous other muscles are also on stretch in the above body position.

Striking Force

Principle: When the angular velocity at the point of rotation remains constant, the velocity at which a lever moves is directly proportional to its length. This principle is based upon the system of levers, meaning that when a body lever is lengthened by extending it, or by adding an implement such as a ball bat or tennis racket, velocity is increased, and distance of movement and striking force are also increased (Figures 11-4 and 11-5).

Example A: When a tennis racket is added to the length of the human lever which rotates around the shoulder joint, the length of the original lever is almost doubled. If the angular velocity at the shoulder remains constant, the velocity at the end of the lever (racket face) will be approximately twice what it was before the lever was lengthened. *Example B*: When a golf club is held in a golfer's hands, the length of the swinging lever is increased. When a golfer strikes a golf ball, the velocity at impact is increased in proportion to the increased lever length, provided that the angular velocity remains constant.

Follow-through

Principle: Emphasis on correct follow-through eliminates the tendency to decelerate a throwing or striking action before its completion. In addition to this, other purposes exist for follow-through: (1) to maintain balance, (2) to avoid boundary-line violations, (3) to place the body in the ready position for the motor movement, and (4) to protect the joints, muscles, and connective tissues by gradually slowing the body parts. In any case, once contact is broken with the object, follow-through actions have no influence on the flight of the object.

Example A: In putting a shot or throwing a discus (Figure 13-4) or javelin, the reversal (follow-through) allows the performer to maintain balance and prevent fouling. If the reversal were eliminated and fouling were to be avoided, the performer would have to discontinue force application sooner, thereby reducing the total force because it would be applied over a shorter distance. *Example B*: In a baseball pitch or a tennis stroke, correct follow-through is essential to both power and accuracy. Conversely, attempts to prevent follow-through result in less final velocity because to avoid follow-through deceleration is necessary before release or strike.

ENVIRONMENTAL FORCES

Several external forces must be confronted. Often they can aid in performance; in such cases their influence should be maximized. But frequently, they are detrimental and must be regulated to exert minimum influence.

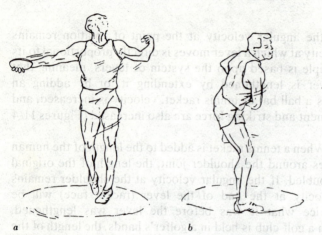

a   *b*

Figure 13-4 Follow-through is essential to maximum force in throwing, putting, and striking performances. The discus throw is an example.

Contending with External Forces

Principle: Among the forces with which we must contend during performance are (1) water resistance, (2) friction, (3) gravity, and (4) air resistance. We attempt to utilize these forces to our advantage. In some cases we will want to minimize and in other cases maximize their effects.

Example A: A swimmer should attempt to increase the water resistance against the power phase of the stroke and kick, in order to increase the propelling force. But at the same time, the water resistance against forward movement should be decreased to a minimum, which is done by using the correct body positions and correct techniques of recovery from the stroke and kick. *Example B:* A water-skier purposely increases the water resistance during the pull-up phase. Once up on the skis, the skier attempts to reduce the resistance to a minimum. *Example C:* While performing in basketball, tennis, track, soccer, and other activities where increased traction adds to stability and maneuverability, friction should be increased between the athlete and the performing surface by the wearing of special footwear. But dancers, skiers, skaters, and swimmers all attempt to reduce friction to some degree in order to improve their performances. The extent to which friction is purposely increased or decreased is determined by the act to be accomplished. *Example D:* The force of gravity on a given amount of mass remains constant, and the wise performer utilizes this force to maximum advantage whenever possible. Gravity is one of the forces which pulls the sprinter forward, especially during the acceleration phase. The gymnast utilizes gravitational force during swinging movements, whereas divers and trampoline performers take advantage of the force of gravity to increase the spring they get from the bouncing surfaces. *Example E*: Air resistance is a force which the performer must reduce to a minimum whenever speed or distance is the goal. This is accomplished by reducing the surface area in the direction of movement to a minimum, streamlining the object, designing a low-friction surface on the object, or using flight dynamics to advantage, as in the discus throw.

Theoretical Square Law

Principle: Air and water resistance vary approximately with the square of the velocity. This means that if the velocity at which a body travels is increased by two, the air or water resistance against it will be increased by four; if velocity is increased by four, the resistance will be increased by sixteen. This law has great application to efficiency, and it is one of the reasons (there are several) why movement at fast speeds expends more energy.

Example A: A swimmer who pulls the arms through the water at the rate of 1.5 meters per second meets a given amount of water resistance, used to propel the body forward. If the rate of pull is increased to 3 meters per second, the resistance is increased four times, resulting in four times as much propulsive force from the stroke. *Example B*: A ball is projected through the air at a speed of 15 meters per second and, therefore, meets a given amount of air resistance. A second ball projected at twice that speed (30 meters per second) will meet four times the amount of air resistance. Even though the second ball leaves the hand at twice the speed of the first ball, it will travel less than twice the distance because initially the air resistance is four times as great as that against the first ball. Similarly, in example A, four times the propulsive force will not increase the swimmer's speed through the water by four times, because the water's resistance also increases proportionately.

Centrifugal Force

Centrifugal force is actually an application of Newton's first law. It is experienced only in rotational (angular) or curvilinear motion, never during linear motion. It results from the tendency for an object to continue in a straight line instead of in a curved path. It is counteracted by forces (usually muscular) which, if effective, equal or exceed the centrifugal force and tend to maintain the object in its curved path. This counteracting force is centripetal force. In the case of a freely moving body, such as a sprinter running around a curve, as velocity increases, centrifugal force increases. Additional weight also increases centrifugal force. The smaller the radius of the curved path, the greater the centrifugal force with the same velocity.

Principle: More centrifugal force demands more centripetal force to

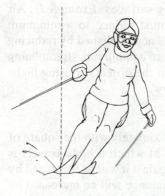

Figure 13-5 When moving at high speeds, the skier must lean into the turn to compensate for the centrifugal force. This also applies to turning movements while running.

counteract it. In human performance, body lean and banked surfaces or both counteract centrifugal force.

Example A: A 200-meter sprinter running around a curve must lean in the direction of the curve. The faster the sprinter runs or the sharper the curve, the greater the lean. *Example B (Figure 13-5):* A slalom skier who increases speed must also increase body lean in the direction of the turns, in order to compensate for the increased centrifugal force. *Example C*: In gymnastics or diving stunts involving angular or swinging motions, the effects of centrifugal force must be considered. Centrifugal force (1) is used to help the performer clear the apparatus by properly timing the release in apparatus dismounts; (2) is nonexistent at the ends of pendulum-type swings, thus allowing maneuvers without danger of flying off the apparatus; (3) tends to straighten the body during a somersault in a tuck, demanding that the performer increase the forces holding the tuck as the rotational velocity increases. *Example D*: The objective in the discus throw is to achieve a maximum velocity of the discus in a curvilinear direction before release. The release allows the centrifugal force to take over and propel the discus away from the body.

FORCE ABSORPTION

In certain activities it is important to dissipate the force of impact. The impact becomes greater as the moving object has more weight and moves at a greater speed; in other words, impact is determined by the combination of weight and speed. If speed is reduced gradually, the performer's chances of incurring injury are decreased. Therefore, when *landing* from a fall or a jump or when *catching* an object, it is important to *absorb* the force. This becomes increasingly important as the speed of the moving object becomes greater. But, recall, it has already been established that in activities such as diving and trampolining (rebound tumbling), the objec-

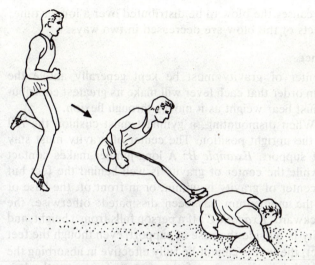

Figure 13-6 Controlled flexion of the joints during landing absorbs the force over a longer time, thus reducing the chance of injury. A soft landing surface, such as a sand pit, also causes absorption of force over a longer time.

tive is to cause the body to rebound, and consequently, force absorption must be avoided.

In general, the performer prepares for an impact by placing all shock-absorbing joints in *extension*. As contact is made, the extended joints flex, owing to the force of impact. This force must be gradually reduced ("apply the brakes") by an opposing force, provided by the extensor muscles. The joints move through flexion, but the extensor muscles contract eccentrically and control the action by gradually increasing their contractile forces, thereby dissipating the impetus of the moving object and absorbing the force (Figure 13-6).

Absorbing a Blow

Principle: A force from a blow can be diminished by distributing the force over either a greater time (and distance) or area, or both.

Example A: As a person lands after jumping, the shock-absorbing joints move through flexion in order to distribute the force over a longer time (and distance). *Example B*: A person falling to the ground attempts to distribute the impact over the hands, arms, and larger fleshy areas of the body as opposed to the point of the elbow. Distributing the force over a greater area results in less force per square centimeter of surface. *Example C*: When a boxer is struck with a 16-ounce glove as opposed to an 8-ounce glove, the blow is distributed over a larger surface, resulting in less force per square centimeter. The increased ability of the larger glove to compress causes the blow to be distributed over a longer time; therefore, the effects of the blow are decreased in two ways.

Landing with Balance

Principle: The center of gravity must be kept generally above the supporting levers in order that each lever will make its greatest contribution. Each lever must bear weight as it moves through flexion.

Example A: When dismounting, a gymnast must cushion the fall while maintaining the upright position. The center of gravity must stay within the base of support. *Example B*: A long-jumper makes contact with the surface while the center of gravity is well behind the feet but must be sure the center of gravity is within, or in front of, the base of support after all the momentum has been dissipated; otherwise, the jumper will fall backward. *Example C*: If a person falls from a height, and the center of gravity is outside the base of support, even though the feet make initial contact, the levers cannot be fully effective in absorbing the shock. The further the displacement of the center of gravity, the less effective the joints can be in absorbing the force.

Transferring Momentum from Vertical to Horizontal

Principle: After achieving some absorption by the levers, transferring the body's momentum from the vertical to the horizontal can reduce force over a longer time and a greater surface area.

Example A: When thrown from a moving car, falling during fast locomotion, or falling from a great height, a rolling action is necessary to prevent injury. *Example B*: The football coach tells players to "fall and roll," which simply means absorb the force over a longer time (and distance), and more surface area.

Catching Objects

Principle: Catching objects is accomplished by following many of the principles already presented. Regardless of the object being caught, the sequence of catching follows a similar pattern: (1) a body part, such as the fingers, makes initial contact; (2) the object's velocity is dissipated by eccentric muscular contractions allowing the joints to move through controlled flexion; and (3) while velocity is being reduced, body parts (usually fingers, sometimes arms) grasp the object securely (Figure 13-7).

Example A: The "cradling" action often used to catch a football which passes over the receiver's shoulder involves the use of shoulder, elbow, wrist, and finger flexors working in eccentric contraction in order to dissipate the ball's movement. This action is opposite the usual catching action and uses the opposite muscles, but the principle is the same. Finally, the ball is secured by finger, wrist, and elbow flexion

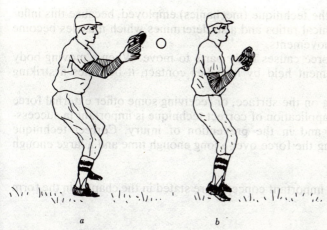

Figure 13-7 Absorbing the force of a fast-moving object (baseball) allows the receiver more time to grasp the object and reduces the chance that it will rebound from the hands.

(concentric action of flexors) to pin the ball to the catcher's torso. *Example B*: When the catching action is continuous with a throwing action, such as the quick release of the ball by the second baseman in a double play, the force dissipation and the preparation for the throw can be accomplished in the same motion. In baseball an infield grounder is often handled this way. *Example C*: If no "give" takes place, and the object has sufficient velocity, it will rebound. The football receiver who allows the first contact of the ball to be on his chest must move his arms with great accuracy and speed to trap the rebounding ball. He has reduced the chances of a successful catch by not cushioning the ball.

IMPORTANT CONCEPTS

1 Motion occurs only as a result of application of *force* great enough to overcome the resistance. In human performance, the force comes from the contraction of muscles (except for some instances involving the forces of gravity and momentum).

2 Efficiency in movement is dependent upon both the *rate* of force application and the *direction* of the force. Unnecessarily rapid forces, misdirected forces, and extraneous forces contribute to inefficiency.

3 Power, which is very important in athletic performances, is a combination of *amount* and *speed* of force application (force times velocity).

4 The rate at which an object can be accelerated is directly related to the amount of force applied, whereas the final velocity of the object is related to the amount of force and the distance over which it is applied.

5 The amount of force that can be applied by the body is strongly dependent upon the technique (mechanics) employed, because this influences the mechanical ratios and also determines which muscles become involved in the movements.

6   Muscle force causes body parts to move. When a moving body part or an implement held by it makes contact, it becomes a striking force.

7   In landing on the surface, or receiving some other external force to the body, the application of correct technique is important in successful performance and in the prevention of injury. Correct technique involves absorbing the force over a long enough time and a large enough surface.

Note   Other important concepts are stated in the chapter in the form of principles.

STUDENT LABORATORY EXPERIENCES

Additional conceptual development will accrue to the student by considering and solving the following problems.

1   Consider muscular strength of the biceps brachii (see Figure 11-2c). A 39-newton weight is held in the hand with the forearm at the horizontal (muscle angle of pull is 90°, weight of hand and forearm is 10 newtons). The center of gravity of the weight, hand, and arm is 30 centimeters from the elbow joint. The insertion of the biceps is 5 centimeters from the elbow joint. (a) What force must the biceps exert to support the arm and weight? (See formula 31.) (b) If the cross section of the biceps at the belly is 18 square centimeters, what is the average force in newtons per square centimeter?

$$\left(\text{Pressure} = \frac{\text{force}}{\text{area}}\right)$$

2   If a person attempts a quadriceps lift when a 343-newton resistance bar is 30 centimeters from the knee joint and is barely moved, the patellar tendon inserts 10 centimeters below the knee joint at an angle of 25°. Find (a) the rotary component of muscle force (see formula 32); (b) The stabilizing component of muscle force ($F_s = F_r/\tan \theta$); (c) The true muscle force ($F_t = F_r/\sin \theta$).

3   A football lineman of 105-kilogram mass makes contact after 0.61 meters of movement. His acceleration is 21 meters per second squared. With what force does he hit his opponent? (See formula 42.)

4   A shot has a 7.27-kilogram mass. It is put at a velocity of 11 meters per second. If the velocity is attained in 0.29 seconds, what is (a) The acceleration of the shot? (b) The applied force on this shot? (See formulas 3, 42.)

5   A lineman gets low and in close to his opponent and charges. He charges through a distance of 0.46 meters before he makes contact. His mass is 95 kilograms and he achieves a velocity of 3.6 meters per second at impact. What is his hitting force? (See formula 41.)

6   A gymnast of 70-kilogram mass is doing the giant swing. The body's center of gravity is 1 meter from the bar. The tangential velocity of the center of gravity at the bottom of the swing is 6.26 meters per second. What is the centrifugal force at the bottom of the swing? (See formula **50**.)

7   How much work is done in meter-newtons in lifting a 70-kilogram barbell from the floor to a position 2 meters above the floor? (See formula **35**.)

8   (*a*) What is the potential energy of a 60-kilogram gymnast 1.5 meters above the trampoline bed? (*b*) What is the kinetic energy when the gymnast hits the bed? (See formulas **37**, **38**.)

9   How much power is expended by a person of 75-kilogram mass running up a stair with a vertical rise of 15 meters if it is done in 5 seconds? (See formula **36**.)

10 If a baseball which weighs 1.4 newtons is traveling 30 meters per second and is caught by a person who recoils the hands 46 centimeters while stopping the ball, what is the force of impact on the hands? (See formula **41**.)

11 A basketball player of 86-kilogram mass drives off his shoe at an angle of 40° with the vertical. At this point he does not slip, but at 41° he does slip. What is the coefficient of friction of the shoe sole? (See formulas **51**, **52**.) (*Note*: force of lean =tan θ × weight)

Chapter 14

Projections

Objects are projected through space in athletic activities by throwing, striking, or kicking actions of the human body, and the body itself becomes a projectile in jumping and leaping activities. Obviously, knowledge about principles related to projections is of vital concern to teachers and performers. To cover this subject adequately, this chapter is divided into four major divisions: (1) forces which affect flight, (2) angle and height of projection, (3) impact, and (4) spin.

FORCES WHICH AFFECT FLIGHT

When the body or an object is projected through space, three forces influence the course of flight (Figure 14-1):

1 The propelling force, which puts the object in flight
2 The force of gravity, which tends to pull the object downward
3 Air resistance, which retards the object's flight

The latter two forces work in opposition to the first force.

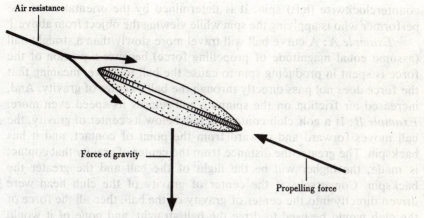

Air resistance

Force of gravity

Propelling force

Figure 14-1 There are three forces acting on an object in flight (discus). The flight pattern is changed by altering any of the forces.

Propelling Force

Principle: The propelling force produces certain effects depending upon its point and direction of application (Figure 14-2). If the application is directly through the projectile's center of gravity, only linear motion results from the force. As the projecting force is moved farther from the center of gravity, rotary motion of the object increases at the expense of linear motion. If the force is below the object's center of gravity, backspin results. Forward spin results when the force is above the center of gravity. When the force is off center to the left, clockwise spin results, and when it is off center to the right, counterclockwise spin occurs. [A point of reference is needed to differentiate clockwise (right) spin from

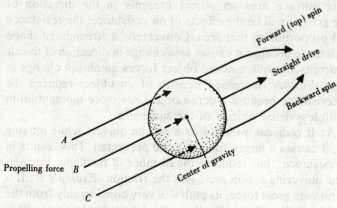

Forward (top) spin

Straight drive

Backward spin

A

Propelling force B

Center of gravity

C

Figure 14-2 The motion of a projected object is influenced by the exact point of application of the propelling force.

counterclockwise (left) spin. It is determined by the orientation of the performer who is applying the spin while viewing the object from above.]

Example A: A curve ball will travel more slowly than a straight ball (assume equal magnitude of propelling force) because a portion of the force is spent in producing spin to cause the ball to curve, meaning that the force does not pass directly through the ball's center of gravity. And, increased air friction on the spinning ball retards its speed even more. *Example B*: If a golf club contacts a ball below its center of gravity, the ball moves forward and upward from the point of contact, and it has backspin. The greater the distance from the center of gravity that contact is made, the higher will be the flight of the ball and the greater the backspin. Conversely, if the center of gravity of the club head were driven directly into the center of gravity of the ball, then all the force of the club would be used to drive the ball straight, and none of it would contribute to rotary motion.

Force of Gravity

Principle: As soon as contact is broken with a projected object, the force of gravity begins to diminish the upward velocity of the object. Finally, gravity overcomes the effects of the upward component of the projectile, and the object begins to descend. The factors that determine how soon gravity will cause the object to descend are (1) weight (mass) of the object, (2) amount of force driving it upward, and (3) the effects of air resistance on the object (see Figure 14-1).

Effects of Air Resistance

Principle: As the speed of an object increases, air resistance has a greater retarding effect. This is true in accordance with the theoretical square law. Also, the more surface area an object presents in the direction of movement, the greater will be the effects of air resistance; the resistance varies in direct proportion to that area. Conversely, a streamlined shape reduces air resistance because it causes less change in direction of the air the object confronts. A square-nosed object forces an abrupt change in direction of air. Further, increased density of an object reduces the effects of air resistance because a dense object has more momentum in comparison with less dense objects of the same size.

Example A: If a discus wobbles or a javelin quivers while moving through space, it causes a larger surface to be presented. This results in increased air resistance, thus reducing the distance of the flight. Further, the wobbling or quivering action increases the friction. *Example B*: If a shuttlecock is hit with great force, its path will vary considerably from the usual path an object takes. Generally, the path of descent of a projectile is similar to the path of ascent, but in this case, the object will fall almost vertically from its peak, owing to the light weight and odd shape of the "bird." It meets a great amount of air resistance relative to its weight.

Example C: When a streamlined object such as a discus or javelin is hurled into a head wind, the object should present as little surface as possible, and its usual angle of flight should be reduced. If a tail wind is encountered, the angle of flight should be increased. In a tail wind, a discus would be thrown at an angle greater than 45°, with the nose pointed slightly upward, whereas with no wind the angle would be about 40°.

ANGLE AND HEIGHT OF PROJECTION

If the propelling force is constant, the angle at which an object is projected determines the height it reaches. In turn, if the speed at which an object travels is constant, the height that it reaches determines the distance it travels because the height determines how long the object remains in flight.

Angle of Projection

Principle: When the beginning and ending points are on the same level, the optimum angle of projection with which to gain maximum distance is 45° from the surface (Figure 14-3). Since most projectiles are above the surface at the time of release, the angle of flight is usually reduced slightly from 45° to compensate for this. If the angle is less than optimum, the projectile will not be in the air long enough to travel a maximum distance, and if the angle is greater than optimum, too much of the propelling force is wasted in vertical rather than horizontal flight.

Example A: A place-kick in football begins and ends at ground level; so for maximum distance the kick should be made at a 45° angle from the surface. Often maximum distance is not the main objective; distance might be secondary to the time in flight (height) or the roll of the ball.

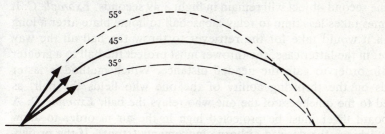

Figure 14-3 The relative horizontal distance covered when an object is projected at angles of 35, 45, and 55°. The propelling force is constant.

Example B: When putting the shot or when long-jumping, the angle should be less than 45°, because the center of gravity of the projectile is lower at the completion than at the beginning of the flight. The shot is usually put at 38 to 41°, and the long jump should be performed at about 40°; however, the horizontal speed of the jumper makes this impractical. The usual angle of projection among long-jumpers is about 30°. *Example C*: When hitting a golf ball from a lower to a higher elevation, the golfer should select a club with a greater pitch (higher number) than would be used if the terrain were level. In this case, the ending point is higher than the beginning point; so the angle would be greater than 45°. *Example D*: In a baseball throw, the quickness of the ball's arrival to a teammate is almost always more important than maximum distance. With this objective in mind, the ball should be thrown as horizontally as possible within the limits of the force the thrower can muster. Obviously, if the thrower has insufficient force, the needed distance will not be obtained unless a high angle of projection is used. But the higher angle will waste time in flight.

Time in Flight (Height of Projection)

Principle: The length of time an object remains in flight depends upon the height it attains, because an object remains in flight only as long as it takes to move through the vertical plane. The horizontal component of force applied to an object is not related to the time of flight.

Example A: If a ball is projected at shoulder height in a perfectly horizontal path, it will strike the surface at exactly the same time as a similar ball simply dropped from the same height. If the ball is projected downward, it will strike the surface sooner than the dropped ball; if it is projected upward, it will strike the surface later than the dropped ball. The greater height the ball attains, the longer it remains in flight. *Example B*: If two identical objects are projected at different angles, causing the first object to reach a height of 30 meters and the second to reach a height of 15 meters, the first object will remain in flight 4.94 seconds while the second object will remain in flight 3.49 seconds. *Example C*: It sometimes takes less time to relay a baseball to home plate after a long hit than it would take for the retriever to throw the ball all the way because, in the latter case, the thrower must project the ball to a greater height in order to gain the needed distance. Which method is faster depends on the throwing ability of the one who fields the ball, as opposed to the quickness of the one who relays the ball. *Example D*: A springboard diver must be projected high in the air in order to allow time to achieve the desired airborne movements (stunt). If the projection is chiefly horizontal, the diver has insufficient time to complete a complex maneuver in good form.

IMPACT

Objects receive impact when they are struck by various implements or when they contact stationary surfaces. In either case a rebound of the object from the surface results, provided resistance of the surface is greater than the momentum of the object. A rebound will occur if (1) the object moves, and the surface does not move, such as the basketball dribble or a handball shot; (2) the object does not move, but the striking surface does move, as in the golf drive; and (3) the object and surface both move, as in striking a moving ball with an implement as in tennis or baseball. The angle and magnitude with which the object rebounds are influenced by several factors.

Angle of Rebound

Principle: The angle at which an object will rebound from a surface can be predicted except for modifications which occur as a result of (1) irregular shapes of the two colliding surfaces, (2) the force resulting from elasticity of the object, and (3) the spin of the object both during and after the contact. When these factors are discounted, the angle of incidence will equal the angle of reflection—that is, the angle at which the object approaches a surface is equal to the angle at which it leaves that surface.

Example A (Figure 14-4a): If a handball player drives a ball into the front wall at an angle of 60°, the ball will reflect from the wall at an angle of 60° in the direction opposite that of the approach (assuming that there is no spin on the ball) and neglecting the coefficient of elasticity (or assuming perfect elasticity). *Example B (Figure 14-4b):* A basketball which strikes the backboard will rebound at an angle equal to the angle at which it approached the board. *Example C*: If a tennis ball strikes the court at an angle of 30°, it will theoretically rebound at the same angle, except as modified by spin and elasticity.

Sufficient Striking Force

Principle: The magnitude of the striking force must be sufficient to overcome the inertia of the object being struck and the striking force is determined by the momentum of the moving object or objects that are involved in the impact.

Example A: A football blocker may be unable to develop enough momentum to overcome the inertia of a heavier opponent. In such a case, the opponent (object) will not be caused to rebound from the striking surface. *Example B*: The striking force of a baseball bat on a ball is determined by the momentum of both the bat and the ball. A fast-moving ball will rebound with greater velocity than a slower ball, provided the bat has enough momentum to overcome sufficiently the inertia of the ball.

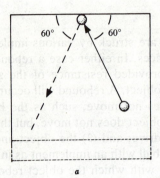

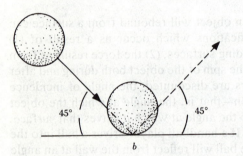

Figure 14-4 (a) A handball approaching a wall at an angle of 60° will rebound at 60°, unless spin influences the rebound. (b) A basketball bounced at an angle of 45° will rebound at 45°.

Example C: A golf club with a heavy head will have greater momentum than one with a lighter head, if velocity is the same. Therefore, the heavier club will exert greater force on the surface of the ball.

Elasticity of the Striking Surfaces

Principle: A highly elastic object will quickly spring back to its original shape after being compressed. Some substances compress easily but are not elastic enough to reassume shape quickly. Other substances are difficult to compress, but once compressed, their ability for restitution to original shape (elasticity) is great. Still other substances are neither highly compressible nor highly elastic. The greatest rebound occurs when the object is greatly compressed and possesses a high degree of elasticity (Figure 14-5).

Example A: Connection with the ball at the middle of a tennis racket produces a faster rebound of the ball because the strings are the most compressible at that point. The movement of the strings back to original position depends upon the quality of the strings and how tightly they are strung. *Example B*: To add to the elasticity of the strings, the tennis ball compresses upon contact with the racket. Then, because of its elasticity,

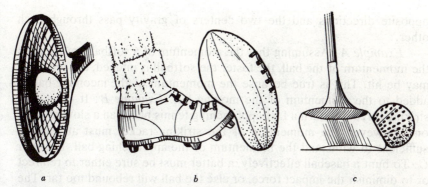

a *b* *c*

Figure 14-5 The ability of an object to react to a force (rebound) depends on the object's compressibility and elasticity. (*a*) Both the tennis ball and racket face have compressibility and elasticity. (*b*) The football is difficult to compress, but it has great elasticity. (*c*) The golf ball is very difficult to compress, but it has great elasticity.

it immediately rebounds from the racket. A "dead" tennis ball is one which has partially lost its elasticity. *Example C*: A metal shot (shot put) lacks the ability to be compressed and is not elastic. Therefore, it rebounds very little upon landing on a hard surface. The same could be said of a rock. *Example D*: A softball is harder to compress and has less elasticity than a tennis ball; therefore, a softball has less rebound ability. *Example E*: Both a handball and a golf ball are highly elastic, but the golf ball is more difficult to compress. If the two balls were dropped from the same height (shoulder height) onto the same surface, the handball's rebound would exceed that of the golf ball. The reason is that the impact would be insufficient to produce enough compression of the golf ball to allow its elastic quality to function. When struck hard with a golf club, the golf ball compresses a considerable amount, thus allowing its elastic quality to function. As a result, the golf ball responds better than a handball to the impact of the club. *Example F*: A basketball with insufficient air will compress easily when bounced, but lack of air pressure within causes the ball to have little elasticity; therefore, its rebound ability is poor. When properly inflated, the ball is more difficult to compress, but it has increased elasticity and thus rebounds farther.

Rebound of Two Moving Objects

Principle: When both the object and the striking surface are moving, the momentum with which the object will rebound equals approximately the sum of the two momenta, minus the momentum retained by the striking surface. A slight additional loss of momentum will result from friction and heat. The direction of the rebound will be the same as the direction of the greater of the two momenta, provided they are moving exactly in opposite directions and the two centers of gravity pass through each other.

Example A : Assuming that the momentum of a softball bat exceeds the momentum of the ball, the faster the softball is pitched, the farther it may be hit. This is true because the momentum of the incoming ball is added to the momentum of the moving bat. *Example B* : It takes less striking force to return a fast-approaching tennis ball than a slow-moving one; however, the momentum of the striking racket must at least be sufficient to withstand the momentum of the approaching ball. *Example C* : To bunt a baseball effectively, a batter must be sure either to redirect or to diminish the impact force, or else the ball will rebound too far. The faster the ball is delivered, the greater the batter's concern must be for this factor.

It should be obvious that maximum rebound is not always the greatest concern. In fact, reducing the rebound is sometimes the objective, as in the bunt. The basketball player attempts to control the speed of his approach when shooting a lay-up to prevent too much rebound from the backboard. Some baseball hitters sacrifice some momentum of their swing to achieve greater accuracy or more frequent contact. A well-placed shot in tennis, handball, volleyball, badminton, and other games is generally more effective than more forceful shots that are not well placed.

SPIN

Application of spin to an object may result from contact with either a moving surface (implement) or a stationary surface. Following are important facts relating to the effects of spin and how to achieve the desired amount of spin on an object.

Effects of Spin on Flight of an Object

Principle: An object propelled without spin tends to waver because of air resistance against the object's irregular surface. The amount of waver varies with the density of the object; denser objects are less influenced by air resistance. A small amount of spin on an object produces a stabilizing effect which tends to hold it on its line of flight. Increased spin will tend to cause the object to curve in the same direction as the spin because of unequal air pressure caused by the spinning. The amount that an object will curve in a given distance is determined primarily by (1) the density, (2) the amount of spin, and (3) the speed at which the object travels. Further, the amount and direction of wind and the shape and surface of the object are important influences.

Example A : A volleyball served with slight spin follows a true course of flight determined by the propelling force, but if the ball is contacted decidedly off center, the resulting increase in spin will produce a curve. If the ball is hit directly through its center of gravity, the ball receives no rotary motion, and it tends to waver. *Example B*: In baseball pitching, a knuckle ball is thrown with the intention of causing a wavering action. In this case the amount of waver is related to the speed the object travels. The faster it moves, the more it will waver. *Example C*: A counterclockwise spin (golf hook, baseball outside curve, and volleyball or tennis serve where the ball is contacted on its right side) will cause a ball to curve to the left. A clockwise spin (golf slice, baseball inside curve, and volleyball or tennis serve where the ball is contacted on its left side) will cause a curve to the right. *Example D*: If a golf ball is hit with topspin, the distance it travels in flight will be reduced because it will tend to dive rather sharply to the surface. This action will be followed by a long roll, enhanced by the forward spin. If the ball is given backspin, it will tend to rise higher; therefore, it will stay in flight longer. Upon landing, the length of its roll will be reduced by the backspin.

Spin Resulting from Striking

Principle: To cause an object to spin in the desired direction, the striking implement should be drawn across the object in the direction of the desired spin. Forward (top) spin is caused by an implement striking forward-upward. Backspin is produced when the strike is made forward-downward. Right spin (clockwise) is generated by drawing the implement across the ball from right to left, and left spin is developed from contact of the implement in a left to right direction.

Example A: In tennis driving strokes, the ball should usually be hit with a forward-upward motion (the racket face tends to roll over the ball) in order to apply topspin to the ball. Topspin causes the ball to drop, producing a tendency for it to land within the opponent's court rather than to be too long. Also, topspin causes the ball to move faster on the rebound and to bounce at a lower angle. *Example B*: If the tennis stroke is a "cut" or chop shot, the ball will backspin. A backspinning ball will "hang" in the air longer and rebound from the surface at a sharper angle, tending to rebound higher. *Example C*: If a golf club is drawn across the ball from right to left on contact, right spin (clockwise) will result. The ball will slice (right-handed golfer). The slicer also tends to "pull" his shots to the left when this "outside-in" swing contacts the ball dead-center. If the heel of the club leads the toe of the club at contact (face open), a slice results, even though the swing may be straight through. *Example D*: If a golf club is swung "inside-out" (club head contacts the ball from left to right), the right-handed golfer will create left spin (counterclockwise), which causes the ball to hook.

Spin Resulting from Contact with a Surface

Principle: A moving object develops spin in the direction of its motion as a result of contact with a surface.

Example A: A bowling ball gains an increasing amount of forward spin as it progresses, owing to friction between it and the surface. The additional spin reduces the friction against forward movement of the ball. If the ball is projected with backspin, it loses its velocity more rapidly.

Example B: When a golf ball or tennis ball lands from its forward flight, it will develop forward spin upon contact. The amount of spin will relate to the ball's horizontal velocity at contact, the angle of approach, and the amount of friction between the ball and the contact surface. If the ball has backspin, the spin tends to be neutralized upon landing. If the backspin is excessive, its effects will supersede the effects of landing, and the ball will discontinue forward motion.

Effects of Spin on a Ball Landing on a Horizontal Surface

Principle: A change may be expected in the rebound angle, in the distance of the bounce, and in the distance of the roll as a spinning ball contacts a horizontal surface (Figure 14-6):

1 *Topspin* causes a lower angle of rebound, a longer bounce, and more roll.

2 *Backspin* causes a higher angle of rebound, a shorter bounce, and less roll.

3 *Sidespin* causes the angle of bounce to change toward the

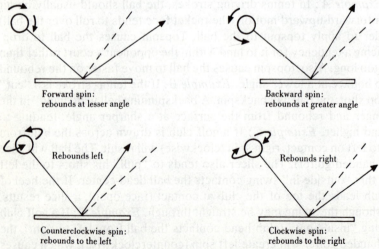

Forward spin:
rebounds at lesser angle

Backward spin:
rebounds at greater angle

Rebounds left

Rebounds right

Counterclockwise spin:
rebounds to the left

Clockwise spin:
rebounds to the right

Figure 14-6   Influence of spin an angle of rebound from a horizontal surface.

direction of the spin (left spin, left bounce). The smaller the angle of the approach of the ball to the horizontal surface, the greater is the effect of sidespin. If the approach is perpendicular (90°), sidespin has no effect.

Example A: A basketball bounce pass may be given sidespin to change the rebound from the floor. If the ball is spinning to the right (clockwise), it will tend to bounce to the right on the rebound. The lower the pass (smaller angle to the floor) and the greater the spin, the greater the ball will deviate from its normal path of rebound. *Example B*: An opponent in tennis is often deceived by spin of the ball; for instance, the cut shot (backspin) results in a higher and shorter bounce than anticipated, while a slice shot (clockwise spin) will cause the ball to bounce toward the right. *Example C*: The effect of a spin on a football is difficult to predict because of the shape of the ball; as a general rule, a longer roll can be expected when a ball turns end-over-end forward than when it rotates around its long axis (a spiral). Hence the quick kick is usually more successful when projected low and end over end. Although with such a kick the ball travels less distance through the air, the long roll may result in more total distance, provided the ball is airborne beyond the deepest receiver.

Effects of Spin on a Ball Striking a Vertical Surface

Principle: The vertical surface which a moving object strikes may be stationary (basketball backboard, billiard-table rail, or handball front wall) or may be a moving implement (paddle, racket, bat, or hand). The following may be expected from contact with a vertical surface (Figure 14-7):

1   *Topspin* causes a higher rebound.
2   *Backspin* causes a lower rebound.
3   Right or clockwise spin causes a rebound to the left.
4   Left or counterclockwise spin causes a rebound to the right.

(It is interesting to note that an object with sidespin responds to a vertical surface in a direction opposite from its response to a horizontal surface.)

Example A: If a tennis opponent delivers a forehand drive with topspin on the ball, compensation in position of the racket face should be made to avoid a return that is too high and too long. If a cut shot (backspin) is approaching, the performer should adjust the racket face to avoid the tendency of the ball to rebound downward into the net. *Example B*: A basketball backboard shot from the front will have a better chance to rebound into the basket if it has backspin, because it will rebound at a lower angle. *Example C*: A table-tennis ball served with left spin (counterclockwise) will rebound from the receiver's paddle to the server's

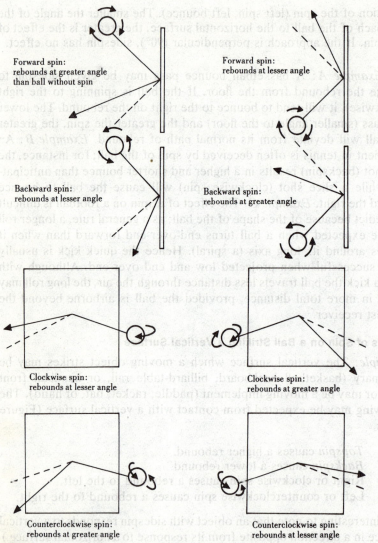

Forward spin:
rebounds at greater angle
than ball without spin

Forward spin:
rebounds at lesser angle

Backward spin:
rebounds at lesser angle

Backward spin:
rebounds at greater angle

Clockwise spin:
rebounds at lesser angle

Clockwise spin:
rebounds at greater angle

Counterclockwise spin:
rebounds at greater angle

Counterclockwise spin:
rebounds at lesser angle

Figure 14-7 Influence of spin an angle of rebound from a vertical surface.

right (receiver's left). *Example D*: A baseball pitched with excessive backspin will tend to rebound downward upon contact with the bat. The batter would need to swing forward-upward in order to hit a fly ball. *Example E*: The curve ball from a right-handed pitcher has a combination of left spin and top spin, which creates a tendency for the ball to be hit high and to the pitcher's right (left field line).

Reducing Effects of Spin by Increasing Striking Force

Principle: The more forceful the contact between an implement and an object, the less will be the effects of spin. The rebound path of the object will be dominated more by the path of the striking implement as its momentum increases. Spin produces greater effects as the force of impact becomes less.

Example A: The effects of spin produced by the baseball pitcher will be greater for a bunt than for a full swing. *Example B*: Tennis players often make errors by attempting to "baby" critically placed shots, because they fail to realize that reducing the force of their stroke increases the effects of spin on the ball.

IMPORTANT CONCEPTS

1   When an object is projected, its course of flight is determined by the combination of three forces: the *propelling* force, the force of *gravity*, and the force of *air resistance*.

2   If maximum speed and distance are desired, it is important for the propelling force to drive directly through the center of gravity of the object being projected.

3   The distance an object will travel in flight is dependent upon the combination of the vertical height it travels and its horizontal speed. The higher it goes the longer it will remain in flight, whereas the faster it moves horizontally the farther it will travel during its period of flight.

4   The angle of projection influences both the height and the horizontal speed. Therefore, the optimum angle is a fundamental consideration in achieving maximum distance.

5   Spin of an object in flight can influence the path of flight in several ways depending on the amount and direction of spin.

6   When a projected object strikes a surface, it will respond in different ways depending on the amount of compressibility and elasticity of the object and the surface, and the amount and direction of spin on the object.

Note   Other important concepts are stated in the chapter in the form of principles.

STUDENT LABORATORY EXPERIENCES

It is suggested that the student try all of the ball spins discussed in the chapter. In addition, the following projection problems should be solved to quantify projections in terms of human performances.

1   If a golf ball is dropped from a height of 2 meters to a concrete floor and rebounds 1.4 meters, what is its coefficient of elasticity? (See formula **53**.)

2   If the coefficient of elasticity of a Superball is 0.89, how high will it rebound if dropped from 3 meters? (See formula **53**.)

3   A football, kicked at an angle of 55° with the horizontal, carries 50 meters where it is caught at the same level from which it as kicked. Neglecting air resistance, find (*a*) the vertical height attained and (*b*) the time of flight (See formulas **6**, **11**, **13**.)

4   The radius of rotation of a tumbler in a lay-out position is 42 centimeters. In the tuck position it is 25 centimeters. The speed of rotation is 2 turns per second from the lay-out position. Will the tumbler, springing 2 meters into the air from the bed of the trampoline, be able to complete a somersault from the lay-out position? How many somersaults could be made from the tuck position? (See formulas **20**, **22**, **10**.)

5   At the moment of takeoff, a long-jumper has a forward velocity (v_x) of 9.14 meters per second. The vertical velocity (v_y) is 3.05 meters per second. (*a*) What is the angle of takeoff? (*b*) How high (*s*) does the jumper's center of gravity rise? (*c*) What is the velocity in the direction of takeoff? (See formulas **17**, **8**, **19**.)

6   A baseball is thrown with an initial velocity of 28 meters per second at an angle of 35° with the horizontal. Neglecting air resistance and assuming the ball is caught at the same height from the ground at which it was released, find (*a*) the distance thrown and (*b*) the time in flight. (See formulas **11**, **13**.)

7   The length of a runner's stride is 2.44 meters and his velocity is 9 meters per second. Each foot is in contact with the ground for 0.6 meters of his stride. (*a*) What is the vertical distance his center of gravity rises? (*b*) At what angle with the horizontal is his center of gravity projected? (See formulas **13**, **12**.) (Note: solve for θ)

8   A shot is put at an angle of 39° with a velocity of 10.67 (v_θ) meters per second in the direction of the put. (*a*) What will be the upward velocity (v_y) at the moment of release? (*b*) What will be its forward velocity (v_x)? (*c*) What will be its time of flight (*T*) from the point of release to the return to the same level from which it was released? (*d*) How high will the shot rise from the point of release? (*e*) If it is released 2.13 meters above the ground and 0.3 meters in front of the toeboard, how far will the shot travel horizontally from the toeboard? (See formulas **16**, **15**, **11**, **8**, **14**.)

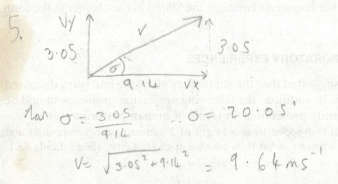

Chapter 15

Equilibrium

Figure 15-1 Center of gravity in the human body

When the body is in equilibrium, an even adjustment exists among all opposing forces, and the body is in *balance*. The state of balance may be secure or precarious. When it is secure, the body is said to possess a high degree of *stability*. Stability is firmness of balance, or the ability to resist forces which may destroy balance. This chapter deals with important facts about equilibrium as it relates to performance. The chapter covers: (1) center of gravity, (2) balance and stability, and (3) posture.

CENTER OF GRAVITY

The center of gravity of the human body (Figure 15-1) may be defined as (1) the point of exact center, around which the body may rotate freely in all directions; (2) the point around which the weight is equal on all opposite sides; or (3) the point of intersection of the three cardinal (primary) body planes—sagittal, frontal, and transverse. The center of gravity in the body is located at a point along the midline, at about 55 percent of the person's height. However, its exact point varies from one

255

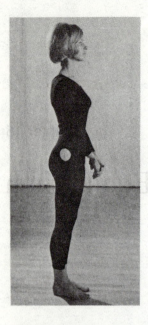

Figure 15-1 Center of gravity in the human body.

individual to another, depending on body proportions. An analysis of the following factors is important to understanding center of gravity and its effects on performance.

 1 Because of the differences in body structure between men and women, center of gravity is usually proportionately lower in women than in men. This gives women a structural advantage in stability, but it gives them a disadvantage when they are required to raise the center of gravity, as in high-jumping.

 2 On the average, center of gravity is proportionately higher in children than in adults as a result of the change in body proportions as one progresses from childhood to adulthood.

 3 The center of gravity is affected by amputations and other structural changes which cause the body to deviate from normal.

 4 In addition, the center of gravity is temporarily influenced by specific body positions; for instance, in diving, a person's center of gravity shifts forward in the move from a lay-out to a pike or tuck position, and it moves away from the midline of the body when the trunk is laterally flexed.

 5 Further, the addition of external weight, such as a backpack, will relocate the center of gravity.

 The human body rests on a base of support defined by the area of contact between the body and the supporting surface. If the base of

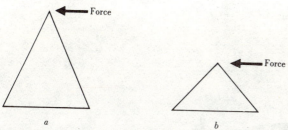

Figure 15-2 The taller triangle (a) is less stable than the shorter (b).

support and other factors remain constant, then, as the center of gravity is lowered, the stability of the body is increased. This can be demonstrated by comparing two triangles with equal bases and different heights, one twice as tall as the other. The shorter triangle is considerably more stable than the taller one (Figure 15-2).

When a body is in balance, an even adjustment exists between opposing forces. A balance center located in the inner ear, the kinesthetic sense, and the eyes all play a role in maintaining balance.

Location of the Center of Gravity

Two methods of locating the center of gravity are given. The first is for a *static position* of the human body and locates the transverse plane of the center of gravity. The illustration given uses the body as if it were in the anatomical position. It is called the *reaction board method* (**19, 64**). The second method is suitable for use in locating the center of gravity of a body in motion. It is called the *segmental method*.

Reaction Board Method This is a way of locating quite closely the transverse plane of the center of gravity above the soles of the feet. A board of suitable strength, which has two knife-edges mounted on the underside about 2 meters apart (one near each end), is used. A vertical footboard is mounted on top, with the inside edge exactly over one of the knife-edges. The other knife-edge is placed on the platform of a set of scales. The footboard end is placed on a block so as to make the reaction board level (see Figure 15-3).

In order to make the procedure clear, assume that the block of wood under one knife-edge is a second set of scales. If a subject now lies on the board in the anatomical position with the soles of the feet flat against the end board centered over one knife-edge, then the total weight of the board and subject is reflected by the combined force registered on the two scales. Mathematically the transverse-plane center of gravity for the board and subject is the balance point between the two

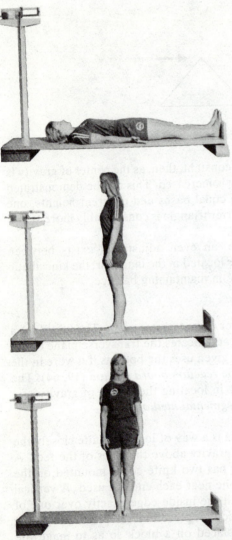

Figure 15-3 Reaction board method of locating center of gravity.

knife-edges or scales. This is represented by the force reading (F_1) on the first scale times the distance (X) to the balance point, and is equal to the force reading (F_2) on the second scale times the distance $(\ell\text{-}X)$ (where ℓ is the distance between knife-edges) from the second scale to the balance point. Since we do not know X, solve the formula $F_1X = F_2(\ell - X)$. When the force resigistered on the two scales is measured for the board only, these amounts can be subtracted from the readings on each scale when the subject is on the board. This net reading can then be used for F_1 and F_2. Assume a 60-kilogram person 170 centimeters tall lies on the board (as in Figure 15-3). The net reading on scale one is 29 kilograms and the net reading on scale two (under the feet) is 31 kilograms. The length (ℓ) between knife-edges is 200 centimeters (2 meters). Then,

$$F_1X = F_2 (\ell - X)$$
29 kilograms X = 31 kilograms (200 centimeters $- X$)
29 kilograms X = 6,200 kilogram centimeter $-$ 39 kilograms X
60 kg X = 6,200 kilogram centimeters
X = 103.33 cm

The center of gravity is 103.33 centimeters from the first knife-edge or ($\ell - X$) 96.67 centimeters above the soles of the feet. This is 56.9 percent of body length above soles of the feet for the 170-centimeter-tall person.

Consider the above using only one scale and the block as in Figure 15-3. Since the net reading on the second scale will always be the total weight of the subject (reflected as a force reading on the scale) minus the net reading on the first scale, the following equation can be used for only one scale:

$$F_1X = (\text{weight} - F_1) (\ell - X)$$
29 kilograms X = (60 kilograms $-$ 29 kilograms) (200 centimeters $- X$)
29 kilograms X = 31 kilograms (200 centimeters $- X$)
29 kilograms X = 6,200 kilograms centimeters $-$ 31 kilograms X
60 kilograms X = 6,200 kilograms centimeters
X = 103.33 centimeters from the knife-edge over the scale
or $\ell - X$ = 96.67 centimeters from the footboard

This method can also be used to find a person's center of gravity in the frontal and sagittal planes. These measures are often important in postural work for corrective assessments in weight bearing. While being measured, a person should avoid swaying sideward, forward, or backward, as this distorts the location of the center of gravity. The same formula given above is used; the person faces away from the toeboard, or stands sideward to it, in about the center of the board. A point is marked at the toe, heel, or side of the foot and is used as reference to measure the resulting difference from that point and the computed X. (See Figure 15-2.) Cooper and Glassow (**19**) have an interesting chapter (see chap. 4) on this material, and it is recommended reading.

Segmental Method   A second *method* of locating the center of gravity, the segmental method, is suitable for dynamic measurement, is, that for measurement of a person in motion and in varying body positions. Consider a simple example. Figure 15-4 is an enlargement of the third image in Figure 12-2 of a man doing a one-and-one-half pike dive. To locate the center of gravity of this diver, the subsequent steps are followed (**32**):

1   The reference points associated with each segment are located and marked as on Figure 15-4. (See Table 15-1, left-hand column.) These points are joint centers in most cases, or extremities of other segments such as the head and feet.

2   These reference points are connected with straight lines, except in the case of the curved trunk in which a curved line approximately parallel to the body curvature connects the points. This essentially results in a stick figure.

3   Using the information in Table 15-1 (right-hand column) the appropriate distance is computed from the superior reference of each segment, then a short line perpendicular to the segment stick figure line is drawn. This represents the center of gravity of the segment.

4   Lines OY and OX are used as the left and bottom frame borders for Figure 15-4. These are the vertical and horizontal reference axes.

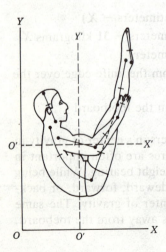

Figure 15-4 The segmental method for locating the center of gravity.

Table 15-1   Weight of Body Segments Relative to Total Body Weight and Segment Center of Gravity Location from Superior Reference

Segment (greatest % to least)	Relative weight	C of g location of segment (% of segment length)
Trunk	0.507	38.0 to suprasternal notch
Combined thighs	0.206	37.2 to hip axis
Combined calf	0.086	37.1 to knee axis
Head	0.073	46.4 to vertex
Combined upper arm	0.052	51.3 to shoulder axis
Combined forearm	0.032	39.0 to elbow axis
Combined foot	0.030	49.9 to heel
Combined hand	0.014	82.0 to wrist axis
	Total 1.000	

Source: Adapted from Charles E. Clauser, John T. McConville, and J. W. Young, *Weight, Volume, and Center of Mass of Segments of the Human Body,* AMRL Technical Report, 1969–70, Wright-Patterson Air Force Base, Ohio, 1969.

5   In Table 15-2 note the segment name at the left of the table. The first column has the appropriate segmental relative weight value. Column 2 lists the perpendicular distance in millimeters from the respective segmental center of gravity to the OY axis.

6   The moments about OY are computed as values in the third column by multiplying values in column 1 by values in column 2. The sum of column 3 represents the total body moment about OY and is 35.65 millimeters.

7   Column 4 lists the perpendicular distance in millimeters from the respective segmental center of gravity to the OX axis.

8   As in step **6** the moments about OX are computed as values in the fifth column by multiplying values in column 1 with values in column 4. The sum of column 5 represents the total body moment about OX and is 50.66 millimeters.

9   To locate the body center of gravity a line $O'Y'$ is drawn parallel to OY and 35.65 millimeters to the right, and line $O'X'$ is drawn parallel to OX and 50.66 millimeters above it. The intersection of these lines $O'Y'$ and $O'X'$ represent the location of the body's center of gravity in Figure 15-4.

The procedure given here can be used with a photograph of any participant in any activity.

If legs and arms are not in the same sagittal position, the table of relative weight should be adapted to account for separate segment values rather than combined values. More computations will be needed for the separate limb segments.

This method is quite accurate but time-consuming; in modern

Table 15-2

Body segment	Col 1 Segment relative weight	Col 2 Distance to OY (mm)	Col 3 Moment about OY (col 1 x col 2)	Col 4 Distance to OX (mm)	Col 5 Moment about OX (col 1 x col 4)
Trunk	0.507	24.0	12.169	39.0	19.773
Comb. thighs	0.206	50.0	10.300	45.5	9.373
Comb. calf	0.086	62.5	5.375	83.5	7.181
Head	0.073	17.5	1.2775	74.2	5.4166
Comb. upper arms	0.052	34.5	1.794	51.5	2.678
Comb. fore-arms	0.032	52.5	1.68	56.0	1.792
Comb. feet	0.030	68.0	2.176	106.5	3.408
Comb. hands	0.014	63.0	.882	74.5	1.0403
Total 1.000			Sum of Moments = 35.6535		Sum of Moments = 50.6646

Source: Adapted from James G. Hay, The Biomechanics of Sports Techniques, Prentice-Hall, 2d ed., 1978, pp. 136–138.

practice it is handled by computer, even in three dimensions by use of x, y, and z coordinates. A sample problem is given at the end of the chapter.

PRINCIPLES OF BALANCE

For balance to be maintained in any stationary position, the center of gravity must remain over the base of support. Whenever the center of gravity passes outside the base of support, the body is off-balance in that direction. This applies to all body positions, including upright, inverted (where the hands form the base of support), and three-, four-, or six-point positions. For balance to be maintained in a standing position, continuous forward body lean is necessary. This results in constant tension on the large calf muscles, and it places the center of weight approximately over the center of the feet.

To perform balance skills effectively (as in Figure 15-5), the performer must develop two primary qualities: (1) adequate strength to support the body in the given positions and (2) ability to shift the body weight

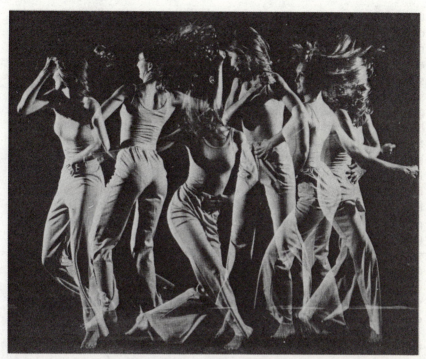

Figure 15-5 Balance is very important in fast and complex dancing movements.

quickly into the correct positions at the right time. The first quality (strength) is dependent on the three factors which compose it, namely, contractile force of the mover muscles, ability to coordinate all the muscles involved in the act, and mechanical ratio of the different levers. The second quality (shifting body weight) depends on several factors, namely, kinesthetic perception and visual perception (the awareness of the positions of the body and its parts), function of the balance center of the inner ear, quick reactions, good neuromuscular coordination, agility, and possibly flexibility.

Recovery of Balance

Principle: If the center of gravity moves outside the base of support, a quick adjustment must be made in order to regain balance. The base of support may be moved or enlarged, or a body part may be adjusted in order to return the center of gravity to a position over the base of support. After the adjustment is made, a lowering of the center of gravity makes the performer more stable and therefore less susceptible to another loss of balance.

Example A: A loss of balance in the handstand may be regained if the performer handwalks (moves the base) in the direction of the overbalance until the base is again beneath the center of gravity. Balance might also be regained by shifting one or both legs in the opposite direction, causing the center of gravity to move back over the base of support. Overcompensations after the balance has been regained can sometimes be avoided by bending the arms (lowering the center of gravity). *Example B*: In the head- and-handstand, the area of the base can be enlarged by increasing the distances between the points of the triangle formed by the points of support, the head and the hands. Often the least stable performers place their hands alongside their ears (head and hands in a straight line), thus reducing the area of their base in the forward-backward direction. If these three points truly represent the area of the base, each must bear approximately equal weight. *Example C*: When the performer is working on a balance beam, the movement of body segments (such as the arms) can shift the center of gravity back over the base of support. While the movement of a segment may be effective immediately after a loss of balance, the same movement may be ineffective if the center of gravity has been allowed to move too far outside the base of support or if too much falling speed has developed. For this reason, very quick and correct adjustments are essential for recovering balance.

Sensory-Receptor Adjustments

Principle: The reduction of unfamiliar sensations associated with balance receptors often reduces dizziness which may lead to a loss of balance. For instance, the eyes have been oriented to certain spatial relationships in an upright world, and deviations from the upright positions often affect sense of balance negatively. Also, fast-twirling head movements produce movement of fluids in the inner ear which give rise to the sensation of dizziness. These negative results can be partially controlled.

  Example A: When bouncing on a trampoline, the performer should focus the eyes on a distant object which is relatively level with the head position, such as a point on a distant wall. This will reduce the up-and-down visual sensation and eliminate dizziness. *Example B*: When spinning rapidly in place during a dance or skating maneuver, the performer should select a fixed point upon which to keep the eyes focused as long as possible during each turn. If the performer returns concentration to this point as quickly as possible in each succeeding turn, the head can be kept stationary during a portion of each turn; this reduces the sight-motion sensation and produces the least possible disturbance of the inner-ear fluids. *Example C*: Beginners often feel dizzy when performing gymnastic turning movements. Even simple stunts like a forward roll can produce this effect until the performer becomes accustomed to unfamiliar positions and movements of the head. Practice helps overcome this dizziness, because kinesthetic adjustments become keener as unfamiliar positions are repeated.

Carrying Postures

Principle: When external weight is applied to the body, as in lifts and carries, the body weight must be shifted in order to maintain balance around the line of gravity (a vertical line passing through the center of gravity to the surface).

Example A: If a 20-kilogram weight is held under the right arm, the line of gravity in the body must be shifted toward the left edge of the base to support in order to compensate for the change in the center of weight. *Example B* (*Figure 15-6*): If, when lifting a heavy object, the performer keeps the object close to the body's center of gravity, less adjustment will be needed and there will be less likelihood of a loss of balance.

PRINCIPLES OF STABILITY

Stability is firmness of balance. The stable body is less apt to be disturbed by any upsetting influences. The physical makeup of a person exerts a

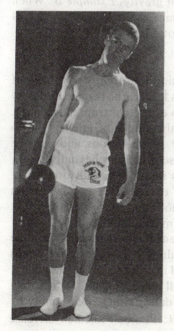

Figure 15-6 External weight added to the body calls for an adjustment in posture. The body's center of gravity must be shifted in a direction away from the external weight.

strong influence on his or her stability, but within the bounds of this limitation, one can purposely assume positions which influence stability in any given situation.

Position of the Center of Gravity

Principle: For maximum stability in all directions the center of gravity of the body should be placed over the center of the base of support, or as near to it as possible. This applies to both foot-supported and arm-supported positions, as well as to three-point and four-point positions.

Example A: A gymnast performing a handstand is most stable in all directions when the weight is directly over the center of the base of support, the hands. *Example B*: A modern dancer in a half-crouched position or a wrestler in a standing position is most stable when the center of weight is directly over the base of support, which, in these cases, is determined by the exact positions of the feet.

Lowered Center of Gravity

Principle: Stability may be increased by lowering the center of gravity (Figure 15-2).

Example A: The wrestler, basketball player, football player, and modern dancer all increase their stability at certain times by assuming a crouched position which lowers the center of gravity. *Example B*: When in an unstable craft, such as a canoe, the chances of tipping become less as the center of gravity gets closer to the bottom.

Enlarged Base of Support

Principle: Stability is enhanced by increasing the area of the base of support (Figure 15-7). As the base becomes larger, the center of gravity must be moved through a greater distance in order to disrupt the balance. (The principles relating both to lowering the center of gravity and to enlarging the base of support are subject to limitations and may be self-defeating. If the performer applies these principles beyond reason, he or she may produce undesirable angles of support and force weak muscular actions. Further, it is generally true that beyond a certain point, an increase in stability reduces mobility; thus, if mobility is important, it may be desirable to sacrifice maximum stability.)

Example A: The baseball batter broadens the base of support in the direction in which the ball is to be hit. Similarly, when the golfer drives with greater force, a wider stance is assumed in order to increase stability. Basketball, tennis, badminton, and volleyball players all spread their feet apart to broaden the base of support, and dancers increase stability by properly positioning their feet. *Example B*: Football linemen increase

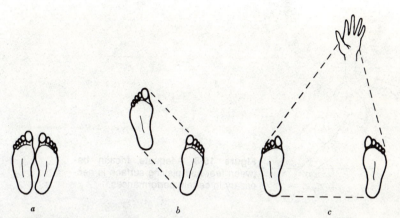

Figure 15-7 As the base of support is enlarged, the object becomes more stable. (*a*) Unstable position. (*b*) More stable position. (*c*) Very stable position.

stability by moving from a two- to a three-point stance. The four-point stance provides a still larger area of support.

Body Size and Proportions

Principle: All else being equal, the greater the weight the more stable the object is against external forces; in fact, the stability is proportional to the weight. Thus in performances where stability is important, weight becomes a consideration. Concentration of weight also influences stability. A larger proportion of body weight concentrated in the upper part of the body raises the center of gravity, which is a disadvantage in activities requiring balance and stability in an upright position but is an advantage in arm-support skills requiring balance.

Example A: A heavy basketball rebounder or post man, a heavy football player, or a heavy wrestler is more stable (harder to move) than a light one. *Example B*: A heavy concentration of weight in the upper portion of the body is a stability disadvantage for the skier, dancer, or skater, who may, however, compensate for it by other qualities. This same structure, though, would enhance performance in most gymnastic skills.

Friction

Principle: The greater the friction between the supporting surface and the body parts in contact with that surface, the greater the stability.

Example A: The use of gymnasium shoes on hard surfaces (Figure 15-8) and the use of baseball, football, and running spikes on their respective surfaces all increase stability by creating increased friction.

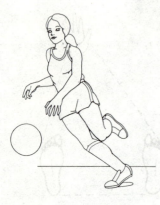

Figure 15-8 Adequate friction between feet and playing surface is necessary in certain performances.

Example B: When traction is insufficient, forces which are applied must have more of a vertical and less of a horizontal component. The performer runs more "up and down" on a slippery or loose surface.

STABILITY AGAINST A KNOWN FORCE

Some of the principles included in the preceding section are not entirely useful when the direction of the force with which the performer must deal is known.

Moving the Center of Gravity toward the Force

Principle: If a known force is approaching, and the performer wishes to maintain balance, the center of gravity should be very near the edge of the base of support on the side nearest the oncoming force. The performer is most stable under these conditions because the center of gravity will need to be moved a maximum distance before it goes outside its supporting base. The effects of the oncoming force may be further diminished by developing momentum in a direction opposite that of the force (Figure 15-9).

    Example A: The football lineman widens his base by stepping toward an oncoming blocker, and he moves his center of gravity in the same direction. (He also lowers the center of gravity.) If the blocker is to upset the lineman, he must move the lineman's center of gravity all the way through the increased distance of the base of support. *Example B*: The boxer or the wrestler usually carries the center of gravity toward the forward edge of the base of support in order to be prepared for potential force from the opponent. The wrestler must be sure not to overdo the forward weight shift in case the opponent pulls him off-balance in the forward direction.

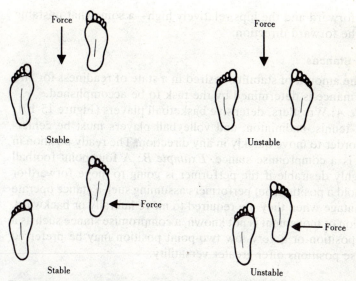

Figure 15-9 The position of the feet should be determined by the direction in which stability is needed.

Destroying the Stability of an Opponent

Principle: A person can be moved off-balance most easily if pushed or pulled toward the nearest edge of the base of support or in the direction of the narrowest part of the base.

Example A: In wrestling, an opponent can be taken off-balance most easily if pushed or pulled in the direction at right angles to the line connecting his feet. *Example B*: In any two-point stance, as in football, an opponent will be least stable in one direction depending on foot placement, because the measurement of the base in one direction can be only as great as the length of the feet.

Tasks Requiring Instability

Principle: Some positions of readiness require instability in a certain direction. The shorter distance the center of gravity must move to clear the base of support the more rapidly the body can be put into motion in that direction.

Example: A performer who wishes to start quickly in a given direction should move the center of gravity close to the edge of the base of support in the direction of movement. A swimmer leans forward as much as possible in the starting stance in order to shift the center of gravity quickly past the forward line of the base of support when the gun goes off. The track sprinter assumes a set position with the body weight shifted well forward and the hips relatively high—a somewhat unstable position in the forward direction.

Compromise Stances

Principle: The amount of stability desired in a state of readiness for any given performance is determined by the task to be accomplished.

Example A: Wrestlers, defensive basketball players (Figure 15-10), boxers, and tennis, badminton, and volleyball players must be center-balanced in order to move quickly in any direction. The ready position in these cases is a compromise stance. *Example B*: A four-point football stance is highly desirable if the performer is going to move forward or attempt to hold a position, but performers assuming such a stance operate at a disadvantage when they are required to move laterally or backward. If the direction of movement is not known, a compromise stance such as a three-point position or a very low two-point position may be preferred because these positions offer greater versatility.

BALANCE AND STABILITY WHILE IN MOTION

Many principles of balance in motion are the same as those applied to stationary postures. Important differences are (1) the base of support is constantly moving, (2) the base of support is often only as large as the one supporting foot, and (3) recovery movements must be especially quick and precise when the body is in motion.

Use of Gravity

Principle: Many locomotor activities depend upon a deliberate loss of balance to enable gravity to combine with muscular forces to move the body in the desired direction. The base of support is then moved beneath the moving body to support it for a brief period of time. This action is repeated rhythmically.

Example A: When a person leans forward to start walking or

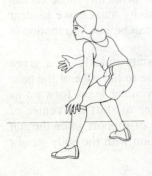

Figure 15-10 The basketball defensive player keeps a low center of gravity and a wide base of support for stability in his or her position and readiness to move quickly in any direction. Similar "ready positions" are employed in tennis, badminton, wrestling, and other sports.

running, the center of gravity is shifted outside the base of support and then a forward step must be taken to regain balance, thus establishing a new base of support. The center of gravity, which is in motion, passes over the new base of support and continues its forward motion. Subsequently, the base of support is moved by stepping forward with the feet, and locomotion (walking) results. When walking, a person is supported simultaneously by both feet for a brief moment between steps, but when running, only one foot contacts the surface at a time. At any time during the run, the base of support is provided by only one supporting limb, which demands intricate timing. *Example B*: When a swimmer or runner starts a race, the center of gravity is shifted forward of the base of support in order to utilize the force of gravity to help moving in that direction.

Increasing Stability while in Motion

Principle: Stability can be gained while in motion by lowering the center of gravity and enlarging the base of support.

Example A: The ballcarrier in football has a low center of gravity and a wide base when running through a congested area. He adds lateral stability by widening his running stance. He may also run with short, choppy steps, which allow him to establish his base of support more often, and, thus he may change direction more quickly. This running technique results in a sacrifice of linear speed. When the runner clears the congested area, he should raise his center of gravity, narrow his stance, and take a longer stride to gain maximum speed. *Example B*: While walking on the hands, a person is most stable in a lateral direction when taking shorter and wider strides. Lowering the center of gravity also aids stability in this particular skill. *Example C*: Automobiles are more stable if they have large wheelbases and low centers of weight.

Control of Momentum

Principle: To stop quickly or change direction when in rapid motion, the performer should widen his base, lower his center of gravity, and slow down in order to control his momentum. This principle is often neglected in teaching skills.

Example A: The basketball player on defense is better able to control momentum and to change direction quickly when the legs are reasonably well spread and the body is reasonably low. *Example B*: If the football pass receiver is to execute sharp and effective cuts, he must observe this principle. If he does not, he will tend to "round corners" and be more easily covered by a defender. The greater his momentum, the more difficult it is to stop or change direction. *Example C*: The offensive basketball player who does not follow this principle is likely to lose balance and "travel." The skier, too, applies the principle when turning sharply, as in slalom racing.

POSTURE

Posture is both dynamic and static, and we must be concerned with both kinds. Static posture (standing, sitting, etc.) is the easier of the two to study. It is relatively easy to establish guidelines for static posture, but it is very difficult to provide guidelines for dynamic posture (body positions during movement) because it takes many different forms. Many of the guidelines for static posture, however, can be applied effectively to dynamic posture.

Correct posture is important because (1) it aids the functioning of the organic systems; (2) it reduces strain on muscles, ligaments, and tendons; and (3) it increases the attractiveness of the person. Further, posture may influence a person's self-concept and thereby have important psychological implications.

It is established that many of the traditional hard-and-fast rules of posture are unjustified. Current thinking is that postural evaluation must be approached from a highly individual and practical point of view. The judgment of how correct a posture is ought be based on physiological, anatomical, and aesthetic considerations.

Physiological Correctness

Posture is physiologically correct when it allows the organic systems to function efficiently. Posture which restricts adequate circulation, respiration, digestion, and elimination is not correct; for instance, a rigid (at attention) standing position restricts circulation.

Anatomical Correctness

Posture is anatomically correct when the body has good balance and alignment, and results in a minimum of muscle strain. In such positions the skeletal structure carries a maximum amount of weight, so that posture demands minimum muscle effort. From the anatomical point of view, the best posture is a position where the bodily structure is vertically aligned and the muscles are as relaxed as possible.

Aesthetic Correctness

Posture is aesthetically correct when it contributes most to the attractiveness of the person. Aesthetically correct posture also tends to be anatomically and physiologically correct. Occasionally, however, the aesthetic point of view tends to lead people toward too much rigidity and too much precision in movement. Figure 15-11 shows good posture.

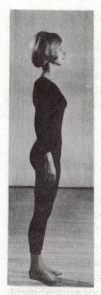 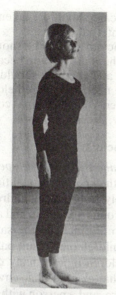 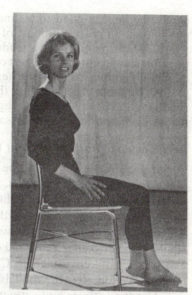

Figure 15-11 Good posture. (a) Standing, side view. (b) Standing, diagonal view. (c) Sitting.

Guidelines for Correct Posture

Whether posture is evaluated from the physiological, anatomical, or aesthetic points of view, there are several guides that should be followed:

1 The weight-bearing segments should be correctly aligned, so that the line of gravity passes through them. This reduces unnecessary muscle strain and contributes to attractiveness.

2 The extension of the weight-bearing joints should be an easy extension not accompanied by strain, tension, or excessive rigidity.

3 The feet should be placed far enough apart to form a base of support over which the body can be balanced easily without excessive muscle use.

4 With respect to inward and outward rotation of the legs, the correct position is the patellae and feet pointed straight forward.

5 Excessive forward tilt of the pelvis should be avoided because it contributes to a protruding abdomen and a swayed back, which in turn can contribute to permanent back problems.

6 The spinal column, when viewed laterally, will naturally exhibit three curves, a convex cervical curve, a concave thoracic curve, and a convex lumbar curve. Efforts to eliminate these curves are undesirable, but it is important not to allow the curves to become excessive. When viewed from the rear, the spinal column should be straight.

7 The abdominal wall, which is composed mostly of muscle tissue, should be kept in good tone, and care should be taken to keep the wall straight and in proper support of internal organs.

8 Many people have a tendency to abduct the shoulder girdles. This position should not become part of habitual posture because the condition commonly known as sunken chest and rounded shoulders will result.

9 In good, erect posture, the neck should be held straight, but not rigid, and the head should be aligned with the spinal column so the neck muscles are not under unnecessary stress.

Relationship of Posture to Other Factors

Postural characteristics may be *inherited* or *developed*, and they may relate to, and be derived from, other personal qualities. A parent with excessive spinal curvatures is likely to produce children with excessive curvatures, whereas a parent with round shoulders and a forward neck tilt will tend to produce children who are inclined the same way. Postural similarities between parents and children may result partly from heredity and partly from environment. Children inherit many qualities, but they tend to develop after the models that exist in their environments.

Nutrition affects body structure, and a person with poor nourishment may have neither the energy nor the muscular endurance and tone to hold the body parts habitually in correct position. Inadequate nutrition may contribute to poor posture, especially during the years of bodily growth when consistently poor temporary body positions gradually become part of habitual posture.

A person's *height* may influence posture. Short people tend to extend their height by standing very straight, and extremely tall people tend to reduce their height by settling at the joints and hunching at the upper back and neck. These people are trying to appear closer to medium height.

Training may have significant effects on posture. Dance, gymnastics, diving, and fencing all contribute to straight and slightly rigid postures and precision in body movements. Wrestling and boxing contribute to a slightly hunched posture. Long-distance running and swimming contribute to a relaxed and, often, slouchy posture. Other activities have specific effects on posture, although many activities are neutral as far as postural development is concerned.

Work conditions also affect posture. For instance, excessive study over a desk tends to develop round shoulders and forward head tilt. The same can be said of high-precision jobs requiring close hand-eye coordination and fine muscle movements, such as the work of a jeweler.

Posture has strong *psychological implications*. It tells much about one's personality. For example, withdrawn and shy persons often display a withdrawn type of posture, as if they are attempting to hide within themselves. The opposite type of personality (highly aggressive) often displays a very straight and outgoing posture.

Correcting Posture

Sometimes correcting posture is a task more for psychiatrists than for physical educators because the deviations sometimes grow out of psychological problems. Well-informed physical educators, however, can often help the student correct poor posture by (1) motivating for correct posture and (2) leading through a corrective exercise program. The program will consist of selected exercises to add strength, endurance, and tone to the muscles which need to apply more tension and to add flexibility to opposing muscle groups.

It has been demonstrated that the following is a successful corrective procedure:

1 Correctly identify the postural deviation and inform the individual of its nature and the importance of correcting it.

2 Attempt to identify the basic causes of the deviation, and control the causes.

3 Motivate the individual to want to correct the deviation. (In the absence of such motivation, postural corrective exercises will probably fail.)

4 Prescribe an exercise program designed to correct the condition.

5 Periodically evaluate the effects of the program.

A well-prepared physical educator should be able to tell which muscle should be exercised and which ones must have increased flexibility in order to bring about the desired posture changes. The educator should also be able to select exercises which will be effective.

IMPORTANT CONCEPTS

1 Balance is important in all motor performances. It is the state of equilibrium where the center of gravity is over the base of support.

2 Once balance is lost, it can be regained by either shifting the center of gravity over the base of support or adjusting the base of support so it is underneath the center of gravity. Both kinds of adjustment are often used simultaneously.

3 The center of gravity of the body is the exact center of weight, or the point about which the body would freely rotate if it were free to rotate, or the point where the weight is exactly equal on all opposite sides, or the point of intersection of the three primary planes of the body.

4 On the average the center of gravity is proportionally lower in women than in men, and proportionally higher in children than adults. This is because of differences in body proportions in the two sexes and differences in children as compared with adults.

5 Balance can be thought of as either static or dynamic, with dynamic balance being more important in most performances.

6 Stability is firmness of balance and is depicted by the amount of

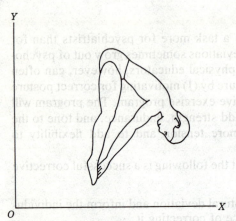

Figure 15-12 Student laboratory experience model for determining the center of gravity by the segmental method.

force necessary to cause imbalance. It is always influenced by three factors; the *size* of the base of support, the *height* of the center of gravity, and the *weight* of the object. In the case of the human body two other factors influence stability: muscular strength, and friction between the body and surface.

7 Posture can be thought of as static or dynamic, with static posture being concerned with sitting and standing positions, and dynamic posture being concerned with body carriage.

8 Posture should be evaluated from practical points of view including *physiological* correctness, *anatomical* correctness, and *aesthetic* correctness.

9 Many postural deviations and poor postural characteristics can be corrected through (*a*) regular concentration on improvement and (*b*) regular participation in a correctly prescribed exercise program.

Note Other important concepts are stated in the chapter in the form of principles.

STUDENT LABORATORY EXPERIENCES.

1 If a scale and reaction board are available, locate your own center of gravity in the three primary planes. Follow the procedure given in this chapter.

2 Using Figure 15-12, work out the center of gravity by the segmental method; follow the same procedure used in the chapter. Table 15-3 has been supplied to help you.

Table 15-3 Work table to help locate the center of gravity in Figure 15-12 by the segmental method.

Body Segment		Col 1 Segment relative weight ♂	Col 2 Distance to OY (mm)	Col 3 Moment about OY (col 1 x col 2)	Col 4 Distance to OX (mm)	Col 5 Moment about OX (col 1 x col 4)
Trunk		0.507				
Comb. thighs		0.206				
Comb. calf		0.086				
Head		0.073				
Comb.	upper arms	0.052				
Comb.	fore-arms	0.030				
Comb. feet		0.030				
Comb. hands		0.014				

Chapter 16

Mechanical Analysis
of a Skill

This chapter is a model to follow in preparing a mechanical analysis. Such a project involves selecting a specific skill of interest to you and performing a thorough mechanical analysis of it. Let the contents of this chapter serve as your guide. Draw heavily from the material in Chapters 11 to 15, but do not necessarily limit yourself to those chapters or to this book.

The golfer is told, "Keep your eye on the ball" and "Keep your left elbow straight" (right-handed golfer). But neither of these coaching tips is necessary for an effective golf shot; they are merely devices to help the performer assume a swing arc which will assure correct contact with the ball. The important factor is the *contact*, and not whether or not the left elbow is straight and the eye is on the ball. These factors do not affect the efficiency of the motion. The stroke will be less effective, however, if the back foot is not securely in contact with the surface upon impact or if the force of the club head does not pass through the center of gravity of the ball. In these cases basic laws of motion and force are violated, thus reducing the propelling force. Such laws are the basis for mechanical analysis of a performance, serving as the foundation upon which correct technique is determined.

The value to the student in doing a mechanical analysis is apparent. The analysis will lend support for many teaching tips and will show that some commonly used tips have no basis for support. Also, the student will understand better the reasoning behind established techniques of performance and why pieces of equipment are constructed and used as they are. A mechanical analysis of one skill has great carryover value in understanding other skills which involve some of the same laws and principles.

After the skill to be analyzed is selected, the logical procedure is to refer to each law, principle, or concept presented in the preceding five chapters and decide whether it is applicable. If the principle does apply to the particular skill, it should be stated and then discussed in light of that skill. Finally, the most important aspects of successful performance of the skill should be summarized.

Mechanical Analysis of the Golf Drive (Right-Handed)

The golf drive (Figure 16-1) was selected because its success depends upon adherence to a wide variety of principles. The purpose of the golf

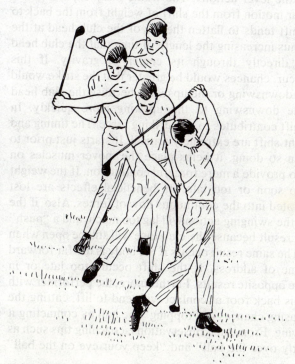

Figure 16-1 Sequence drawings of the golf drive.

drive is to achieve maximum distance and accuracy. The technique may be varied to meet different conditions, especially by a performer of advanced skill, but the purpose remains essentially the same for all golfers. The skill includes (1) the development of a maximum and accurate striking force, (2) control of balance by the performer during the swing, and (3) factors involved in the behavior of the projectile. Essentially, the desired qualities of the swing are (1) maximum club-head momentum at impact, (2) correct position and direction of motion of the club head at impact, and (3) contact of the ball directly through its center of gravity. All the techniques employed should produce these desired results.

Principles of Motion

Principle: Combining of translatory and rotary motion   Successful performance often calls for effectively combining translatory and rotary motions.

Application   Angular (rotary) motion is the only kind that a body lever can experience. The golf drive requires successive actions of several body levers, and the arc of the club head undergoes angular motion as a result of the lever actions. The whole body experiences a limited amount of linear motion from the shift of weight from the back to the front foot. This shift tends to flatten the arc of the club head at the bottom of the swing, thus increasing the length of time that the club head can contact the ball directly through its center of gravity. If this "flattening" did not occur, chances would be greater that the strike would be made on either the downswing or the upswing, because the club head would move from the downswing to the upswing more quickly. In addition, the weight shift contributes to the striking force. The timing and the extent of the weight shift are extremely critical. It starts just prior to the downswing, and in so doing, it helps place the mover muscles on stretch for the swing to provide a more forceful contraction. If the weight shift is completed too soon or too late, its beneficial effects are lost because it is not integrated into the continuous flow of forces. Also, if the shift occurs too soon, the swinging action will lag too much, and a "push" or possibly a slice will result because the club face will still be open when the ball is contacted. The same result occurs if the body is too far forward of the ball at the time of address. If the shift occurs too late or in insufficient amount, the opposite results. Furthermore, the performer with too much weight on his back foot at contact will tend to lift, cutting the swing short and increasing chances of "topping" the ball by contacting it decidedly on the upswing. From such observations, coaching tips such as "keep the head directly over the ball" and "keep your eye on the ball" were evolved.

In addition to the body experiencing linear and rotary motions, the ball undergoes both kinds of motions. When struck, the ball undergoes translatory motion which becomes increasingly curvilinear as air resistance reduces its velocity. At the same time, the ball usually encounters rotary motion (spin), applied either purposely or inadvertently. The amount and direction of the spin may influence the flight of the ball a significant amount.

Principle: Continuity of motion When performing activities in which two or more consecutive motions contribute toward movement in the same direction, the performer should not pause between motions.

Application Each successive motion of body parts should occur so that the club head undergoes constant acceleration. The appearance of a swing which develops in this manner is smooth and flowing; the smooth swing will produce a greater final momentum than the jerky swing because inertia against the action is less. Also, energy is conserved when the forces are smooth and consistent in intensity.

Principle: Effects of momentum When a moving object strikes another object, the greater its momentum at impact, the greater will be its force.

Application Because momentum is the product of velocity and mass, the increase in either of these factors results in increased momentum. In the golf swing it would appear that a heavier or longer club would produce greater momentum, and thus a greater impact. This is true provided velocity is not sacrificed; however, the key factor here is whether the performer has adequate strength to handle the heavier or longer club so that the same final velocity results as would with the lighter or shorter club. Theoretically, as strength increases, a heavier club can be handled at the same velocity; therefore, the momentum of the drive is increased. It should be noted that the momentum developed in the backswing must be overcome before the downswing can begin, which explains the reason for a slow backswing, especially with a heavy club. It is obvious, then, that additional strength in the correct muscles is one key to more distance off the tee.

Control is another aspect of momentum. The club movements may destroy the balance of the performer or may alter the swing arc, causing inaccuracies in the contact. A greater club momentum tends to magnify these tendencies. A golfer who swings harder (faster) or who uses a heavier club becomes more susceptible to such inaccuracies. Any performer will be able to cope better with these conditions if the muscles controlling the club and body balance are stronger.

In conclusion, the performer needs adequate strength in muscles that produce striking forces and in muscles that maintain balance. Usually, additional strength is needed in these muscles to increase the distance of the drive either by swinging harder or by using a heavier or longer club.

Principle: Transfer of momentum   Momentum developed in a body segment is transferred to the rest of the body only while the body is still in contact with the supporting surface.

Application   The momentum of the club and the movements of the body in the direction of the swing will tend to pull the body off balance in that direction. Maintenance of balance is discussed more fully in Chapter 15.

Principle: Maximum acceleration and efficiency of motion   All available forces should be applied sequentially with proper timing, and as directly in the intended line of motion as possible. Body movements extraneous to the desired motion should be reduced to a minimum.

Application   The major forces of the golf swing in proper sequence follow:

1   Inward rotation of the front hip (a reversal of customary muscle function—the pelvis rotates on the fixed leg)
2   Left rotation of the thoracic spine
3   Abduction and outward rotation of the left shoulder (this may vary some from true abduction), coupled with scapular adduction to the left side and extension of the right elbow
4   Ulnar flexion (adduction) of the left wrist and flexion of the right wrist (the right wrist may also tend somewhat toward ulnar flexion)

These forces are in addition to the total body-weight shift, which has already been discussed. Each of the forces makes a particular contribution to maintaining the accuracy of the swing. If too much or too little motion results from any one force, inaccuracies result. If the timing of any force is too early or too late in the sequence, the result will be inaccuracy, reduction of momentum, or both.

Few extraneous movements are seen in golf swings, but a common one is too long a backswing, which tends to pull the golfer off balance. Another common undesired motion is extension of the trunk, which pulls the golfer away from the ball just before contact, causing him or her to top, slice, or completely miss the ball. Overeagerness to watch the flight of the ball also contributes to this mistake.

It appears that extra force would become available for generating momentum if the left elbow were flexed in the backswing and extended just before contact. But this movement has not been advocated; in fact, golfers are cautioned to keep the left elbow straight throughout the swing. In a way, this can be compared to punting a football without using the extension of the knee. The reasoning behind this restriction is twofold: (1) the timing between forces 2, 3, and 4 above is so precise that the inclusion of another force would be impossible to control consistently; and (2) if the elbow did not return to complete extension prior to contact, the length of the lever would be shortened, and a complete miss could result. It appears prudent to sacrifice some possible additional momentum for consistency and accuracy.

Principle: Rotational speed　If a constant force causes a body to rotate, then as changes in the radius of rotation occur, variations in the speed of rotation (the term angular and rotational speed can be interchanged) will result. As the radius is lengthened, the body rotates more slowly; as the radius is shortened the body rotates more rapidly.

Application　We can assume the available muscular force is constant and the distance from the shoulders to the club head represents the radius of rotation. The point of grip on the handle can be varied slightly to alter the radius of rotation. It will take less force to achieve a given angular velocity if the grip is farther down the club; however, unless there is considerable increase in angular velocity, the performer can expect less club-head momentum at contact because of the shorter radius of swing. The shorter grip will probably aid accuracy at the expense of speed of the club head.

Principle: Counterforces in striking activities　The amount of force a striking implement imparts to an object depends upon the combined momentum of the implement and the object at the moment of impact. Any "give" in the implement at impact reduces the propulsive force.

Application　Obviously, strong contractions of the agonist and stabilizing muscles are essential for reducing loss of force due to "give" at the moment of impact. Foot contact with the surface must be secure, and the grip must be firm. Instructions to relax in the swing refer to antagonist muscles and muscles not directly involved in the action or support of the action.

Principle: Direction of the counterforce　The counterforce is directly opposite and equal to the applied force.

Application　The applied forces in the golf drive are the push with the right (back) leg, the strong body rotation to the left, and the arm actions in the downswing. The first force requires firm footing to avoid the tendency of the feet to slip backward, and the second force requires firm footing against the tendency of both feet to turn to the right in reaction to the striking force to the left. Cleats of golf shoes are designed to hold the feet firmly in place; without proper footwear, it is likely that reduction in the force of impact will occur, because of slippage (give). A slippery surface exaggerates this effect.

A stance with the feet wider than shoulder width increases the tendency to slip, because forces are directed farther away from a line perpendicular to the surface and the body weight is less concentrated directly over the two points of support (the feet).

Principle: Temporarily stored counterforce If a surface, implement, or object used in a performance has elasticity, then an applied force produces bend or compression, which represents stored energy.

Application The shafts of golf clubs vary in flexibility; a more flexible shaft bends with the forces of the downswing, only to snap back to original shape at impact. This energy adds to the striking force, but at the same time, it makes accuracy more difficult. Some golfers prefer a stiffer shaft rather than contend with the possible loss of accuracy.

Principle: Leverage By changing the amount or type of leverage, either speed (and distance) or force can be gained at the sacrifice of the other.

Application Practically all the body levers used in the golf drive are in the third class. This type provides speed and range of motion (distance) at the expense of force. Class three levers are especially effective in producing a fast striking force with a relatively light object. These levers require great amounts of muscular force to accumulate momentum because of their short effort arms, but this problem is rectified by the successive application and precise timing of the numerous separate levers, each adding to the same motion. To obtain the optimum effect, the total range of motion must be great enough to allow time for each lever to make its fullest contribution.

Principles of Force

Because of the direct relationship between force and motion, some of the principles of force have been touched upon under Principles of Motion above. Those principles of force not yet identified are:

Principle: Total force The final velocity (or force) is the sum of the velocities of all contributing movements, if the movements are applied in a single direction, in the proper sequence, with proper timing.

Application At the moment of contact, the club head has a velocity approximately equal to the sum of the velocities of the contributing levers. In order to accumulate the greatest velocity, a particular movement in the sequence of movements should be applied at the peak velocity of the preceding movement. Because so many levers operate in such a short time in the golf swing, the importance of timing becomes apparent. Much practice is needed to develop correct timing, and conscious attempts to intensify forces without regard to timing in the swing ("pressing the swing") are often disastrous. This principle explains why the strongest person may not necessarily hit the ball the farthest if ability to time the individual forces correctly is inadequate.

Principle: Duration of force application If a constant force is applied to a body, the body develops greater acceleration as the duration (distance) over which the force is applied increases.

Application For maximum duration of force application, the backswing should be as long as possible without destroying the swing arc or pulling the body off balance. It should be understood that the backswing is only to gain correct position for an effective downswing and to place on stretch those muscles used in the downswing. If optimum backswing and optimum total body shift are used, the optimum duration of force will result.

Principle: Follow-through Emphasis on a correct follow-through eliminates a tendency to decelerate the striking action before contact.

Application Adequate follow-through is vital to a forceful and complete swing. Lack of follow-through contributes to a "chopping" or "punching" action. Also, an adequate follow-through allows the golfer to select a "point of aim" on the ball and to drive with full force toward that point. The coaching tip is "throw the club head toward the target." Concentration on the follow-through may also help to control the consistency of muscular contractions during the downswing.

Principle: Effects of spin on the ball The flight of an object is influenced by the direction and amount of its spin.

Application We know that a spinning ball curves from an accumulation of air resistance on the forward spinning side of the ball and from a reduction of air resistance on the opposite side. The curve is magnified if the ball remains in flight for a longer time as a result of a slowing of the ball, which allows a greater effect of the spin. Therefore, inaccuracies in the club-ball contact (causing spin) are of greater concern when the driver is used because it produces greater linear velocity, which results in long flight. The ball will slice, hook, rise, or drop to a greater extent for a given amount of spin if it is driven farther.

Principle: Centrifugal force   Centrifugal force creates the tendency for an object to continue momentum in a straight line instead of in a curved path.

Application   During the swing, the golfer feels the results of the force attempting to pull the club head away from the desired arc. Applying the precise amount of opposing force to counteract this effect is extremely difficult, and it is one of the keys to accuracy of the swing. If the grip is not secure, the club may fly from the hands. The golfer who pulls back too far will miss the ball or top it. The need to contend with this force also illustrates the importance of assuming an address stance which is relatively close to the ball (no need for reaching), which is rather upright (reduces tendency to straighten up), and which distributes weight over the whole foot (reduces tendency to shift weight forward or backward during swing).

The greater the momentum of the club, the greater the centrifugal force. This again points to the driver as a difficult club to master, and it illustrates that the relatively unskilled golfer will experience more accuracy by not attempting to drive too hard. Some professionals advocate hitting with all available force, but this appears to be good advice only for certain exceptionally skilled golfers.

Principles of Balance and Stability

The principles of balance and stability related to the golf drive have influenced the adoption of techniques which provide a relatively stable base of support.

Principle: Enlarged base of support   Balance and stability are enhanced by increasing the body's base of support.

Application   Because the total body shift is from right to left and the momentum of the swing is basically in the same direction, the stance must be broadened in the lateral direction. This keeps the center of gravity over the base throughout the swing. Care must be taken to avoid developing so much momentum on the backswing that balance is adversely affected. Also, the feet must not be spread too far apart because hip rotation (a powerful force) will be restricted.

From the standpoint of balance, the least room for error is in the forward-backward direction, because the size of the base in this direction is only as great as the length of the feet. For this reason, it is very important for the golfer to place the center of gravity as near the middle of the base as possible. Consequently, the weight should be distributed evenly over the feet rather than on the balls of the feet, as recommended for many other activities. For this stance, the coaching tips given are "keep the weight on your heels" or "pretend you're sitting on a high stool."

The back foot must be perpendicular to the line of drive for purposes of adequate support. The front foot may deviate slightly from the direction of the back foot, but any significant deviation will affect hip rotation adversely.

It is recommended that a slightly closed stance be used; that is, the left (front) foot should be slightly forward of the right foot. The ball should be placed well forward, directly outward from the inside edge of the left foot. This lengthens the swing before contact. The swing should move slightly from the inside (close to the body) at the backswing to the outside at the point of contact.

The obvious check to determine whether poor shots are caused by loss of balance is to see that the shot is completed in a balanced position and that the feet have not moved to correct loss of balance.

Principle: Lower center of gravity   Stability is increased by lowering the center of gravity.

Application   The correct address position includes slight flexion at the ankles, knees, and hips. This flexion lowers the center of gravity and increases stability. It would appear that an advantage could be gained by bending the knees even more, but such is *not* the case. The correct address position establishes exactly the right relationship for club-ball contact. If any additional flexion of body joints occurs during the swing (bending of the knees is a common error), this correct relationship is lost. It is important to maintain the same stance throughout the address and the swing.

Principles of Projection

Some of the important principles of projection apply to the golf drive. They are as follows:

Principle: Angle of projection   When the beginning and ending points are on the same plane, the optimum angle of projection to gain maximum distance in flight is 45° from the surface.

Application   When only the distance in flight is considered, the 45° angle is the optimum angle of projection. But in the golf drive, there are two factors which change this condition and cause the optimum angle to be less than 45°. First, the great air resistance encountered by the ball moving at high velocity favors a lower angle of projection. Second, the total distance of the drive is a combination of the flight and the roll, and an angle of considerably less than 45° will produce a longer total distance (flight plus roll), provided the terrain is suited to a long roll, as fairways usually are. Also, the amount and direction of wind must be considered in selecting the most desirable angle.

Principle: Force causing the projection　The force causing the projection produces varying effects depending upon its point of application.

Application　Off-center contact produces rotation. If this contact is below the ball's center of gravity, backspin results; if it is above the center of gravity, the ball gains top spin. If the ball is struck on the right side, it curves to the left; if struck on the left side, it curves to the right. Except under specific conditions, these spins are unwanted because they detract from the linear direction the ball will travel. Obviously, force in the desired direction is greatest when the club face is square to the ball and the line of swing is directly through the ball's center of gravity. The angle of the face of the club head, then, determines the angle of flight, and it also determines how much of the force contributes to the linear motion of the ball.

Summary Statements

Much detail was omitted in this analysis that could have been included. For instance, Chapter 14 contains much additional material that could be applied in special situations. Such principles as time in flight, magnitude of the rebound, elasticity of the striking surfaces, intentional spins, and the effects of spin present fertile ground for a more detailed analysis. Also, the analysis could have included points specific to the golf drive, such as a comparison of popular gripping methods and their effects. Recall that the only reference to the grip in this analysis was in relation to firmness throughout the swing and extra firmness upon impact.

Additional material could have been brought into the analysis from popular articles which stress certain styles or techniques. Do their contents stand up to a thorough mechanical analysis?

Another approach is to question popular coaching tips, such as "keep the left heel on the ground," which is obviously violated by almost all professionals. Why is it still found in the literature? Another approach is to select a common error, investigate the causes, and suggest the possible corrections.

In the present analysis, the movements producing the major forces were identified, and their correct sequence and timing were emphasized. The contributions of the swing technique and the maintenance of balance to the production of force and accuracy were stressed. Other important factors related to equipment, flight, and special effects and conditions were observed.

Some words of caution seem to be in order. (1) Just because the teacher is aware of the factors necessary for successful performance, it does not necessarily follow that the performers should be bombarded with a multitude of instructional points. It is pathetic for a performer to try to concentrate on a multitude of individual aspects of a skill when the skill requires one fluid motion. The mechanics of the total motion must be gradually improved by improving specific points, one at a time. (2) Balance principles are easily recognized in a skill whose primary objective is balance, but often the principles are unrecognized and unheeded in throwing, striking, jumping, or locomotor activities, even where balance may be of vital importance. Correct balance is basic to almost all athletic performances, and it is very important in the golf drive.

STUDENT LABORATORY EXPERIENCES

Select three different sport or dance skills and analyze them mechanically. Follow the pattern of this chapter, drawing heavily on Part Three and on outside materials. Do analysis in brief outline form only so as to practice the thought pattern in mechanical analysis.

Part Four

Application of Kinesiology to Basic Performance Patterns

In Part Four physical education performances are conveniently grouped into five general patterns. One chapter is devoted to each performance pattern. In each of the chapters the more important facts are identified relative to (1) the general nature of the performance pattern, (2) the major actions and muscle groups involved, (3) the application of natural laws and principles, and (4) generally how to improve performances included in that group. Some sample problems are given for each pattern; solution of these problems will help the student to quantify the performances.

Chapter 17 deals with the most basic and frequently used skills, locomotion. Chapter 18 has to do with performance involving jumping, leaping, and hopping (projecting the body). Chapter 19 is the application of kinesiology to throwing, putting, and striking skills (projecting objects). Chapter 20 deals with arm-supported skills. Chapter 21 covers skills performed in the water, and Chapter 22 is a summary of the important considerations involved in improving performance.

Chapter 17

Locomotive Skills

Any self-produced movement that transports the body from place to place is locomotive. Some locomotive skills are discussed in other sections of the text (i.e., body projections, arm-supported skills, and locomotion in water). The most common forms of locomotion, walking and running, are discussed in this chapter along with other forms, including skating and skiing.

WALKING

A person walking at the rate of 120 steps per minute for 8 hours would take 57,600 steps. If the person weighed 882 newtons, the bottoms of the feet and the muscles would bear 50,803,200 newtons in the 8-hour period. In walking at 120 steps per minute with 1-meter stride, one moves at a rate of 7.2 kilometers per hour. Many persons may walk inefficiently, but regardless of the level of efficiency for each of us, walking is probably our best-learned skill. It has been practiced since infancy, and, consequently, neural pathways used in walking are deeply ingrained.

Walking results from successive losses of balance of the two alternating feet. Each balance loss is followed by a newly established base of support and a regaining of balance. Forward progress in walking results from a combination of three forces: (1) muscular force causing pressure of the foot against the surface, (2) force of gravity which tends to pull the body forward and downward once it is off-balance, and (3) force of momentum which tends to keep the body moving in the same direction and at a constant speed. Limited additional force may result from the transfer of momentum from the arm swing, which is performed primarily to aid balance.

In walking, the leg movements (stride) occur in three phases (Figure 17-1): (1) *propulsion*, (2) *swing*, and (d) *catch and support*. The propulsion phase starts with the push-off leg in a flexed position. The joint actions during propulsion are simply extension at the hip, knee, and ankle (plantar flexion), and flexion of the toes. The main muscles involved in this phase of the stride are the hip extensors, knee extensors, ankle plantar flexors, and toe flexors. These muscles must be well conditioned if extensive walking is done. Hip rotation inward (medial) accompanies the propulsive phase of the stride.

During the swinging phase, the hip, knee, and ankle of the swinging leg flex to allow clearance for the foot to swing forward. The hip flexion movement is especially ballistic in nature, and the other flexion movements are also ballistic, but to a lesser extent. This means that the initial movement is caused by muscle contractions and that the remainder of the movement results from momentum of the moving segment. Hip rotation outward (lateral) accompanies the swinging phase to keep the toes

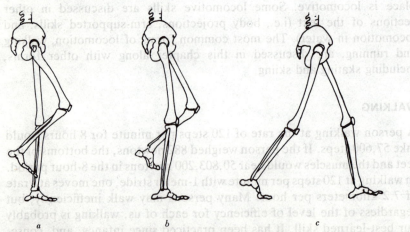

a   b   c

Figure 17-1 The three phases of the walking stride (right leg). (a) Swinging phase. (b) Support phase. (c) Propelling phase.

pointing in the line of progress. Hip rotation results in the pelvis twisting in the direction of the stride. The outward hip rotator muscles cause the movement, but as the femur rotates to a point near the correct line of direction, the inward rotators contract to hold the leg in line. The longer the stride, the greater is the amount of outward hip rotation.

The catch and support phase of the walk begins by dissipating the force of the landing. The ankle, knee, and hip joints absorb the shock by gradually flexing, but the force for flexion is provided by the body's momentum and the force of gravity. As a result, the extensor muscles of these joints contract eccentrically to reduce the forces slowly; the muscles "apply the brakes." When the forces are sufficiently reduced, flexion is halted, and there is a momentary isometric contraction of the leg extensors, during which no apparent changes in the positions of the joints are noted. This does not mean the body is motionless, as it still maintains its horizontal momentum. The support phase smoothly flows into the propulsion phase, and the cycle is completed. Figure 17-2 shows the pattern of foot contact during walking.

Besides the three phases of the stride, *other body movements* are important in walking. With each stride, the pelvis twists toward the lead leg to the point diagonal to the line of progress. If the right leg is providing the force (trail leg), the left hip leads and the right hip trails. This pelvic twist contributes significantly to the length of stride and to smoothness of the gait. Rotation occurs at both hip joints to keep the feet and legs pointing straight ahead. The back hip rotates medially while the lead hip rotates laterally. Actually, the pelvis rotates on the support leg, and the lead leg rotates on the pelvis. Therefore, the hip rotator muscles are important contributors to walking.

As the pelvis turns, the upper trunk turns in the opposite direction to keep the upper body on line with the forward movement. Therefore, the trunk rotator muscles are important contributors. The rotation of the upper trunk occurs primarily in the thoracic region of the spine.

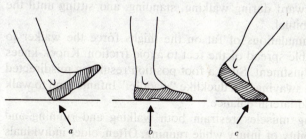

Figure 17-2 Foot-contact pattern during walking. The body weight rolls from the heel across the sole of the foot and onto the toes. The arrows *a*, *b*, and *c* indicate the direction in which the force is applied during each phase of foot contact.

In both walking and running, the arms swing diagonally forward and inward. Diagonal movement should not be so excessive that the arm swing appears awkward. The arm movements are opposite the leg movements, thus aiding the upper portion of the trunk to rotate counter to the rotation of the pelvis.

Speed of Walking

Walking speed is determined by the combination of the *length* and *frequency* of the strides. As length of stride increases, the lead leg flexes more. This puts the leg in better position for application of force, allows propulsion in a more horizontal direction, and thus permits a longer stride. As frequency of stride increases, the period of double support decreases slightly; as the frequency continues to increase, the double-support phase disappears, and the walk becomes a run. With the reduction of double support, there is a corresponding proportionate increase in the swing phase of the stride.

For adult males the optimum walking speed in terms of energy cost is about 4.83 kilometers per hour. When the pace exceeds this speed the walk becomes more fatiguing. Adult females experience optimum energy usage at a slightly slower speed than males.

Incorrect Mechanics of Walking

Many people walk with the feet in a slightly "toed-out" position, which results from outward rotation at the hip joints. This walking style is very undesirable. Toeing out results in a diagonally directed propulsive force, and it almost eliminates the use of the four small toes. In addition, the length of the foot as a lever is reduced, and the stride is shortened.

Some people walk with the feet "toed in" (pigeon-toed). This practice does not reduce efficiency a great amount unless the toes turn in excessively. Usually the main concern about this deviation is its awkward appearance. Both toed-in and toed-out deviations can be corrected to some extent by the individual if he concentrates on keeping the feet pointed straight forward during walking, standing, and sitting until the change becomes habitual.

Excessive accumulations of fat on the thighs force the walker to assume an undesirable spread of the feet to avoid friction. Knock-knees require a similar adjustment. Such a foot position results in misdirected forces resulting in a swaying or a ducklike "waddle." Infants tend to walk in this manner to aid lateral balance.

Tight hamstring muscles restrain both walking and running and increase the probability of injury while running. Often, older individuals suffer from this affliction unless a special effort is made to maintain the flexibility of this muscle group.

Ascending and Descending

Adjustments must be made for walking on inclines. A walker who wishes to locate the center of gravity properly for an uphill grade leans farther forward than usual. Such leaning places the body in a position where applied force will propel the body forward, helping to bring the powerful gluteus maximus muscle into hip extension (not ordinarily effective in the last 15° of extension). However, this forward lean has some detrimental effects. It reduces the length of the stride and increases the work of the back extensor muscles which support the trunk in a forward-leaning position. The adjustment in forward lean is made primarily at the ankle and hip joints. A flat-footed landing is most efficient when walking upstairs, because rest is provided for the calf (plantar flexor) muscles when the heel is supported.

In walking down an incline, a backward lean from the lumbar area of the spine and from the ankle joints causes the center of gravity to align over the supporting base (foot). Gravity provides all the necessary force for the descent, and the walker's efforts are mainly limited to controlling the effects of gravity. The knee extensor muscles (front of thigh) are used the most and usually tire from walking downhill. These muscles contract eccentrically to lower the body through controlled movements during the descent. The hip extensors are also important contributors, and they also contract eccentrically.

RUNNING

Running not only is an athletic event itself (track events) but is also a very important part of other sports. Speed and maneuverability in running are very important in almost all court and field games. Running and walking are similar except the *actions are greatly accentuated in running.* Two other apparent differences are:

1 In running, there is a brief period during which there is no contact with the surface (body totally suspended).
2 In running, there is no period in which both feet are in contact with the surface at the same time.

In running, the support phase is a much smaller portion of the total cycle than in walking, and the propulsion phase can begin almost immediately after the foot contacts the surface because the center of gravity is moving forward rapidly. Because the body is moving at a fast rate, the propelling force must be perfectly timed, and it must develop quickly. This means the hip, knee, and ankle extensor muscles and the toe flexors must be able to contract rapidly and with great force.

The direction of the driving force is more horizontal in running than in walking, and the push-off leg inclines much farther forward before surface contact is broken. In a sense, this is another way of saying the stride is much longer in running (about 1.83–2.13 meters for the adult male). It should be emphasized that overstriding increases the resistance provided by the lead leg upon contact; thus overstriding is mechanically inefficient. On the other hand, chopping the stride too much is inefficient because it prevents each stride from making its optimum contribution.

Generally, in running, the body has a greater forward incline than in walking, the rotary actions in the spine and pelvic regions are greatly increased, and the arm actions are higher and much more vigorous.

Running Speed

Speed is determined by the *length of stride* and *frequency (speed) of stride*. For increased running speed, one or both of these factors must be increased. Length of stride is dependent primarily upon leg length and the power of the stride. Leg speed (frequency) is mostly dependent upon speed of muscle contractions and neuromuscular coordination (skill) in running.

Running mechanics vary from one person to another, and they vary in the same person running at different speeds (Figure 17-3). More specifically, running mechanics change with speed in the following ways:

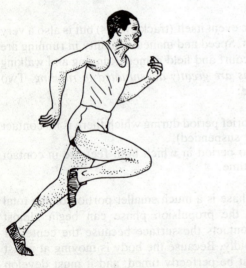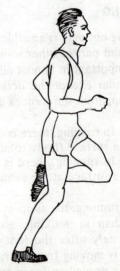

Sprinter   Distance runner

Figure 17-3 Differences in running styles at different speeds. When compared with the sprinter, the distance runner typically runs with shorter strides, less vigorous and lower arm actions, a more upright body position, and more foot-surface contact.

1 Amount and type of foot contact with the surface
2 Amount of joint flexion and extension
3 Amount of body inclination

At a slow running speed, complete foot contact is used. The foot-surface contact with each stride goes from the ball of the foot to the heel and back to the ball (restful to calf muscles). As running rate increases, the amount of foot contact becomes less, until finally at full speed only the forward part of the foot contacts the surface. The sprinter "runs on the toes."

At a slow running speed, a relatively small amount of action occurs in the joints throughout the body, and the runner tends to run with the arms low. As speed is increased, more flexion and extension occur in the arm and leg joints, and other joint actions increase accordingly. Also, the arm action is higher.

At slower speeds, runners tend to run more erectly, whereas at full speed, the typical sprinter leans forward at about 15° from the perpendicular. Forward lean usually comes naturally with the increased propulsive forces, and conscious attempts to increase lean are not usually necessary. However, on occasion it is necessary to teach a runner to increase forward lean.

Sprinting Sprinting is essentially a power performance. It depends on one's ability to project the body forcefully and rapidly from alternate feet. Developed to a peak relatively early in life, about age twenty for men and about eighteen for women, running speed is a quality that can be improved a limited amount. The best possibilities for increasing speed are (1) to increase the power (force times velocity) of the leg extensor muscles, thus causing more powerful propelling forces, and (2) to practice running at top speeds, which should improve sprinting technique and the specific coordinations involved in sprinting. In certain instances, errors in the mechanics of sprinting may be corrected, which may improve speed.

Middle-Distance Running Middle distances are run at a fast pace and with a style that is somewhat more relaxed than the sprinting style. Of course, the speed and running form varies with the length of the particular race. But, generally speaking, when compared with sprinting, middle-distance running requires less joint action, less forward inclination, and more complete foot-surface contact. Pace is very important, and physiologists generally agree that an even pace over the entire distance is the most economical. In middle-distance races, success is determined by the correct combination of (1) running speed, (2) running efficiency, and (3) running endurance. Circulorespiratory endurance exerts the greatest influence in middle distances where a relatively long distance must be covered at a fairly fast pace.

Long-Distance Running   Long distances are run at a slower pace, with great emphasis placed on a relaxed and easy running style, which conserves energy. As compared with middle-distance running, the long distances require still less joint action, less forward lean, and maximum foot-surface contact. Here again, an even pace over the entire distance is recommended. Whereas endurance (especially of the circulorespiratory system) has limited influence on sprinting, it is very important in distance running. Research shows that the long-distance runner assumes about 80 percent of his or her maximum oxygen uptake and attempts to maintain this level throughout the race. In long distances another prime factor is the ability to conserve energy. Of course, a reasonable amount of running speed is always beneficial.

Running in Sports Other than Track   Field and court games like football, basketball, and baseball often require changes in direction, changes of pace, stability from lateral forces, and other changes which demand agility-type movements while running. These maneuvers are always made at a sacrifice to straight-ahead speed. Under such conditions, the location and movement of the center of gravity need to be more precisely controlled. The length of stride is often reduced so foot-surface contact will be more frequent, enabling quick changes in direction. Also, more lateral spread of the feet is often desirable. The trunk is usually carried with less forward lean than in sprinting. The typical even cadence of the running strides may be interrupted as adjustments are made in speed and direction. Energy patterns are specifically developed in response to demands. One trains energy sources by specific duplication of the kinds of requirements encountered in each sport.

Incorrect Mechanics of Running

Even some champions run incorrectly, and if their running styles could be corrected, some of them would run faster (see Figure 17-4, for example). If running mechanics deviate from the following important guides, incorrect mechanics are used, resulting in some loss of running efficiency:

1   The knees and toes should point straight in the line of progress. Deviations from this in either direction result in loss of power.
2   The middle of the body should pass directly over the inner sole of each footprint. Any lateral deviation from this results in loss of power and a weaving action of the total body (Figure 17-5).
3   The total body should incline forward at about 15° from perpen-

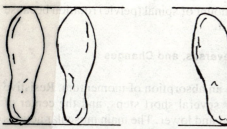
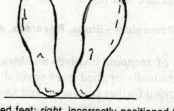

Figure 17-4 *Left*, correctly positioned feet; *right*, incorrectly positioned feet. A loss of distance on each stride results from turning the feet slightly outward. (*Clarence Robison, Clayne Jensen, Sherald James, and Willard Hirschi, Modern Techniques of Track and Field, Lea & Febiger, Philadelphia, 1974.*)

dicular at top running speed. The amount of incline will gradually reduce as running rate is reduced. If the incline is too far forward, the propelling forces will be too horizontal. Too little incline will cause the forces to be too vertical. If, when viewed from the side, a runner's head moves up and down excessively with each stride, misdirected propelling forces are indicated.

4 The arm swing should be close to the body, and the hands should swing forward to a point in front of the chest. Almost all arm action should occur at the shoulder joint. There should be only slight movement at the elbows.

5 Rotary movements in the spine and at the hip joints should be reasonably free, because these movements can greatly enhance the length of stride. In a way, the rotation of the pelvis substitutes for the limited amount of hyperextension available at the hips (restricted by the strong anterior capsular ligaments). Any excessive spinal curvatures (lordosis,

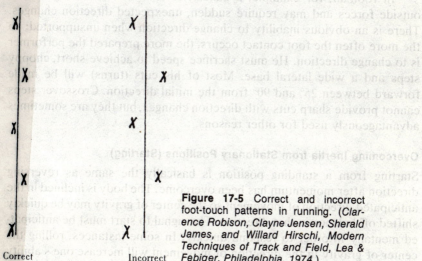

Correct   Incorrect

Figure 17-5 Correct and incorrect foot-touch patterns in running. (*Clarence Robison, Clayne Jensen, Sherald James, and Willard Hirschi, Modern Techniques of Track and Field, Lea & Febiger, Philadelphia, 1974.*)

kyphosis, scoliosis) restrict the amount of spinal (pelvic) rotation because the bone structure will not allow it.

Controlling Momentum—Stops, Reverses, and Changes of Direction

The process of *stopping* involves an absorption of momentum. Resistive forces are gradually applied over several short steps, and the center of gravity is carried farther backward and lower. The main muscular actions involved are eccentric contractions of the hip, knee, and ankle extensors. The ability of these muscles to resist force (their strength) is very important to stopping quickly.

A *reverse* is a stop with an immediate reversal of momentum. After the momentum has been dissipated as described above, the body is immediately turned, led by upper body rotation, and put into motion in the opposite direction. The body should already be inclined in the new direction of movement; however, some additional lean may be needed at the moment the reversal occurs. The same muscles (hip, knee, and ankle extensors) that contracted eccentrically to stop the body now contract concentrically to put it into motion in the new direction. The toe flexors are also important contributors. Both reversing and sharply *changing direction* with a jab-type step while running involve essentially the same actions. The force for direction change is always applied at about right angles to the length of the foot. For a 90° turn, the planted foot continues to point along the initial line of direction. If a 45° turn is desired, the foot is toed out about 45°. If more than 90° is desired, the foot is toed in a corresponding amount.

In football, for example, a ballcarrier is in constant danger from outside forces and may require sudden, unexpected direction changes. There is an obvious inability to change direction when unsupported; so the more often the foot contact occurs, the more prepared the performer is to change direction. He must sacrifice speed to achieve short, choppy steps and a wide lateral base. Most of his cuts (turns) will be made forward between 25° and 90° from the initial direction. Crossover steps cannot provide sharp cuts with direction changes, but they are sometimes advantageously used for other reasons.

Overcoming Inertia from Stationary Positions (Starting)

Starting from a standing position is basically the same as reversing direction after momentum has been overcome. The body is inclined in the anticipated direction of movement so the center of gravity may be quickly shifted off-balance in that direction. The signal to start must be anticipated mentally in order to respond quickly. In some instances, rolling the center of gravity in the direction of movement will increase one's ability to move quickly once the signal is given. However, in racing starts, such action is illegal. In other activities, such as baseball, tennis, football, and basketball, this procedure often makes the difference between success and failure. However, occasionally it results in error when a quick adjustment in the intended direction of movement must be made, and the body is already off-balance in the anticipated direction.

The position of the crouch, track, and football starts were discussed in Chapter 15, but the process of gaining acceleration following the start has not been discussed (Figures 17-6 and 17-7). The short and powerful strides used in accelerating are energy-consuming; however, they are necessary to accelerate rapidly. One reason for the short strides is that the base must be reestablished often because of the excessive amount of forward body lean. A second reason for short strides is that the leg joints

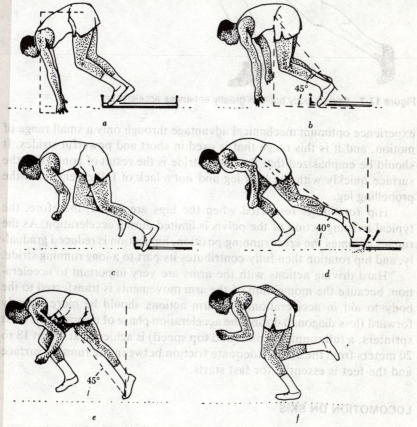

Figure 17-6 A sprinter must design his starting technique so that the forces are correctly directed. The above illustrations show the former world-record-holder Bob Hayes at the start. Illustration a shows him in a high hip position with his shoulders 8 or 10 centimeters beyond his hands. Illustrations b and c show his low body position (body at 45° angle, back parallel to the track). Illustration d shows the extreme horizontal components of his initial drive. Illustrations e and f show him a few meters from the blocks.

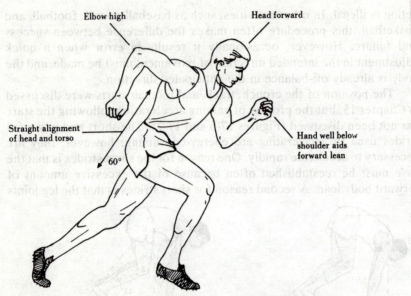

Elbow high

Head forward

Straight alignment
of head and torso

60°

Hand well below
shoulder aids
forward lean

Figure 17-7 Correct body position greatly enhances acceleration.

experience optimum mechanical advantage through only a small range of motion, and it is this range that is used in short and powerful strides. It should be emphasized that the short stride is the result of contacting the surface quickly with the lead leg and *not* a lack of full extension in the propelling leg.

Hip rotation is restricted when the hips are flexed; therefore, the typical twisting action of the pelvis is limited during acceleration. As the runner assumes the erect running position, hip flexion is reduced gradually, and hip rotation then fully contributes its part to a long running stride.

Hard driving actions with the arms are very important to acceleration, because the momentum of the arm movements is transferred to the body to aid in acceleration. The arm actions should be more directly forward (less diagonal) during the acceleration phase of a sprint. For most sprinters, a full running stride (and top speed) is achieved at about 18 to 20 meters from the start. Adequate friction between the running surface and the feet is essential for fast starts.

LOCOMOTION ON SKIS

In downhill skiing the propelling force is provided by the force of gravity. Skis are especially designed to provide a minimum amount of friction against the snow, and waxing the skis may reduce the friction even more. The various body segments are used to support and balance the body and to perform maneuvers.

Skis enlarge one's base of support in the forward-backward direction, thus making greater lean possible without loss of balance. The base of support in the lateral direction is determined by the width at which the skis are placed from each other. Beginning skiers tend to keep the base wide so they can maintain balance. Expert skiers narrow the base because this aids in maneuvering.

The typical body position of the skier (Figure 17-8) is (1) skis parallel and close together, (2) partial flexion at the ankles, knees, and hips, (3) elbows close to sides and bent to about 110° angle, and (4) the whole body leaning forward so the center of gravity is over the balls of the feet. Generally, the steeper the slope, the more flexion there should be in the lower extremities. The flexion of the legs provides the skier with several advantages: (1) it lowers the center of gravity, and this aids in balance; (2) it places the skier in a position of readiness so quick adjustments in body position can be made; and (3) it provides the opportunity to cushion over rough spots.

As the skier extends the legs, the weight is temporarily lifted from the skis, which allows them to move faster over the snow. Flexing the legs has an opposite effect on speed because it weights the skis. The muscles used mainly in supporting body weight on skis are the hip, knee, and ankle extensors. These are also the muscles used in weighting and unweighting the skis. In weighting (leg flexion), the extensor muscles contract eccentrically; in unweighting (leg extension), the extensor muscles contract concentrically. Other muscles of great importance to skiing are the hip and spinal rotators. In downhill racing the hip and back extensor muscles also get a good overload in the skier's aerodynamic position, where the trunk is basically held in a position parallel to the snow surface.

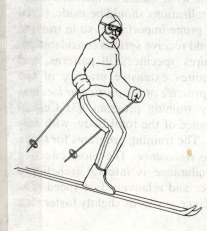

Figure 17-8 Side view of a good straight-run skiing position. Joint flexion and forward body lean are essential.

The forces used to effect a change in direction (turns) are (1) deflecting force—resistance against the side of the ski, which is caused by the snow and results from the correct edging of the skis during a turn; (2) turning force—moving one ski at an angle to the direction of descent and using a transfer of body weight to that ski, thus causing the turn, as in snowplow and stem turns; (3) turning power of the body—counterrotation of the body to cause the skis to turn, as in the short swing and the wedeln techniques.

LOCOMOTION ON SKATES

Skating action is much like walking action. The support phase of the walk becomes the skating glide. During the glide, the skate blades are placed approximately in the line of progress because this position presents minimum resistance against forward movement. The propelling foot must have the toes turned outward at the time of the push (outward rotation at the hip) in order to utilize the sharp edge of the blade and to present as much of the blade edge as possible to the ice. This foot position is necessary to gain sufficient friction between the blade and the ice, but it results in glides that, of necessity, must be somewhat oblique to the line of direction. Sharp blades add a great deal to propulsion. Forward momentum is greatly aided by forward lean at the hips and sweeping arm actions with the arms fairly straight. Diagonal movement of the arms is emphasized. At high skating speeds air resistance is reduced by a horizontal body position.

TRAINING FOR LOCOMOTIVE SKILLS

Locomotive skills vary so much in their nature that it is necessary to analyze each skill separately to determine what should be included in the training program. However, a few generalizations should be made. (1) In most locomotive skills, leg power is of prime importance; so in training for such skills, *increasing leg power* should receive serious consideration. (2) Each method of locomotion requires specific skill patterns, and development of the skill patterns requires extensive practice of the correct technique. Therefore, *extensive practice of the particular locomotive skill* is an important part of any training program. (3) Certain locomotive events require much endurance of the total body, with emphasis on circulorespiratory endurance. The training programs for these events must concentrate on *increasing endurance.* The most effective means known for developing such endurance is interval (repetition) training with emphasis on underdistance and relatively fast speed (distances shorter than the competitive distance at speeds slightly faster than the competitive speed). The ideal number of repetitions for a practice session is not established; this number can be greatly influenced by the length of each repeated distance, the speed at which it is performed, and the condition of the performer. For additional information on interval training, refer to Chapter 9.

STUDENT LABORATORY EXPERIENCES

Consider and solve the following problems to gain quantitative experience with the concepts presented in this chapter.

1. What is the distance covered by a walker who has 1.2-meter stride with a frequency of 150 strides per minute during a 10-minute interval? (See formula **1**.)

2. In running a 400-meter race, an athlete toes out on each stride so that her foot length is 2 centimeters shorter than if she toed straight ahead. If her stride length averaged 2 meters per stride, how much more distance could she cover in the same length of time (50 seconds) if she toed straight ahead? (See formula **1**.)

3. A runner starts from the blocks. After 0.3 meters of movement he has a velocity of 3 meters per second. (*a*) What is his acceleration? (*b*) If at 0.6 meters his velocity is 4 meters per second, what is the new acceleration? (*c*) If at 1 meter his new velocity is 5 meters per second, what is the new acceleration? (See formulas **1, 2, 3**.)

4. A runner at maximum velocity runs 20 meters in 2.2 seconds. Her stride length is 2 meters. (*a*) What is her velocity? (*b*) What is her stride frequency? (See formula **1**.)

5. A runner rounds a curve in a 200-meter oval track. The curve radius is 20 meters. (*a*) How much centrifugal force would an 80-kilogram runner have at a velocity of 10 meters per second on the curve? (*b*) What angle of lean with the vertical must be achieved to keep the runner in the lane? (See formulas **50, 51**.)

6. A basketball player with good shoes who weighs 882 newtons requires a 490-newton horizontal pull at the ankles to make his shoes slide. What is the coefficient of friction of shoes with the floor? (See formula **51**.)

7. If the player in problem 6 changes direction while running, what is the maximum angle of lean with the vertical he can manage without slipping? (See formula **51**.)

8. Upon what factors does a skier's acceleration depend?

Chapter 18

Body-Projection Skills

Jumps are defined as body projections characterized by landing simultaneously on both feet. Takeoffs for jumps can be from either one foot or both feet. *Leaps* and *hops* occur only with takeoffs from one foot and landing on one foot. The leap differs from the hop in that in the leap the landing foot is not the same as the takeoff foot, whereas in the hop the same foot is used for takeoff and landing.

Several mechanical principles are common to all jumps, leaps, and hops: (1) They all depend upon the counterforce available from the supporting surface. All factors which reduce maximum counterforce, such as insufficient friction between the performer and the surface or "give" in the supporting surface, in any of the performer's joints, or in both, are detrimental to a maximum projection. (2) They all involve similar patterns of sequential muscular actions. In each case the main propulsive force comes from the supporting leg (or legs), beginning with hip extension, followed by knee extension, ankle and foot extension (plantar flexion), and toe flexion. (3) In each case the "transfer of momentum" principle is applied when nonsupporting body parts (arms,

308

shoulders, and often the free leg) are thrust in the direction of projection; these motions are initiated prior to the application of the propulsive force. The transfer of momentum (thrust of body parts) exerts its maximum influence only if the body segments are moving rapidly in the direction of the projection when the performer leaves the surface. If deviations from this ideal timing occur, the effectiveness of the thrust is reduced.

In addition to the mechanical factors already mentioned, the following influence body projections:

1 Individuals possessing high centers of gravity enjoy an advantage when the purpose is to project their bodies vertically over barriers, such as high-jumping or hurdling, or when reaching height is important, such as basketball rebounding or the basketball lay-up shot. These individuals also have an advantage, though less obvious, in horizontal projections for distance, such as barrel-jumping on ice skates, long-jumping, and triple-jumping. This advantage results from the principle that a body remains in flight only as long as it takes to move through its vertical plane of flight, regardless of the horizontal distance the body covers. A lower center of gravity is one reason why women cannot equal men in body-projection performances. On the average, women are shorter and their centers of gravity are proportionately lower than men's. Other more important factors are involved, however.

2 Another advantageous anatomical feature is longer levers. If bones are longer, more linear velocity can be developed at their ends, provided that angular velocity remains constant. Long-geared performers enjoy this advantage if they have sufficient power to achieve comparable angular velocity.

Physiological factors which contribute significantly to body projections are *strength* and *speed of movement.* Projections performed for maximum distance are tests of power. Power is a combination of force (strength) and velocity (speed of movement). Therefore, the force and speed with which the mover muscles contract will greatly influence projections. Antagonist muscles must relax to reduce resistance to the development of power.

Excessive weight, especially weight due to fat which does not contribute to performance, hinders projections of the body. Weight due to additional muscle also adds resistance, but its contribution to the action may exceed its detrimental effects. Small dumbbells held in the hands have been shown to improve long-jumping performances significantly. Such devices are outlawed in the rules of competition but do demonstrate the important contribution of the transfer of momentum.

Inflexibility at certain joints may restrict the needed range of motion for a maximum projection. By analyzing the mechanics of a performance, the body regions which need unusual flexibility can be identified, and specific exercises can be used to develop the flexibility necessary for maximum performance.

STATIONARY TAKEOFFS

Projection of the body from a stationary position depends almost entirely upon two factors: (1) explosive power from leg extension and (2) ability to transfer momentum from other body parts. The momentum of the swinging body parts (arms and shoulders) overcomes part of the body's inertia, and this action aids in shifting the center of gravity to a position where the forces from the legs can be directed through it. The leg-extension action must encounter the center of gravity when it is located in the best position for optimum results.

If the objective is to project the body forward for a maximum horizontal distance, then leg extension must occur when the center of gravity is well forward of the feet, and the arm and upper-body thrust must be directed partly toward the horizontal. If, at the time of leg extension, a line were drawn from the feet through the center of gravity, that line would create nearly a 45° angle with the surface. The pressure of the feet on the surface is both downward and backward. If the objective is to project the body vertically, thrust is made upward, and leg extension occurs when the center of gravity is directly above the base of support.

Double-Leg Stationary Projections

The use of both legs in stationary takeoffs affords two advantages over single-leg projections: (1) the projecting force is increased about twofold and (2) the larger supporting base enhances balance. The feet should be spread about the width of the shoulders in order to aid balance and ensure that the forces will be properly directed. The two legs must contribute about equally. If one leg generates more force than the other, or if the two legs do not extend simultaneously, the projection will not be in the intended direction. Similarly, the two arms must produce momentum of about equal amounts simultaneously. Check points in leg and foot positions include feet below the shoulders, toes pointing in the intended line of flight, and knees directly above and pointing in the same direction as the toes.

The optimum amount the legs should flex to develop maximum force depends upon the strength of the extensor muscles. If the crouch is deeper, force can be applied over a greater distance to develop more acceleration. Conversely, the greater depth of crouch signifies that more work must be done to lift the body, and as the joint angles become less, the muscles must "pull around corners" at the joints. Strong muscles are more effective when joint flexion is slightly less than 90° (deep crouch); weak muscles contribute best with lesser amounts of flexion (shallow crouch).

Greater muscle forces are developed when the stretch reflex adds nerve impulses to those impulses voluntarily provided. Recall, the stretch reflex is initiated by sudden stretching of the agonist muscles, provided the stretch is followed immediately by contraction of those muscles. (Refer to discussion of stretch reflex in Chapter 4.) Basically, this means that a slight, sharp dipping action (sudden crouch) should immediately precede and flow into the leg-extension action. If a pause occurs at the bottom of the dip, the effects of the stretch reflex are lost. If the dip is extensive, too much downward momentum develops, which wastes contractile force in the reversing of such momentum.

Standing Long Jump   This skill depends greatly upon leg power, and is often used to measure that trait. However, correct technique is very important to success. Studies show that at takeoff inferior jumpers do not have their centers of gravity as far forward as better jumpers. Upon landing, the feet of the inferior performers are usually not as far forward of their centers of gravity as the feet of better performers. When a jump is correctly performed, the angle of projection with the surface is slightly less than 45°, because the center of gravity is at a lower level upon landing than it was at takeoff.

The driving force is initiated with an arm swing directed forward and upward, which is combined with thrusting actions of the shoulder girdle and trunk. Momentum from these movements is transferred to the total body during the jump—this momentum can add greatly to the distance of the jump. However, the primary driving force comes from hip, knee, and ankle extension and toe flexion. The center of gravity should be well ahead of the feet at the time of leg extension in order that the force from the legs may be correctly directed.

During flight, leg joints must quickly be flexed so the lower body can swing through rapidly, resulting in the feet reaching as far forward as possible upon landing. Care must be taken not to reach too far with the feet, because loss of balance backward may result from insufficient momentum to carry the center of gravity forward to a position above the base of support.

The main muscles contributing to the projection are the shoulder flexors, shoulder-girdle elevators, back extensors, hip, knee, and ankle extensors, and toe flexors. Note that the gluteus maximus, the strongest hip extensor muscle, contributes only when the hip is flexed beyond 15°; therefore, deep flexion at the hip is important. During flight, the abdominal muscles must contract strongly to stabilize the pelvis, which enables the hip flexors to lift the thighs during the flight.

Common errors in this skill are (1) incorrect angle of projection, (2) lack of precise coordination of the swinging parts with leg extension, and (3) loss of distance resulting from improper positioning of the feet upon landing. The landing errors occur when the feet fail to reach forward enough or when too low a projection does not permit sufficient time in flight to achieve a correct landing position.

Racing Dive This skill (see Figure 18-1) is different from the standing long jump in only three ways: (1) The center of gravity shifts much farther forward before leg and trunk extension occurs, in fact, so far forward that the projection is almost horizontal. (2) The toes curl around the pool's edge so that the last push may be perpendicular to the resisting surface (the pool's vertical edge). If this situation did not exist, the lack of friction between the two surfaces would detract a great deal from the projection. (3) Projected into a prone position, the body is as straight and slender as possible in order to reduce water resistance against forward motion upon entry into the water. Upon landing, the body should be at an angle of only 5 to 10° below the horizontal.

Current practice on college swim teams for the breast stroke is a

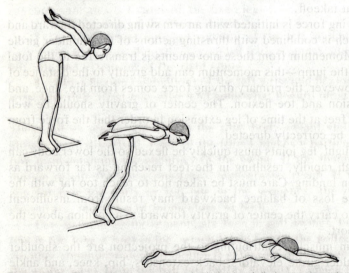

Figure 18-1 The ability to project the body horizontally is very important in the racing dive. The angle of projection and angle of entry must be correct to get maximum horizontal distance.

modification of the above-described racing dive. This new style requires a higher angle of takeoff, a greater distance of projection, a much steeper angle of entry with the body in a semijackknife position. Upon entering the water the arms, trunk, hips, and legs do a body wave by pressing the body from semipike to arch during entry. This results in a giant force-producing dolphin kick which greatly accelerates the swimmer and lengthens the glide (as it takes longer to slow down to swimming speed). Some skilled swimmers do not surface or begin stroking until reaching midpool in a 25-meter pool.

Vertical Jump   The vertical jump for height (see Figure 18-2) is dependent upon leg power, and it is highly correlated with the standing long jump. The widest use of the vertical jump is in basketball, volleyball, and dance activities, but it is also used in many other performances. The basic technique is similar to that of the standing long jump, except that the forces are directed upward and the projection takes place with the center of gravity directly over the base of support. Some individuals achieve better results when they assume a stance with one foot slightly forward of the other. This position provides improved stability in the forward-backward direction; however, it should not be overdone so that less advantageous joint angles appear.

After initiation of the upward movement of the arms, the movements that follow in very close sequence are hip, knee, and ankle extension and toe flexion. The combined forces from these movements determine how high the body will be projected.

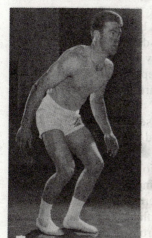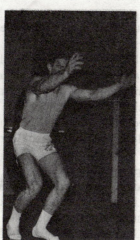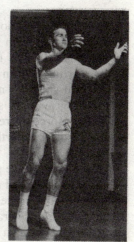

Figure 18-2 Source and direction of projecting forces in the vertical jump.

Trampoline Bounce   The trampoline bounce is a unique kind of vertical bounce performed on a mat with elastic qualities due to springs. The important body actions necessary to create and utilize the energy stored in the mat are discussed in Chapter 12, under stored counterforce. The arms and shoulders are used to transfer momentum, as in the vertical jump, but they have an additional use when great heights are attained. They maintain balance while the body is in flight, and they serve this purpose best when abducted to a horizontal position with elbows flexed horizontally. When the arms are in the abducted position, their weight is farther from the body, and thus the movements of the arms are more effective in controlling balance. The tightrope walker uses this effect by selecting a long balance pole. Balance during flight is essential, because if the base of support is not directly under the center of gravity in the landing, little can be done to control the direction of the subsequent bounce.

The performer should contact the mat with the legs straight and rigid, which causes maximum depression of the trampoline mat, allowing the mat to store more energy. Near the bottom of the bounce (mat almost fully depressed), the arms and shoulders should be thrust downward to add a final bit of downward momentum, and the legs should assume slight flexion. As the mat responds (releasing its stored energy), the arms and shoulders are thrust upward, and the legs are extended. These body movements must be correctly timed to the response of the trampoline mat. It is important to land near the center of the mat to get maximum benefit from its elasticity, and to avoid being thrown off-balance by its response.

Back Dive   Various back dives and some backward projections in tumbling begin from stationary stances and depend upon double-leg projections. Most of the same principles apply to these projections as apply to projections in a forward direction. Exceptions are (1) the transfer of arm and shoulder momentum is more upward and backward, (2) the center of gravity is shifted behind the base of support, and (3) the projecting force is reduced somewhat because a major force (ankle plantar flexion) is partly eliminated in backward projections.

Rotations   Some projections require rotation of the body in either a forward or backward direction (diving and trampoline stunts). It should be understood that the force for the rotation is created at takeoff and only accelerated or decelerated by body positions in flight. For example, if one wished to perform a backward somersault from a diving board, the amount of rotation produced would depend on the timing of the leg extension in relation to the position of the body's center of gravity. If the line of force is directly through the center of gravity, no rotation occurs; however, if the center of gravity is off center from the line of force, the body will tend to rotate in the direction in which the center of gravity is displaced. For the performer to accomplish a forward somersault, the center of gravity must be slightly forward of the line of force. A backward somersault requires that the center of gravity is slightly behind the line of force. After a given amount of rotating force has been applied, the speed with which the body rotates depends upon its weight and the position of its segments. The less it weighs and the closer its segments are to its center, the faster it will rotate. This is the reason a diver rotates relatively slowly in a lay-out position, faster in a pike position, and still faster in a tuck position.

Single-Leg Stationary Projections

Single-leg projections from stationary positions are not often used. A few movements may qualify as single-leg projections, but they appear more as exaggerated weight shifts. Among these movements are dodging actions from stationary positions and standing leaps in dance. In any case, such activities are limited in use, and the principles involved do not differ from the principles already discussed.

MOVING TAKEOFFS

The principles discussed in the preceding section, stationary takeoffs, also pertain to skills found in this section. The primary difference between projections involving a stationary takeoff and those involving a moving takeoff is that the latter includes an approach used to develop additional momentum of the whole body. In a projection involving an approach, the key to success is to add a correct vertical component of force to the horizontal momentum. This involves correct positioning of the center of gravity in relation to the line of the projecting force, as was the case with stationary takeoffs. But with the running approach, the skill becomes more intricate and the timing more precise. In moving takeoffs, balance is harder to control, the muscles must act with greater speed and more precise timing, and the projecting forces must act in concert with the momentum of the approach; these actions, along with power, project the body a maximum distance at the desired angle.

Double-Leg Moving Projections

Only a few double-leg projections are used in combination with a moving takeoff because the double-leg takeoff requires that velocity be carefully controlled in order to assume the double-leg position.

Tumbling, Gymnastic, and Diving Skills   Double-leg moving takeoffs are used in various gymnastic performances on the long horse and in such tumbling performances as the forward roll and dive-and-roll. In these performances, considerable horizontal speed is necessary to carry the body through the performance. At the same time, it is necessary to project the body forward in a position square with the direction of movement, a position which can be accomplished only by using moving double-leg takeoffs. Following the run, a short and rather high hurdle step is taken. The hurdle step checks the horizontal speed and converts some of it to the vertical direction. Also, the hurdle step allows the performer time to position the body for a double-leg landing. Upon landing on both feet simultaneously, the performer assumes a position similar to that at the beginning of the standing long jump, and the subsequent movements are practically the same as those discussed earlier in the standing long jump. The body is moving forward rapidly; therefore, the projecting movements must be precisely timed.

In springboard diving (Figure 18-3), the approach is terminated with a hurdle step. The main objective of the approach is to gain height and correct body position during the hurdle. The more height the performer gains, the more force he can apply downward to depress the board. The farther the board is depressed, the more energy it stores, and the stronger will be its reaction. The body actions during the double-leg projection in diving are almost identical to those in the vertical jump. In the dive, the body actions must be perfectly timed with the rebound of the board. Placement of the feet in relation to the end of the board is very important to the responsiveness of the board. For best results, the toes should be near the end (within 2.5 or 5 centimeters), but not beyond the end. The objective of the spring is to gain as much height as possible to allow time to perform the desired dive. *Remember* that a body remains in flight only as long as it takes to move through its vertical plane of flight.

Ski Jump   The development of velocity for the ski jump is provided by a push-off at the top of the runway followed by acceleration due to gravity. The skier can develop even greater velocity if he can reduce friction and air resistance as he moves down the runway. The technique of the takeoff is about the same as for double-leg takeoffs, except that the skier is less concerned with the powerful extension and more concerned with balance and perfect timing. Because of the excessive speed of the jumper, excessive forward lean is necessary.

The airborne phase requires the use of some principles of aerodynamics as the jumper utilizes air resistance to prolong his flight by correctly positioning his body and skis. The ski tips are angled slightly

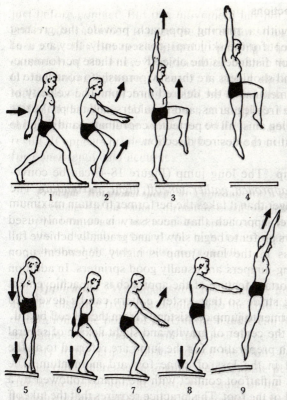

Figure 18-3 Body actions during the hurdle and takeoff in springboard diving. The body thrust must be perfectly timed with the response of the board. The transfer of momentum by the arms and swinging leg is very important to the height of the hurdle; transfer of momentum downward from the arm and shoulder action to depress the board is equally important.

upward to catch the wind, and the total body is angled forward and upward for several reasons, one of which is to increase upward air lift. The arms are held close to the sides with the hands slightly back of the hips. Air resistance has unusual potential in this event because of the long period of time the jumper is airborne and the great velocity attained during the approach. The jumper must maintain balance and good form upon landing (this is included in the judging); it is done by (1) increasing the forward-backward base of support by placing one ski slightly forward of the other, (2) absorbing the landing shock with controlled flexion at several joints (eccentric contraction of extensor muscles), (3) maintaining the center of gravity well forward but within the base of support, and (4) spreading the arms sideward to aid lateral balance (the skis should be spread very little).

Single-Leg Moving Projections

Single-leg projections with a running approach provide the greatest amount of velocity (except for the ski jump); consequently, they are used when maximum height or distance is the objective. In these performances, the free leg, arms, and shoulders are thrust vigorously to contribute to the development of momentum in the desired direction. The velocity of the run, the thrust of the free leg, arms, and shoulders, and the projecting force from the push-off leg must all be perfectly coordinated and timed to provide maximum thrust in the desired direction.

Running Long Jump The long jump (Figure 18-4) can be conveniently divided into the *approach, gather, takeoff, flight*, and *landing*. The approach need be no longer than it takes the performer to attain maximum running speed. A longer approach than necessary is commonly used because most performers prefer to begin slowly and gradually achieve full speed. Because success in the long jump is highly dependent upon running speed, good long-jumpers are usually good sprinters. In addition to speed, the other important feature of the approach is the achievement of a consistent running stride so that a step pattern can be developed which will aid the performer to jump consistently from the takeoff board.

The positioning of the center of gravity and slight flexion of several joints (sinking action) in preparation for the jump are referred to as the gather, and they result in the loss of some forward momentum. The gathering action results in flatfoot contact with the board, followed by a rolling action to the ball of the foot. This practice requires that the takeoff heel be afforded special protection from heel bruises.

The takeoff itself results from the combination of three forces: (1) velocity from the run; (2) push-off from the leg; and (3) thrusting actions with the swinging leg and arms. Each of these forces must make its maximum contribution, and the three forces must be perfectly timed. The major muscle groups involved in the takeoff are the hip, knee, and ankle extensors of the takeoff leg, the hip flexors of the swinging leg, and the shoulder flexors.

Optimum angle of projection at takeoff varies slightly with individuals depending upon their jumping styles. Even though the optimum angle would seem to be about 40°, the rapid horizontal speed from the run makes it impractical to project the body at an angle greater than about 30° from the surface. Most inexperienced performers tend *not* to jump high enough. The takeoff and flight involve most of the principles of projections discussed in Chapter 14.

The "run-in-air," or hitch-kick, flight is the most widely used. Actions while in flight are used to aid balance and to assume a good body position for landing, and the move may be either change the angle of flight to prolong the

The swinging leg is very important to success of the jump, for it must be brought back so that it is possible and will allow the center of gravity to move up over the base of support as the jumper lands in a position where position with feet spread apart buttocks as between them. He cushions the landing by flexing the knees, allowing each of the body at the points of support.

Running High Jump This discussion refers specifically to the "osbury flop" technique (Figure 18-5). Many of the basic principles involved apply to other techniques, but not exactly in the same way. The tall, long-legged person has a definite structural advantage in the high jump. To properly execute technique the body's center of gravity must be raised to within 2 centimeters of the crossbar height. Because

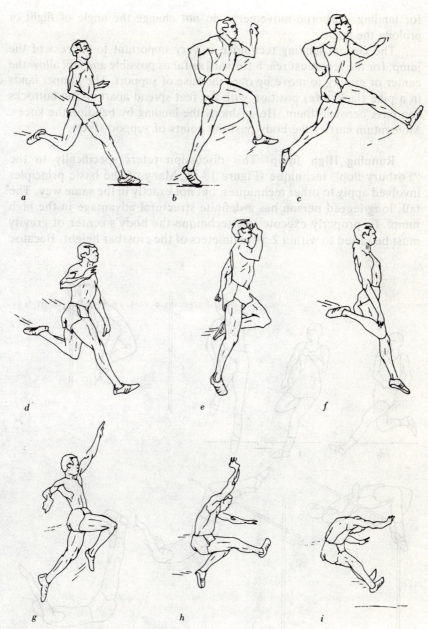

Figure 18-4 Illustration of good technique in the running long jump.

for landing. Airborne movements do *not* change the angle of flight or prolong the flight.

The correct landing technique is very important to success of the jump, for the feet must reach forward as far as possible and still allow the center of gravity to move up over the base of support. The jumper lands in a pike (jackknife) position with the feet spread apart so the buttocks can pass between them. He cushions the landing by bending the knees. Momentum carries the body past the points of support (feet).

Running High Jump   This discussion refers specifically to the "Fosbury flop" technique (Figure 18-5). Many of the basic principles involved apply to other techniques, but not exactly in the same way. The tall, long-legged person has a definite structural advantage in the high jump. To properly execute this technique the body's center of gravity must be raised to within 2.5 centimeters of the crossbar height. Because

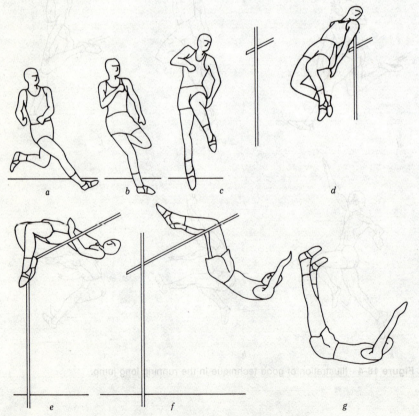

Figure 18-5   Illustration of Dick Fosbury in the flop technique.

of this, the person with a relatively high center of gravity needs to attain less distance upward to clear the bar.

Location of the center of gravity above the soles of the feet generally varies between 55 and 56 percent of total body height in adult males. If a man 183 centimeters tall has long legs in comparison with his height, his center of gravity could be located about 107 centimeters above the surface in his normal standing position. This means that if he raised his center of gravity another 10 centimeters in a tiptoe takeoff position, then projected his center of gravity vertically an additional 107 centimeters with the best possible crossing in the flop style (with his center of gravity 2 centimeters below the bar), the total height that could be reached would be 226 centimeters, or 7 feet, 5 inches. A man whose center of gravity is 10 centimeters lower would have to project his body an additional 10 centimeters to achieve the same height.

For purposes of analysis the high jump can be conveniently divided into the *approach*, the *lift*, the *crossing*, and the *landing*. The approach is designed to serve three purposes: (1) to counteract centrifugal force created in the curved approach by body lean away from the bar during the last three steps before takeoff (the velocity is considerably greater than in the straddle style); (2) to develop horizontal speed which can be converted to the vertical direction by backward lean on plant; and (3) to place body parts in position to contribute best to the vertical thrust at takeoff. With the horizontal distance (takeoff to landing) stored in the curved approach, the jumper can devote all the momentum possible to raising the body vertically. It is important to develop a step pattern to make the point of takeoff and the velocity at takeoff consistent. The last stride should be a bit longer (Figure 18-5a), placing the center of gravity well behind the planted foot, while still maintaining inward lean. The angle of crossing should be about 30° to the bar (the tangent to the circular approach at the point of plant).

The lift occurs simultaneously with the loss of body lean and requires precise coordination; hip and knee extension plus plantar flexion of the takeoff leg must be timed to coincide with the passing of the center of gravity over the takeoff foot. The lift also requires correct timing of movement of the shoulders, arms, and nonsupport leg to contribute upward thrust (Figure 18-5c). On leaving the ground, centrifugal force pulls the jumper toward the bar along the aforementioned tangent line; while the force of the jump carries him up, the body rotates a quarter turn to present the back to the bar. This is accomplished by moving the nonsupport leg away from the bar, thus causing a rotation of the body. At this point the jumper is able to see the bar by looking over his shoulder (Figure 18-5d).

The crossing occurs with the back arched, hips extended, and knees flexed (Figure 18-5e). Arms are kept at the sides. The body is perpendicular to the bar with only a small segment over the bar at one time. During the jump the body is following a rotation about the center of gravity. As the head and shoulders drop below the bar and the lower legs approach it, the hips are flexed and the knees are extended. This causes a reaction, reversing the rotation of the trunk toward the thighs, permitting a safe landing on the upper back on a foam pad (Figure 18-5f and g). It also permits the legs to clear the bar.

A common error of "flop-style" jumpers is that they fail to maintain the circular approach with lean into the final stride before takeoff. This causes the loss of the stored centrifugal force and also forces the jumper to cross the bar with the body at about 20 to 30° angle. Such an angle requires a high position of the center of gravity with respect to the bar, since more of the body mass is above the bar at the critical time. With this lapse in technique, the flop style becomes similar to the straddle style, but with the back, instead of the anterior body surface, facing the bar. As a result it becomes less effective as a jumping technique than the straddle style (see Figure 18-6).

An alternate style based on the "flop" mechanics is suggested. In

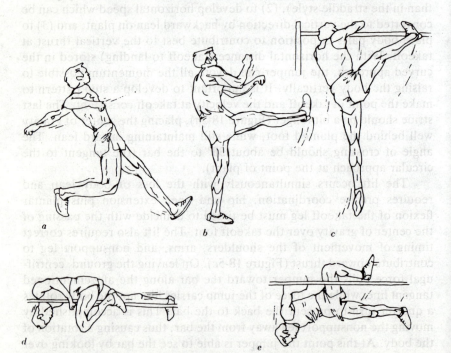

Figure 18-6 Illustration of good technique in the straddle-roll form of high-jumping. (*Clarence Robison, Clayne Jensen, Sherald James, and Willard Hirschi, Modern Techniques of Track and Field, Lea & Febiger, Philadelphia, 1974.*)

this method the position at crossing has the front of the body toward the bar; the body crosses in a deep pike position, then pulls into a tight tuck to rotate the body to a complete somersault. This permits the center of gravity to pass as much as 10 to 12 centimeters below the bar. This method requires a curved approach from the opposite side, a takeoff from the leg nearest the bar, the same angle of approach (30°), and a crossing with the body perpendicular to the bar. Hence, the jumper is able to maintain visual contact with the bar from takeoff to clearance. This style could be dubbed the "flop-flip."

Triple Jump (Hop, Step, and Jump)   When performing three body projections successively after a running approach, as this skill requires, it is essential for the performer to place great emphasis on preserving horizontal momentum. Excessive loss of momentum during any part of the performance reduces total distance. This means the hop must be rather low, the step somewhat higher, and the jump the highest of the three. Some of the possible distance from the first two phases (hop and step) is sacrificed in order to conserve horizontal momentum for the third phase (jump).

The landing after each of the first two phases results in precarious balance, and complex coordination and timing are required to maintain good balance for the next phase. Both the hop and step are one-footed landings with the center of gravity moving at a high velocity. Such landing, along wih a subsequent projection, requires very powerful hip, knee, and ankle extensor muscles. As these landings occur, the extensors of the leg must contract eccentrically to cushion the shock and produce joint flexion in preparation for the next projection. Almost immediately, the muscle contractions change to concentric contractions, thus causing the leg to extend. Arm, shoulder, and free leg movements must be perfectly timed and coordinated with extension of the push-off leg. The muscle actions of the total body in the triple jump are essentially the same as in the long jump. Very powerful leg extensors and a good deal of specific skill are required for success in this event.

In both the long jump and the triple jump, air resistance is a significant factor. During the 1968 Olympics in Mexico City, five long-jumpers broke the world record, each exceeding his own best mark by 0.3 to 0.6 meters. Sea-level air pressure is about 1,000 millibars, while at Mexico City it is about 800 millibars. This 20 percent reduction in pressure in part explains the longer jumps. Triple-jump marks at Mexico City also exceeded previous "bests."

Hurdling   Hurdling action is classified as a leap, which in turn can be thought of simply as an exaggerated running stride. Hurdling was analyzed in detail in Chapter 10; therefore it does not receive detailed attention here. But a few additional points of information should be established at this time.

The efficient hurdler attempts (1) to raise the center of gravity as little as possible and yet provide clearance, (2) to remain in the air as short a time as possible, and (3) to land in good balance and in a position conducive to continuing the drive to the next barrier. To keep the center of gravity low when passing over the hurdle, the performer must develop great flexibility of the hip region. The hip adductor muscles of the trail leg and the extensors of the lead leg must be especially flexible.

A person with a high center of gravity has an advantage in hurdling, for the same reason explained in the high jump. Individuals who have this advantage show little change in the vertical position of the center of gravity when leaping a hurdle. Other important attributes of a hurdler are the same as those for a sprinter—a top hurdler must be a good sprinter. For the specific movements and the muscular actions involved in hurdling, refer to Chapter 10.

The Leap in Dance   In order to retain correct form or to create an illusion, in some skills the performer must sacrifice maximal projection. The leap in dance (Figure 18-7) is one such skill. The meaning expressed by a certain posture during a leap may be vital to good form, and certain joint alignments aid the illusion of "hanging." The idea of illusion is best illustrated by the fact that dancers themselves, when questioned, often estimate their leaps to last "about 2 seconds." In such a leap the dancer would attain a height of 3½ meters! That is, in fact, quite an illusion. Though maximum height and/or distance is usually desirable, it is of secondary importance. Transfer of momentum principles (involving the free leg and arms) sometimes must be disregarded to accomplish the more important objectives of the particular leap.

Kick Turns   Essentially, kick turns are hops with varying degrees of twist. Various types of kick turns are widely used in dance and figure skating. In skating they are called axles. Even though kick turns vary from one another in appearance, the basic actions and principles governing them are the same. The takeoff is initiated by a dipping action of the trunk and takeoff leg, followed by the usual trunk and leg extension actions. To supplement the force from the takeoff leg, momentum is transferred to the body at takeoff by actions from the free leg and the arms. Usually this takeoff is preceded by horizontal momentum of the total body; so an important problem becomes one of correctly converting horizontal motion to a more vertical direction. The projection should be high enough to allow time for the necessary movements in the air.

For a turn to the left (left leg takeoff), the takeoff involves two major

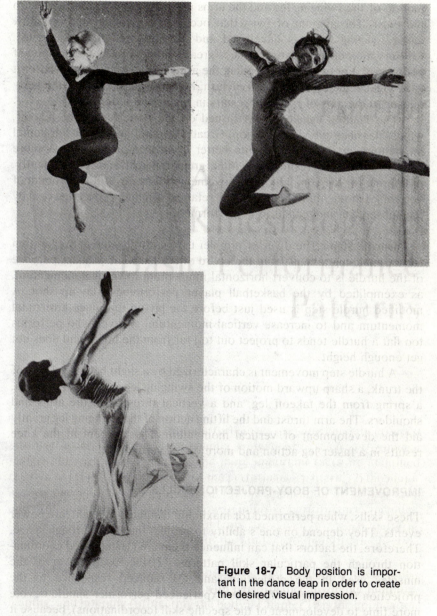

Figure 18-7 Body position is important in the dance leap in order to create the desired visual impression.

twisting actions around the body's vertical axis before the takeoff foot leaves the surface: (1) inward rotation at the left hip (the pelvis rotates on the fixed takeoff leg) and (2) left rotation of the thoracic spine (torso rotation), which results in upper-body rotation to the left. The direction of motion of the swinging leg and the arms may also favor the left to add to the twist. The amount of twist that occurs is dependent upon (1) how much twisting force is developed and (2) how well it is conserved. Conservation of the twisting force is greatly influenced by the position of body parts. For example, extending the arms away from the body after it is in flight reduces the amount of turn, but drawing them near the body (closer to the axis of rotation) results in faster and more turns.

The landing usually is performed on the same leg as the takeoff, which classifies the skill as a hop. Greater vertical and lesser horizontal momentum in the flight permits better control upon landing. A more vertical flight also results in gaining greater height and, consequently, more time for the completion of movements in the air. But the amount of horizontal momentum that should be retained is influenced a great deal by the subsequent movement to be performed.

Hurdle Step   The diver or tumbler uses a hurdle step in preparation for a double-leg takeoff from the board or the mat. The primary purpose of the hurdle is to convert horizontal momentum to vertical momentum, as exemplified by the basketball player performing a lay-up shot. A modified hurdle step is used just before the lay-up to reduce horizontal momentum and to increase vertical momentum. A diver who performs too flat a hurdle tends to project out too far from the board and does not get enough height.

A hurdle step movement is characterized by a slight backward lean of the trunk, a sharp upward motion of the swinging leg in the bent position, a spring from the takeoff leg, and a vertical thrust with the arms and shoulders. The arm thrust and the lifting action of the swinging leg greatly aid the development of vertical momentum. The leg bent at the knee results in a faster leg action and more direct vertical lift.

IMPROVEMENT OF BODY-PROJECTION SKILLS

These skills, when performed for maximum distance or height, are power events. They depend on one's ability to project the body through space. Therefore, the factors that can influence them are (1) improved coordination through the particular skill patterns, (2) increased power of the muscles used in the projection, and (3) reduced resistance to the projection (less weight). The less experienced performer should devote more time to development of the specific skill (coordinations), because it offers the greatest opportunity for improvement. It is very important to practice the correct technique. The more experienced performer should have already developed a high level of skill, and should place greater emphasis on increasing power of the particular muscles involved. But the advanced performer must not forget that sharpening skills as often as possible is still vital. The physiological changes resulting from training may call for frequent reestablishment of timing in the skill pattern.

Upper-body exercises may be beneficial but are of less direct concern. In projections, the hip flexor muscles act with great velocity but not against great resistance; so the development of power in the hip flexors is of limited concern. The prime concern is with the hip, knee, and ankle extensors (plantar flexors) and the abdominal muscles which stabilize the pelvis. Training exercises should include leg presses, squats, step-ups, jumps for height, body curls, sit-ups, and leg lifts. It should be remembered that the objective is not strength alone, but power; therefore, the exercise should be performed with great speed against reasonably heavy resistance. Isometrics may serve as a substitute, but their limitations involving speed of contraction should be obvious.

In performances where a running approach is used, such as the long jump, running speed and endurance and consistency of stride are important; so training programs should be designed to improve these factors.

A lack of endurance will hamper a jumper in practice sessions, preventing the performance of enough repetitions of the skill. The importance of speed and consistency of stride is apparent.

A reasonable amount of flexibility, especially of the hip extensor muscles, is important. Lack of such flexibility may restrict the desired range of motion and contribute to injury. Flexibility can be increased best by repeatedly placing the muscles on steady stretch for short periods of time.

STUDENT LABORATORY EXPERIENCES

Solve the following problems to fix the body-projection concepts presented in this chapter and to note the body-projection parameters.

1 A diver leaves the 1-meter board with a vertical velocity (v_y) of 5 meters per second. (a) How high will her center of gravity rise? (b) How long a time from takeoff until her center of gravity is 1 meter below its takeoff level? (See formulas **6, 8, 10.**)

2 A standing long-jumper leaves the ground with a horizontal velocity (v_x) of 3 meters per second and a vertical velocity (v_y) of 3 meters per second. (a) What is the angle of takeoff? (b) What is the velocity in the direction of the jump (v_θ)? (c) How high does his center of gravity rise? (d) If his center of gravity is 0.5 meters ahead of the toes at takeoff and 0.5 meters behind the center of gravity upon landing, which is at the same height as at takeoff, how far did he jump? (See formulas **17, 19, 6, 13.**)

3 How high would a jumper be able to raise the center of gravity with a vertical velocity (v_y) of 4.2 meters per second? (b) If the center of gravity is 105

centimeters above the ground at tiptoe position and the bar is successfully crossed with the center of gravity 2 centimeters below the bar, how high does the jumper go? (See formula **8**.)

4 Neglecting air resistance, consider the following case of the long-jumper. Horizontal velocity (v_x) is 9 meters per second. Vertical velocity (v_y) is 3 meters per second. Find (a) the velocity in the direction of the jump (v_θ); (b) the angle of takeoff (θ); (c) the height the center of gravity is raised; (d) the total distance of the jump, if the center of gravity is 0.5 meters ahead of the board at takeoff, 0.5 meters behind the heels at landing, and 0.4 meters lower at landing than at takeoff. (See formulas **19**, **15**, **8**, **14**.)

5 A dancer desires to do a double pirouette during a leap. If she can stay in the air for 0.65 seconds, what angular velocity should be achieved? (See formula **20**.)

6 A diver on a 1-meter board can achieve a total flight time of 1.2 seconds. She takes off with a lay-out rotation of 1 revolution per second. Her radius of rotation is 45 centimeters. If she tucks to a radius of rotation of 25 centimeters, can she complete a double somersault dive? (See formula **22b**.)

Skills for Providing Impetus to Objects

Chapter 19

Skills for Providing Impetus to Objects

Throwing and pushing receive more attention in this chapter than striking, because Chapter 16 provides a detailed mechanical analysis of a striking activity, the golf swing. The reader should refer to that analysis for principles which apply to striking activities. The analysis is also partially applicable to throwing, for the movements which develop striking force are similar to those that contribute to velocity of the hand in throwing, and objects in flight behave similarly whether thrown, struck, or pushed.

Throwing, striking, and pushing objects all result in projections, and success in these activities is dependent primarily upon the *velocity* (momentum in striking) or *accuracy*, depending on the objective of the particular performance. The acceleration and control of the projected object are produced by muscle contractions, which cause body movements in correct sequence. These performances are usually initiated by foot pressure against the supporting surface, followed by sequential movements progressing upward through the body, and finally terminating in the object to be projected. Each body segment receives the velocity produced by the preceding movements. A buildup of velocity occurs as

329

each successive body movement adds to the sum of the velocities of the previous movements. For example, in throwing a ball, the velocity of the ball at the moment of release is equal to the sum of the velocities of all contributing body movements, provided the movements are performed in correct sequence and each new movement is timed to add to the peak velocity of the movement which preceded it.

In the case of striking, *momentum* rather than velocity is of prime importance. When a baseball is struck with a bat, the velocity combined with the mass ($v \times m$ = momentum) of the bat determines the amount of impetus given to the ball. The lighter the bat, the greater velocity it must have in order to give an equal amount of impetus.

Several points are common to skills in which external objects are projected, regardless of the method used to set the objects in motion:

1 Lack of firm footing reduces the velocity of body segments necessary to gain maximum final velocity of the projected object. For example, a football jump pass is less forceful than one made from a set position where the feet are in firm contact.

2 As the length of the preparatory phase of the movement (backswing or windup) increases, ability to gain velocity in the action phase increases because the levers move through a greater range of motion and the muscles contract with greater initial force when placed on stretch.

3 Forced attempts to speed up the action in a sequential movement pattern are often destructive to the sequence and timing, which may result in an unsatisfactory performance.

4 Distance magnifies errors in accuracy. More specifically, a longer backswing will increase the effects of errors in movements, and the farther the object is projected, the more apparent inaccuracies become.

5 Denser objects are influenced less by air resistance and air movements than less dense objects.

THROWING PATTERNS

Arm motion at the shoulder joint makes possible these convenient classifications of throwing actions:

Underarm—shoulder, elbow, and wrist flexion

Sidearm—shoulder horizontal flexion, elbow extension, and wrist flexion

Overarm—shoulder inward rotation and horizontal flexion, elbow extension, and wrist flexion

Overhead—shoulder and elbow extension, and wrist flexion

The weight of the object may determine the throwing pattern used; heavier objects are usually projected with the underarm or pushing pattern. But for most people, the overarm and sidearm patterns produce the greatest speed and accuracy. The purpose of the throw and its place in game strategy normally determine the throwing pattern used.

Underarm Patterns

The underarm pattern is characterized by shoulder flexion. Perhaps the most forceful underhand pattern is the softball pitch. Other similar actions are the badminton underarm shot, handball and paddleball underarm shots, horseshoe pitch, and bowling. Most underarm patterns progress with the following sequence of actions—and these actions indicate the muscles involved. In general, the movements flow from the ground upward through the body and out the arm.

1 Initiation of total body-weight shift
2 Left hip inward rotation (right-handed pitch)
3 Left rotation of the trunk (spine)
4 Scapular abduction
5 Shoulder-joint flexion and outward rotation
6 Elbow flexion (slight)
7 Lower-arm rotation outward (in some cases only)
8 Wrist flexion

Cooper, Adrian, and Glassow (19) found that in underarm patterns, shoulder flexion consistently makes the greatest contribution. For example, they found that in the underarm pitch, the relative contributions of the different joints are shoulder flexion 45 percent, wrist flexion 32 percent, hip rotation 15 percent, and trunk rotation 8 percent.

Underarm Pitch A very powerful underarm action, the underarm pitch (Figure 19-1) requires that all contributing body segments make their maximum contribution. This calls for an extensive windup (preparatory action) to allow greater time for acceleration. As explained earlier, extensive windup is conducive to inaccuracy; therefore, the correct combination of velocity and accuracy is of prime concern to the softball pitcher. Major muscle groups which contribute to left-right accuracy are the shoulder-joint adductors and abductors in concert with the left rotators of the trunk. Very fine coordination of these muscles is required. Of greater concern to accuracy, though, are high-low errors, which result from improper timing of the ball's release. The ball should be released at the lowest point of the arc; if it is held too long, the flight is high, and if released too early, the trajectory is low. Although the bottom of the arc is passed almost immediately in a fast pitch, its time can be extended by emphasizing two other body actions. The shoulder girdle moves forward because of scapular abduction, and the whole body moves forward

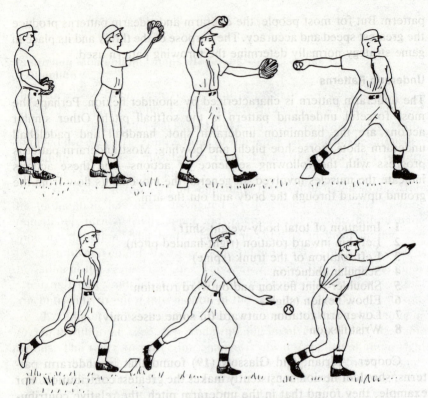

Figure 19-1 Body actions in the underarm softball pitch.

because of the stride (shift of body weight) into the pitch. Extending these actions keeps the ball at its lowest point for a longer period of time (flattens the bottom of the arc), permitting a greater tolerance for errors in the time of release.

Sidearm Patterns

In sidearm throwing, great reliance is placed upon the hip and spinal rotator muscles. Basically, the arm becomes a long lever, lying horizontally, rather than a series of short levers. The arm lengthens the levers which act in hip and spinal rotation. The primary movements for a right-handed pitcher are:

1 Initiation of total body-weight shift
2 Left hip inward rotation
3 Left rotation of the trunk (spine)
4 Scapular abduction
5 Shoulder horizontal flexion and slight medial rotation
6 Wrist flexion

Sidearm Pitch In this method of throwing, the high-low accuracy becomes less of a problem, but errors to the left or right become more prevalent. Here the left-right inaccuracies are caused mostly by errors in the timing of the release. The horizontal arc of the hand movement can be somewhat flattened in the sidearm throw by the same techniques described in the underarm throw. In the sidearm throw, flattening of the arc helps to control left-right errors.

If a baseball pitcher delivers a sidearm throw, the point of release is toward the third-base line (right-handed pitch). If such a ball is thrown to a right-handed batter, the angle of delivery causes the ball to move at an angle away from the batter. This reduces the power with which the batter can meet the ball, and it reduces the area of playing field (left field) to which the batter may hit with maximum power. The right fielder can play especially shallow if the pitcher is effective with the sidearm throw. The sidearm throw is used by ballplayers other than the pitcher when the situation requires quick release and a fast throw for a short distance.

The sidearm pattern is often used when larger and heavier objects are hurled and the arm is to be protected from strain. This pattern ordinarily supplies more speed than the underarm pattern, but less speed than the overarm pattern.

Discus Throw Difficulty in gripping the discus explains, in one sense, why the sidearm delivery is used. But even if its shape were more appropriate for grasping, its weight would still force a sidearm delivery for protection of the arm. Since accuracy is of little concern in discus-throwing, it is advantageous to ulitize a full range of shoulder motion as well as maximum hip and torso rotations.

The discus is put into motion by a total body spin. As the performer spins, the movement is forward across the ring in the direction of the throw. Then the final thrust (throw) is added to these movements (Figure 19-2). The velocity of the discus results from the combination of the three kinds of movements, namely, (1) total body rotation, (2) forward progress of the body, and (3) actions involved in throwing. An increase in force from any of these movements will increase the velocity of the discus at release.

Experienced performers attain 20 to 25 percent additional distance from the spin as compared with a stationary throw. When a very rapid spin is used, the event becomes a real test of body balance, and many mediocre performances are caused by loss of balance during the spin. It is presently common to use $1\frac{1}{4}$ to $1\frac{1}{2}$ turns in the spin. Conceivably, future record breaking will be the result of an additional fraction of a turn.

One problem resulting from the turn is the centrifugal force pulling on the discus during the spin. This tends to draw the arm away from the

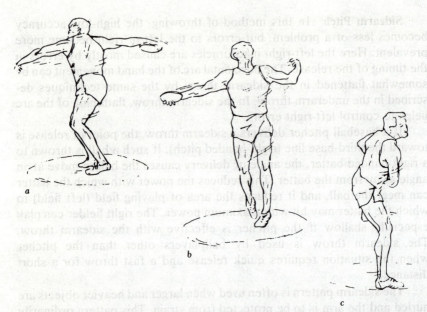

Figure 19-2 Body actions during the last phase (throwing phase) of the discus throw. (*Clarence Robison, Clayne Jensen, Sherald James, and Willard Hirschi, Modern Tecnhiques of Track and Field, Lea & Febiger, Philadelphia, 1974.*)

fully cocked position, thus reducing the length of the action at the shoulder joint when it becomes time to deliver. Another problem of discus-throwing is releasing the missile with its leading edge too high. This occurs when forearm rotation is not properly controlled, causing a "thumb-up" delivery. In this position, pronation of the forearm is insufficient, for the best flight is obtained when the palm of the hand is down and the leading edge of the discus is pointed at the angle of flight. The air pressure then provides aerodynamic lift similar to that of an airplane wing. Still another frequent problem is falling away from the throw. Usually, this is manifestation of balance loss. Almost invariably, if the performer is off-balance at the release, it is in the backward direction. Because discus-throwing is a very complex skill, it requires many hours of practice and unusual neuromuscular coordination.

The muscles which contribute the most during the spin are the hip rotators and the hip, knee, and ankle extensors. During the throw the key muscles are the ankle, knee, and hip extensors of the back leg, hip and trunk rotators (to the left), the shoulder horizontal flexors of the right (throwing) arm, and the horizontal extensors of the left (opposite) arm. Because the discus throw is a power event, muscle-conditioning programs should be designed to increase muscle power.

There are a limited number of two-handed sidearm patterns; the most common one is the hammer throw. Some professional tennis players have popularized a two-hand sidearm pattern as their basic stroke.

Overarm Patterns

We commonly identify the baseball throw as the standard overarm throw; although it does serve as a good standard, some other overarm throws deviate from it slightly. The overarm pattern is distinctive in that the performer often has an incorrect mental image of the mechanics of the arm actions. Many visualize the major arm force resulting from a downward and backward movement (extension) of the humerus beginning from the vertical. In truth, the major force results from inward rotation of the humerus, and the humerus is not vertical; it is usually almost horizontal and parallel with the surface. Even at times when the point of the elbow is higher than the shoulder, the relationship of the humerus to the trunk is changed very little because the higher elbow results mostly from lateral flexion of the spine.

The sequence of movements which are involved in the whiplike action of the overarm throw include (right-handed thrower):

1 Initiation of the total body-weight shift
2 Inward rotation at the forward hip (the pelvis rotates on the fixed leg)
3 Left lateral flexion, and strong left rotation of the trunk
4 Strong inward rotation and horizontal flexion at the shoulder joint
5 Elbow extension, combined with lower-arm rotation, to give correct direction to the throw
6 Strong wrist action, the direction of which depends on the purpose of the throw (Straight flexion is the dominant wrist action, but ulnar flexion is often used.)

Overarm Pitch See Figure 19-3. Among expert throwers, about one-half the force is derived from the movement of the legs and trunk and one-half from the arm actions. (This ratio may be influenced considerably by the size and shape of the object being thrown.) This demonstrates the importance of total body action. The overarm method is the one method which allows the greatest opportunity to utilize all available levers through their greatest range of motion. Therefore, with relatively light objects, this is the throwing method with which the greatest speed can be developed. Cooper, Adrian, and Glassow (**19**) found that in the baseball throw, wrist flexion is the greatest contributing action. Hip rotation, spinal rotation, and medial rotation at the shoulder (humerus) were also very important.

Most errors in accuracy in this pattern are high-low errors. The

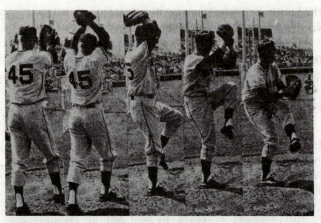

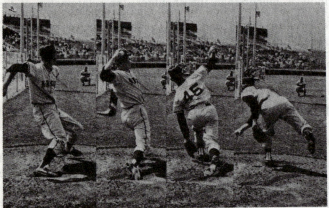

Figure 19-3 Body actions in the overarm baseball throw. (*Athletic Journal, January 1968, pp. 56–57.*)

overarm throw generally produces more left-right errors than the underarm, but fewer than the sidearm throw.

Incorrect technique resulting in loss of force in the overarm throw is most commonly—though not exclusively—observed in young girls. The most serious error occurs when the wrong foot is placed forward; the wrong foot, in this case, is the one on the side of the throwing arm. This action eliminates almost all contributions of trunk rotation, and the shoulder actions begin too soon in the sequence, causing their contributions to be almost fully spent before they can add acceleration to the ball.

Accuracy in the overhand throw develops at the speed at which it is practiced. A person may be fairly accurate at one speed but much less accurate at another speed. In consequence, practicing throws at slow speed appears to be of limited value if the performance must be at fast speed. Repetition in practice is needed at all the velocities to be used.

It has been said that throwing without the use of the fingers is like taking a flat-footed jump. Failure to use these levers limits the opportunity to develop maximum velocity. In order to use the fingers effectively, the performer must hold the ball by the fingers, not in the palm of the hand. If these levers are lengthened by moving the ball closer to the fingertips, effectiveness is increased, but the ball must not be so far toward the fingertips that the force does not pass through the ball's center of gravity. If the object is heavy, finger and wrist flexor muscles may be unable to contend with it when the weight is placed too far toward the fingertips.

The muscles which contribute most to the overarm pitch are the ankle, knee, and hip extensors of the back leg, hip and trunk rotators to the left, shoulder horizontal flexors and medial rotators, elbow extensors, and wrist and finger flexors.

Curve Ball Throwing a curve ball differs from throwing a fast ball in movements of the elbow, wrist, and fingers (Figure 19-4). The elbow extends in either case, but while the forearm is pronated for a fast-ball delivery, it is supinated with a "snap" for a curve-ball delivery. The wrist

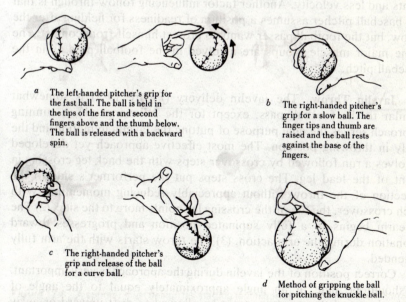

a The left-handed pitcher's grip for the fast ball. The ball is held in the tips of the first and second fingers above and the thumb below. The ball is released with a backward spin.

b The right-handed pitcher's grip for a slow ball. The finger tips and thumb are raised and the ball rests against the base of the fingers.

c The right-handed pitcher's grip and release of the ball for a curve ball.

d Method of gripping the ball for pitching the knuckle ball.

Figure 19-4 Grips used to cause different effects on the flight of a ball. (*After Daniel E. Jessee, Baseball, A. S. Barnes and Co., Inc., Cranbury, N. J., 1939.*)

moves sharply through ulnar flexion for the curve, but the fast ball requires straight wrist flexion. At least two fingers are behind the ball in the fast-ball delivery, whereas for the curve ball the thumb remains behind the ball, and the ball is released by rolling it forward over the index finger. For more information about the flight of curve balls, refer to Chapter 14.

Football Pass The football pass is nearly the same as the overarm baseball throw already described. The forearm position is between that of the fast-ball and that of the curve-ball throws. The wrist action is mostly ulnar flexion. A sharp downward movement at the wrist and the inward rotation at the shoulder produce the spiral flight of the ball. Large hands are an aid to better control.

Compared with the baseball pitch, the football pass involves less action at almost all joints, especially at the hip, and it results in more of a push and less of a whip action, because the football is harder to grip and control and must be released in such a way that it will travel in a spiral. The football throw may be preceded by several sideward shuffle steps, and right lateral flexion of the trunk is used in preparation when more distance is needed. The follow-through actions are less extensive than in the baseball pitch because the football throw involves less action at all joints and less velocity. Another factor influencing follow-through is that the baseball pitcher assumes a position of readiness for fielding after the throw, but the football passer wants to protect himself from contact. The same major muscle groups are involved in the football pass as in the baseball pitch.

Javelin Throw The javelin delivery (Figure 19-5) is somewhat similar to the football pass, except for the following: (1) A running approach serves the dual purpose of putting the javelin in motion and the body in throwing position. The most effective approach yet developed involves a run followed by crossover steps with the back leg crossing in front of the lead leg. The cross steps put the performer's side to the direction of the throw without appreciably reducing momentum. With each crossover, the toe of the crossing leg points more to the side. (2) The forearm begins in a fully supinated position and progresses toward pronation during the arm action. (3) The throw starts with the arm fully extended.

Correct position of the javelin during the approach is very important. It should be held at an angle approximately equal to the angle of projection, and the point must not be allowed to drift upward or away during the approach (it should stay close to the thrower's ear). If it drifts

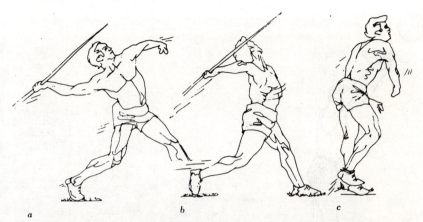

Figure 19-5 Illustration of good techniques during the latter phase of the javelin throw. (*Clarence Robison, Clayne Jensen, Sherald James, and Willard Hirschi, Modern Techniques of Track and Field, Lea & Febiger, Philadelphia, 1974.*)

away from the ear, misdirection will result when the throwing forces are applied.

The balance of the javelin must be in accord with the ability of the thrower. For throwers whose distance will probably be short, more weight is located in the javelin's point, whereas for throwers of longer length, less weight is needed in the point for maximum flight. Only throwers of a long distance can afford this luxury, because when the javelin is in flight for a longer period, it requires less weight in the point to pull the point down in time for a correct (point first) landing.

Expert throwers also concern themselves with the position of the forward leg just before the release. They recognize the importance of the long lever extending from the toe to the lead leg to the javelin; the longer this lever is, the more it will contribute to the speed of the javelin, and the higher the javelin will be at release. Both these factors are favorable to greater distance, and consequently, the experts throw "against" a *straight* lead leg and attempt to rise to the toes and reach high with the hand at release.

The same major muscle groups are involved in the javelin throw as in the baseball throw, and the objective of a conditioning program is also the same—to increase muscle power.

Double-Arm Overarm Patterns Examples of this type of throw are the overhead toss in soccer and the overhead two-handed pass or shot in basketball (Figure 19-6). In these skills, as in other throwing skills, total body action is essential. This involves precisely coordinated extension at

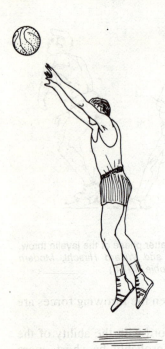

Figure 19-6 Basketball overhead two-handed shot at release.

various joints of the legs, trunk, and arms, which may be accompanied by a jump from both feet or a forward step to add force to the throw. The hands should be held on opposite sides of and partially behind the ball. The hands act as clamps. The elbows should be out front and above the shoulders. If the elbows are too far apart, forward force is sacrificed. During the action, there is slight extension at the shoulders, elbow extension, wrist flexion, ulnar flexion, and finger flexion. When accuracy is desired, the finger and wrist movements are very important because they put the "final touch" on the ball.

Single-Arm Circular Overhead Actions

Few activities can be classified within this category. The most common are the basketball hook shot and hook pass. Accuracy of this technique is less than that of other overarm throwing techniques, mainly because it is not suited for good hand-eye coordination. However, some players become reasonably proficient in shooting basketball hook shots when they shoot from known spots on the floor. The action is most often preceded by a hurdle-step approach which gains height and makes it difficult for an opponent to interfere with the shot. Often a smaller person finds the hook to be the best shot to avoid blocking by a larger opponent. Large hands are obviously advantageous in controlling a hook pass or shot. Most errors in accuracy result from too high a projection, which indicates inadequate control of the ball.

PUSHING PATTERNS

As compared with overarm throwing, pushing patterns involve less arm action and leverage that is less favorable to producing great speed against light resistance. But pushing patterns involve very powerful movements, movements in which the leverage is highly favorable to application of force against heavy resistance. In pushing, the more powerful muscle groups are used, especially in the arm and shoulder movements. Also pushing patterns are conducive to great accuracy in certain performances because the hand moves linearly in the line of flight, which makes timing of the release less critical than in throwing.

Single-Arm Pushes

The most common single-arm pushing actions are shot-putting and the one-handed push shot in basketball. In the first case, the primary consideration is distance, and in the second, accuracy is of prime importance.

When *maximum velocity* of the missile is desired, as in shot-putting, actions of the legs and trunk are greatly emphasized. (They are similar to those of the overarm throw.) When *accuracy* is wanted, as in the basketball push shot, body and leg actions are limited to correspond with the objective of the skill.

Shot Put See Figure 19-7. The shot is put (pushed) and not thrown. The prime objective is distance, and assuming the angle of projection is correct, the distance is dependent upon the velocity at which the shot is moving at release. One's ability to develop velocity of the shot is dependent upon power, which is a combination of strength and speed. The shot-putter, then, is essentially concerned with increasing power and perfecting the specific skill of shot-putting. Because of the importance of power, the shot-putter spends much training time attempting to increase strength and speed of movement against heavy resistance. Adequate attention must also be given to the development of shot-putting skill, because the mechanics of movement and the sequential timing of the movements are of tremendous importance.

Shot-putting combines three kinds of body movements: (1) linear movement of the total body across the 2.134-meter ring, (2) rotation of the total body through about 180°, and (3) the pushing actions of the various body segments. Each type of movement must be correctly timed and fully utilized in order to make its maximum contribution. To

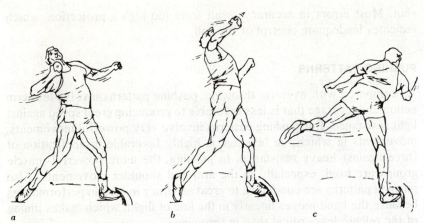

Figure 19-7 Illustration of good technique during the thrusting phase of the shotput. (*Clarence Robison, Clayne Jensen, Sherald James, and Willard Hirschi, Modern Techniques of Track and Field, Lea & Febiger, Philadelphia, 1974.*)

illustrate the importance of each kind of movement, consider "O'Brien style," which revolutionized shot-putting. Its unique feature is that the performer starts the put with the back, rather than the side, toward the direction of flight. This position allows an additional one-quarter turn of the total body, thus increasing the time over which the body rotational forces can be applied. More recently, the "Oldfield style" added still another one-quarter turn to O'Brien's contribution.

After movement across the ring and just before the final thrusting movement, all body segments should be in correct position, the same position as if a stationary put were being made. In consequence, at the completion of movement across the ring, the legs and spine should be sufficiently flexed to provide for optimum effects from extension at those joints. The most effective depth of flexion in preparation is directly related to the strength of the extensor muscles. Certainly the muscles contribute little if the joints are nearly extended after the glide across the ring and before the thrust.

The major force of the thrusting action in shot-putting results from the following body movements: extension at the various leg joints, with emphasis on the back leg; rotation at the hips and trunk; horizontal flexion at the shoulder; elbow extension; and wrist and finger flexion. As in the overhand throw, the movements generally flow from the legs upward. One very important movement often not recognized is horizontal extension and adduction of the opposite arm. This vigorous movement can add greatly to the speed of hip and trunk rotation.

The idea of maintaining contact with the surface is especially important in this event because if foot-surface contact is broken too early, the driving forces of the body are greatly reduced. Holding the shot high on the fingers can provide extra leverage, provided the fingers are strong enough to overcome the resisting force of the shot. If the fingers lack sufficient strength, then placing the shot too high on them will be self-defeating. The reversal (follow-through) at the completion of the putting action is important because it allows the performer to continue the thrusting movements longer, while it places the body in a better position to maintain balance.

Basketball One-Handed Push Shot   The most widely used basketball shot today is the one-handed push shot performed with a jump (jump shot, Figure 19-8). In this performance, accuracy, and not force, is of prime importance.

The jump is usually initiated from a double-leg takeoff which is essentially directed upward, though some performers jump somewhat forward; on occasion, the backward "falling away" jump shot is useful. The main reason for the jump is to provide height to gain clearance over an opponent. In addition to the increased height, two other factors have contributed to the popularity of this technique: (1) the unexpectedness of the time and direction of the takeoff and (2) the delay of the shot, which makes it difficult to anticipate when to block. These factors have led some coaches to label the shot as indefensible. It should be noted that the delay, especially if it extends until the shooter begins the descent, eliminates the

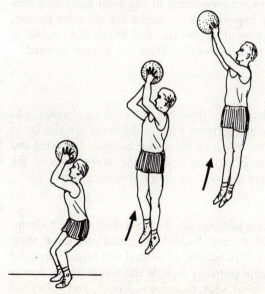

Figure 19-8   Illustration of body actions during the basketball jump shot.

contribution of the legs and trunk to the force of the projection. As the shot becomes longer, shooting earlier in the jump becomes more necessary, and power in the hand, arm, and shoulder muscles becomes more essential.

Aside from the jump, almost all the actions in this shooting technique occur in the shooting arm. They are shoulder flexion, elbow extension, and wrist and finger flexion. Wrist and finger flexion are the final movements, and they are very important because they put the correct "touch" on the ball. For accuracy it is important that the ball be controlled with the fingers; when the ball is held high over the head, less action occurs in the shoulder and elbow, and more reliance is placed on the wrist and finger actions. Some performers shoot with the elbow in front of the shoulder; some shoot with the elbow almost directly to the side; and others have the elbow at some intermediate point between the front and side. There is no evidence that any of these styles is superior in accuracy.

The one-handed free throw shot or the one-handed set shot follows about the same pattern as the jump shot, except the leg and trunk actions are used more to contribute to the force.

Double-Arm Pushes

A few skills involve double-arm pushes. The most common ones are the basketball push pass and the volleyball setup. In these performances, the initial force comes from forward movement of the total body as a step forward is taken. The other important movements are shoulder flexion, elbow extension, wrist flexion, ulnar flexion, and finger flexion. As in other thrusting actions, the movements flow from the ground upward.

STRIKING PATTERNS

Most of the principles which apply to throwing and pushing also apply to striking, and the arm-movement patterns used in throwing are similar to those used in striking. The one essential difference between throwing and striking is that the emphasis in striking is upon the *momentum* of the striking implement rather than the *velocity* of the throwing hand.

Arm Striking Patterns

Examples of *underarm striking patterns* are the volleyball serve, badminton serve, tennis pickup shot, and badminton underarm clear shot. Examples of *sidearm patterns* are batting a baseball and tennis forehand and backhand drives. *Overarm patterns* include the tennis serve, tennis smash, badminton overarm clear shot, badminton smash, and volleyball spike. A *circular arm pattern* is illustrated by the left hook of the boxer.

Boxing also incorporates pushing patterns which produce striking forces. Examples are the jab and cross.

In striking, as in throwing and pushing, movements flow from the feet upward, and the final motion is that of the striking implement. If all the contributing body motions occur in correct sequence with correct timing, the velocity of the implement will represent the sum of the velocities of all contributing levers. The actual magnitude of the striking force is determined by the velocity and weight (momentum) of the implement.

In arm striking patterns, most of the force is provided by the following actions: total body-weight shift (stepping into the strike), hip rotation, trunk rotation, horizontal flexion at the back shoulder, and horizontal extension at the front shoulder. In certain striking actions, elbow extension and wrist flexion, or ulnar flexion, are also important movements.

In Chapter 16 a mechanical analysis of a striking activity (golf drive) was presented. Many ideas relating to the mechanics of striking actions can be gleaned from that chapter. Following are interesting points about striking that were not discussed:

1 An oblique striking surface, an off-center contact, or glancing blows produce spin on the object at the expense of force. The spin may significantly influence the flight of the object in different ways, depending on the direction of the spin.

2 If the object (ball) is moving toward the striking implement, and the momentum of the implement is greater than that of the object, the momentum of the object adds to that of the implement. This means that the faster a ball approaches, the farther it can be hit, as long as the implement's momentum exceeds that of the ball.

3 Maximum distance or force is not always desired, and often accuracy and quickness of movement can be gained by sacrificing maximum force. This concept is especially useful in baseball batting and tennis, where placement of the ball is very important.

4 The length of levers may be altered to suit the strength of the performer. A weaker person must sometimes shorten levers to maintain the desired speed of movement. This performer "chokes up" on the baseball bat or tennis racket in order to be sure to overcome momentum of the ball and still not sacrifice accuracy. A person who is strong enough to lengthen the lever would achieve a longer arc of swing and thereby gain the advantage of a more powerful swing. In the case of the tennis serve, the longer lever would give the ball a better approach angle to the net. When a very heavy implement is used, the performer may have to shorten the levers to achieve any degree of success.

5 In bunting a baseball, either the sacrifice or the drag bunt usually requires that the bat move away from the ball at contact or that a loose grip is used to absorb the striking forces (or both), thus reducing the distance of the rebound. Accuracy in directing the ball downward is also important to reducing rebound distance.

6 If great force is desired, it follows that the grip must be very firm, especially at contact. If the hands are spread in the grip, speed of movement of the implement is sacrificed for accuracy. The closer the hands are to each other, the more they act as a single unit.

Kicking Patterns

In sports performances, kicking is most commonly used in American football, rugby, and soccer. The investigation of kicking reveals that a backward inclination of the trunk almost always precedes a kick in which force or distance is the objective. This backward inclination contributes to the "stretch" of the rectus femoris muscle, a major contributor to the kicking action. The stretch stimulates the stretch reflex and removes slack in the muscle, enabling its contraction to have immediate and strong effect on knee extension. The backward inclination is most obvious in football and soccer punts. In place-kicking it is less obvious but still exists. Another result of backward inclination is that it starts the forward-upward motion of the thigh prior to the time hip flexion begins. This movement contributes to the force of hip flexion which follows. The action of the kick is best described as "whiplike," with the backward swing of the trunk as the initial motion, followed by the lashing action of the leg.

The placement of the supporting foot is very important to the place-kick. If the foot is placed too far forward, sufficient time is not available to build momentum before contact is made with the ball. If it is placed too far back of the ball, the peak force of the kick will be spent before contact is made. For the greatest force and best control, contact should be made at the bottom of the kick arc. The arc is flattened by the forward movement of the whole body and by a slight bending of the knee of the supporting leg. This provides greater tolerance for error.

The instep soccer kick has gained popularity for football place-kicking. It is difficult to assess the potential of each kicking technique in terms of force. The instep kick makes use of hip rotation, along with one long lever (from the hip) in an adducting movement. The adductor muscles are very powerful, and the lever is long. On the other hand, the toe kick utilizes two levers (lower and upper leg), which probably allow a greater development of momentum over a longer range of motion.

For accuracy the area of contact on the inside of the foot appears to be superior to the toe. Not only is a broader area of contact available, but the concave foot fits well with the convex ball. The square-toed kicking shoe partially alleviates this disadvantage of toe kicking.

In summary, it seems that either kick may develop great striking force depending on the development of the musculature and the skill pattern, but greater accuracy is likely with the instep kick. Accuracy may develop more slowly with the instep kick, however, because the line of sight is not along the line of movement as it is in the toe kick. Difficulties with the instep kick are a low angle of projection and a tendency to "pull" or "hook" the kick to the side.

STOPPING MOVING OBJECTS

In catching objects such as a baseball, softball or football, it is important to trade force for distance by recoiling as the catch is made. The formula by which kinetic energy is changed to work is

$$Fd = \tfrac{1}{2}\, mv^2$$

To determine the force of catching the object, the formula is rewritten as

$$F = \frac{mv^2}{2d}$$

where m is mass, v is velocity at impact, and d is the distance through which the object is stopped.

Trading force for surface area is achieved in baseball and softball by the pocketed padded glove.

IMPROVEMENT OF PROJECTILE SKILLS

Most of these activities are power events of a ballistic nature. Therefore, the components of fitness that should dominate the time available for training are (1) muscular strength, (2) speed of muscle contraction, and (3) flexibility in certain body regions. Of course, practice of the correct mechanics and specific coordinations necessary to the performance must not be neglected.

The natural amount of body power is usually insufficient for maximum performance in throwing, striking, and pushing activities. Therefore, each skill should be evaluated in terms of the requirements of power for its success. Then artificial overload (weight training, isometrics, or functional overloads) should be used to provide the needed power-building stimuli. For power, exercises should be performed explosively to improve both strength and speed of contraction. Although increasing power in the upper body should be emphasized, the trunk and lower extremities cannot be neglected, because these areas provide much of the force for throwing, pushing, and striking. Special exercises should be selected to increase flexibility in the areas where muscle tightness restricts the desired range of movement.

It seems to be rarely profitable to break these skills down into parts for practice, because they are so dependent upon correct timing and sequence. Also, it is of little value to substitute similar skills, for these tend to disturb the timing of ballistic movements. For improved coordination of a particular pattern, the skill as a whole should be practiced extensively.

STUDENT LABORATORY EXPERIENCES

The following problems will help the student to apply the concepts presented in the chapter.

1 The sequential segment contributions to a softball pitch, in linear velocity units of meters per second, are as follows: (1) weight shift, 1.5; (2) hip medial rotation, 3; (3) trunk (spinal) rotation, 1.6; (4) scapular adduction, 0.3; (5) shoulder joint flexion, 9; and (6) wrist flexion, 7. If these contributions are correctly timed, with what velocity will the ball be thrown (a) in meters per second? (b) in feet per second?

2 In the discus sidearm throw a performer achieves an angular velocity at release of 26 radians per seconds. If this radius of rotation is 0.9 meters, what is the tangential velocity (v_T) of the discus at release. (See formula 22.)

3 Using the data in problem 1, what would be the final velocity of the softball if the pitcher omitted hip rotation?

4 A baseball player throws the ball from center field to home plate. Neglecting air resistance and supposing that the ball is thrown at a 22° angle with the horizontal at a velocity of 30 meters per second and is caught at the height of release, find (a) the distance of the throw and (b) the time of flight. (c) Can a runner on third base score if the fielder uses 0.5 seconds from catch-to-throw release? (Assume that the runner averages 9 meters per second from third base to home plate.) (See formulas 13, 11, 1.)

5 A shot-putter releases the shot 2.2 meters above the ground and 0.3 meters in front of the toeboard. The velocity of the shot at release is 14 meters per second at an angle of 42° with the horizontal. Assuming a level area, what is the total distance of the put (a) in meters? (b) in feet? (c) Is this a world-class put? (See formula 14.)

6 A thrown baseball weighing 1.4 newtons and traveling 35 meters per second is caught by a player who recoils 40 centimeters during the catch. What is the force the hand must receive during the catch? (a) in newtons? (b) in pounds? (See formula 41.)

Chapter 20

Arm-Support and Arm-Suspension Skills

The category of arm-support and arm-suspension skills is dominated by gymnastic activities. Arm support, however, is also used in several starting stances, and arm suspension is used in the rope climb and pole vault. A great deal of strength and muscular endurance in the upper body are prerequisites to the successful performance of these skills, and precise control of muscular contractions is of utmost importance. Here, precision of the muscular contractions is highly dependent upon incoming information from the kinesthetic sense. In essence, the basic aspects of these skills are (1) sufficient strength to support the body in the desired positions and (2) effective manipulation and control of the center of gravity to maintain balance. In most arm-supported and arm-suspension skills there is little room for error.

When the body is in arm-supported positions, the elbow extensor muscles contract strongly to resist the pull of gravity. Other joints of the upper extremities may either be in movement or be stabilized; therefore, few muscles in the upper body can relax. Unlike that of the lower body, the upper-body bone structure is not well suited for weight bearing, and

349

deficiencies in structure must be compensated for by extensive muscular use.

INVERTED BALANCES

All the principles of stability discussed earlier are applicable to inverted balance skills. In addition, factors pertaining to the base of support apply to these skills. For instance, in the inverted position, it is important to keep the center of gravity of the body over the base and to keep the center of gravity as low as possible within the confines of desirable form. If a performer's weight is proportionately greater in the upper body than in the legs, then the center of gravity is lower in the inverted position. This creates an advantage in balance and stability. Any position which lowers the body toward the surface aids in stability.

Once a balanced position is accomplished, the subsequent problems involve muscular strength-endurance and ability to make adjustments necessary to regain balance when deviations occur. Some necessary, though sometimes undesirable, adjustments to preserve balance include (1) flexion of the elbows (to lower the center of gravity), (2) movement of the legs (to the side opposite the balance loss), and (3) reestablishment of the base of support to keep it underneath the center of gravity.

Handstands on the *floor* involve a base of support which is narrow in the front-back directions. Because of this narrow base, great strength is required in the muscles surrounding the wrist to oppose body sway. Effective stabilization of certain joints (elbows, shoulders, thoracic and lumbar spine, hips, knees, and ankles) may relieve tension on wrist muscles by reducing the amount of body sway. Also, correct movements in those joints will help to maintain control.

A handstand on the *parallel bars* is easier than on the floor, because the wrists are in stronger positions, owing to the fact that (1) forward and backward deviations are now controlled by the wrist adductors and abductors instead of the flexors and extensors and (2) the grip on the bars provides a firmer base of support. The same circumstances are true to a lesser extent on the *rings*. During a handstand on the *horizontal bar*, the wrist flexors and extensors are in control, and the base of support is extremely narrow (diameter of the bar), making this a very difficult balance skill.

One-handed stands are still more difficult, because the supporting muscles carry a double load, and the base of support is reduced to the size of the one-handed contact with the surface. The center of gravity must be held over that small base. As additional body parts come in contact with the surface, the base of support is enlarged. Examples are the shoulder stand on the parallel bars and the head- and handstand on the floor. In the

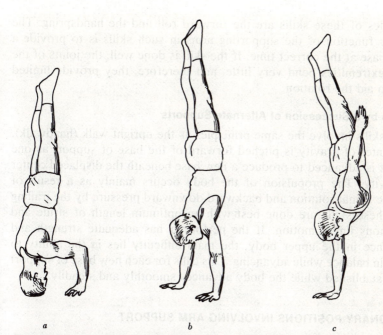

Figure 20-1 In progressing from the head- and handstand to a two-handed stand to a one-handed stand, the performer must demonstrate an increased sense of balance and greater strength, in order to compensate for the smaller base of support and fewer supporting limbs.

head- and handstand, an additional stability advantage is gained because the center of gravity is lowered from the bending of the arms. Also, the head- and handstand affords the opportunity to widen the base of support in the forward-backward direction, as well as in the lateral direction (Figure 20-1).

ARM-SUPPORTED TRAVELS

Skills like the handspring, the cartwheel, the handwalk, and progressing forward on the parallel bars are examples of traveling while being supported by the arms. The first two constitute linear movement accomplished by rotary motion of the entire body, and the last two result from linear movement by a progression of balance losses, each followed by successive reestablishment of the base of support.

Travels by Rotary Motion of the Entire Body

These skills depend upon an approach run to build sufficient forward momentum, followed by a takeoff of sufficient force and in the correct direction to provide enough rotary momentum to complete the skill.

Examples of these skills are the forward roll and the handspring. The primary function of the supporting arms in such skills is to provide a stable base at the correct time. If the skill is done well, the joints of the upper extremities bend very little, and therefore, they provide limited force to aid the rotation.

Travels by a Succession of Alternate Supports

These skills involve the same principles as the upright walk (handwalk). The center of gravity is pitched forward of the base of support as one support is advanced to produce a new base beneath the displaced center of gravity. The propulsion of the body occurs mainly as a result of thoracic spinal rotation and backward-downward pressure by the trailing arm. These skills are done best with an optimum length of stride and continuous linear motion. If the performer has adequate strength and endurance in the upper body, the main difficulty lies in the ability to maintain balance while advancing. This calls for each new base of support to be established while the body advances smoothly and steadily.

STATIONARY POSITIONS INVOLVING ARM SUPPORT

The exact stance used in any position of readiness is determined by the task to be accomplished. *Track and football starting stances* are established for the purpose of moving quickly in a predetermined direction. The stance of a performer in the dash in track is obviously designed to initiate motion in the forward direction as quickly as possible. For this reason, the center of gravity is placed as far forward as possible without sacrificing balance, which results in considerable weight on the arms. The football stance with the center of gravity well forward (Figure 20-2) is desirable only if movement is to be in a forward direction. If the player must be ready to move in any direction, the center of weight should be

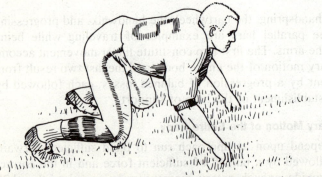

Figure 20-2 The football four-point stance combines two important factors: (1) great stability and (2) ability to move quickly and forcefully in the forward direction.

located near the center of the base. This is a stance of compromise which is not highly suited to movement in any particular direction, but well suited to quick adjustment in any direction.

In a *front-leaning rest position* on the floor, the arms carry most of the weight. This position is used in exercises like the push-up or the squat thrust, and it may also be used during floor exercise routines in gymnastics. Its effective execution depends largely upon muscular strength and endurance of the shoulder-girdle abductors, shoulder flexors, elbow extensors, and wrist flexors. The abdominal and hip flexor muscles bear the special burden of opposing a tendency for the pelvis to sag as a result of the pull of gravity.

An *upright rest (support) position* varies with the gymnastic apparatus on which it is performed. On the horizontal bar or the side horse, the performer need only produce arm support against gravity, because balance is very easy when leaning forward onto the apparatus and maintaining body rigidity. In the support position on the parallel bars (Figure 20-3) and still rings, the shoulder flexors and extensors must actively oppose each other to prevent the center of gravity from swinging forward or backward beyond the supporting hands. The still rings pose an additional problem because of their tendency to spread laterally. This calls for strong contractions of the shoulder adductors.

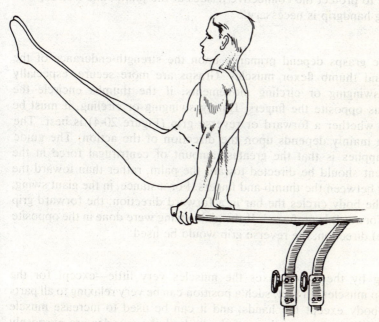

Figure 20-3 Maneuvering in the arm-support position on parallel bars (or similar apparatus) requires great arm and shoulder strength.

MOUNTS AND VAULTS

A good number of mounts and vaults are very much alike during the initial phases. They involve a leg spring combined with a downward-backward thrust by the arms. It is very important that the arm and leg actions are precisely timed so they complement each other. As the center of gravity rises and the arms assume support of the body weight, it is important that the arms are completely straight to achieve the highest possible point of elevation. At this point the mount and the vault differ. The vault requires the momentum of the original thrust to continue in order to provide clearance of apparatus by the body, whereas the mount requires the performer to control the momentum in order to assume (usually) a resting support position. This dissipation of momentum can be aided partially by a direction of thrust slightly different (more upward) from that of the vault, but mostly, it requires controlled absorption of the force of the thrust. This absorption calls for muscle contractions which gradually bring the body to a stop in the desired rest position.

SKILLS INVOLVING ARM SUSPENSION

Suspending the body from the arms tends to separate the joints, especially in the arms and shoulders. Therefore, the muscles must partially contract to protect the connective tissues at the joints; and a strong and enduring handgrip is necessary.

Grasps

Effective grasps depend primarily upon the strength-endurance of the finger and thumb flexor muscles. Grasps are more secure, especially during swinging or circling movements, if the thumbs encircle the apparatus opposite the fingers. During swinging or circling, it must be decided whether a forward or reverse grip (Figure 20-4) is best. The decision mainly depends upon the direction of the action. The guide which applies is that the greatest amount of centrifugal force in the movement should be directed toward the palm, rather than toward the opening between the thumb and fingers. For instance, in the giant swing, where the body circles the bar in a forward direction, the forward grip (palms forward) is preferred. If the giant swing were done in the opposite (reverse) direction, the reverse grip would be used.

Hangs

Hanging by the hands taxes the muscles very little—except for the handgrip muscles. In fact, such a position can be very relaxing to all parts of the body except the hands, and it can be used to increase muscle flexibility in various portions of the body if the muscles are purposely relaxed during the hang.

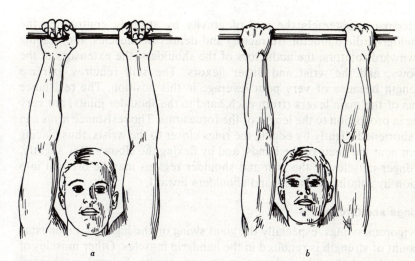

Figure 20-4 Grips. (a) Forward. (b) Reverse.

A special kind of hang, the *iron cross on the rings*, can be accomplished only with very strong and sustained contractions of the muscles of the arms and shoulders (Figure 20-5). The performer starts in an upright support position, slowly spreads the rings sideward until the arms are abducted to the horizontal position, and then holds this position. The

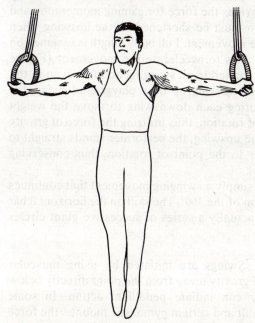

Figure 20-5 The iron-cross hang illustrates poor mechanical ratio and the need for very strong muscle contractions.

performer counteracts the pull of gravity by strongly contracting the shoulder-girdle adductor (retractor) and depressor muscles, the scapula downward rotators, the adductors of the shoulders, the extensors of the elbows, and the wrist and finger flexors. The skill requires extreme strength because of very poor leverage in this position. The resistance arms of the main levers (from each hand to the shoulder joints) are very long in proportion to the length of the force arms. The resistance arms can be shortened slightly by edging the rings closer to the wrists, thus placing them near the heels of the hands, and by flexing the elbows very slightly. Stronger muscles of the arm and shoulder regions may be brought into action by rotating the arms and shoulders inward.

Swings and Circles

In vigorous swings, especially the giant swing on the high bar, an unusual amount of strength is required in the handgrip muscles. Other muscles of the arms and shoulders also must be very strong. Several mechanical factors apply to this category of skills; the most important are concerned with initiating and conserving angular momentum and contending with centrifugal force. In swinging, the body acts as a pendulum which swings as a result of certain muscles contracting and relaxing, causing the body to move toward the bar, then away from the bar at the right times. (In gymnastics these actions are restricted to certain joints, determined by acceptable form.) Gravity provides the force for gaining momentum, and consequently, the body length must be shortened on the upswing when gravity tends to decelerate the movement. Full body length is assumed on the downswing when gravity acts to accelerate the movement (Figure 12-5). This same principle is applied in all swinging actions, even in the case of playground swings. In working up on a playground swing, the performer crouches down during each downswing to move the weight farther away from the point of rotation, thus utilizing the force of gravity to gain momentum. During the upswing, the performer stands straight to move the body weight closer to the point of rotation, thus conserving momentum.

A circle in gymnastics is simply a swinging movement that continues through the full angular motion of the 360°. The skill on the horizontal bar known as the giant swing is actually a series of successive giant circles (see Figure 12-5).

Initiation of the Swing Swings are initiated by using muscular actions to place the center of gravity away from the point directly below the support so that gravity can initiate pendulum action. In some activities, such as the pole vault and certain gymnastic mounts, the force for starting the swing is the result of momentum developed in the approach. In gymnastics, if the performer begins from an arm-suspension or arm-support position on the apparatus, the starting action is called an upstart or a cast-off. Muscular actions project the center of gravity from its normal suspended position. Once this occurs, the force of gravity contributes to momentum of the swing. To begin a swing on the high bar from a hang, for example, the performer pulls upward and forward to move the center of gravity in that direction, and at this point extends the body to lengthen the radius of rotation. The extension enables gravity to exert its greatest force toward the pendulum action of the body.

To do a backward hip circle on the high bar, the performer begins from a front support position. The center of gravity is projected backward and slightly upward away from the bar. This movement provides linear momentum as the hips return to the bar. This momentum is converted to angular momentum as the hips meet the bar at a slightly lower point than the level of the starting position. The hips are then flexed to conserve the angular momentum during the time that the lower portion of the body is moving forward and upward against gravity. This same principle is applied on the parallel bars when the forward cast is used in swinging up to a handstand position. In this case, the forward-upward movement of the lower body from the support position leads to the position from which gravity can act on the body to produce momentum for the swing.

Kip The kip is a movement from a swing (suspension) in which the center of gravity is raised to a point that enables the performer to pull up to a support position in a single thrust. It may be done on the rings, parallel bars, or horizontal bar. The principles are essentially the same, regardless of the apparatus on which it is performed. Its success is highly dependent upon precise timing.

At the end of the forward swing, forceful shoulder extension, trunk flexion, and hip flexion elevate the center of gravity to a level comparable with that in the support position. As the backswing begins, trunk and hip extension are quickly and powerfully applied when the body's center of gravity passes below the bar. This is the critical time. The hip extension at the bottom of the backward swing shortens the radius of the angular motion and brings the center of gravity close to the handgrip (Figure 20-6). The force of hip extension produces angular motion of the total body at the time when the handgrip and the center of gravity are at about the same height. The hips are kept close to the handgrip, and if the force of momentum is great enough, the arms can shift from suspension to support so the performance will be successful.

Regrasps and Dismounts While Swinging At either end of a swing the velocity and centrifugal force are zero, and the body is weightless; at about the middle of the swing, velocity is maximum. It is obvious, then, that all regrasping (adjusting or changing the grip) and most dismount-

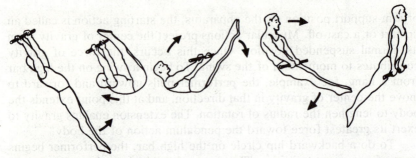

Figure 20-6 Kip on the high bar illustrates importance of quick and correctly timed weight shifts.

ing maneuvers are easier at either end of the swing where there is no need to contend with the body's momentum. If the grip release is inappropriately timed and too much momentum from the swing is retained, maintaining balance upon landing is difficult, if not impossible.

Travels While Suspended

Travel in an arm-suspended position may be in a horizontal direction, as in hand travel on an overhead horizontal ladder, or in a vertical direction, as in the rope climb. Progression in a horizontal direction is accomplished by trunk rotation to the left as the right hand reaches forward and the left hand maintains the grip. The lower body naturally turns in the opposite direction (Newton's third law of motion), becoming a preparatory movement for the development of momentum for the succeeding reach. The succeeding reach brings a reversal of the actions of the previous reach. The longer the reach, the greater is the momentum resulting from the swing. Within reason, then, longer strides are more efficient. Shorter strides may be advantageous to a weak person because of the shorter period of time needed to support the body with one arm during each swing. However, the slower progress results in additional taxing of the muscles.

Most of the same points apply to vertical travels (climbing) that apply to horizontal travels. A high reach is advantageous provided the elbow does not fully extend. A fully extended elbow places the flexors of that joint under a severe mechanical disadvantage. The reaching action should come primarily from shoulder-joint flexion, shoulder-girdle elevation, spinal rotation (to the side opposite the reaching arm), and a slight lateral pendulum action of the body, which adds to the vertical momentum. The major propelling force should be provided by the large back muscles (especially the latissimus dorsi), which contribute to shoulder-joint extension, adduction, and inward rotation. Shoulder-girdle depression and elbow flexion are also very important. Hip flexion of the leg opposite the pulling arm results in a transfer of momentum which contributes to the upward body lift. Much skill is needed for efficiency in the rope climb, and the more skillful climbers require less strength. If the legs are used in contact with the rope, they wrap around the rope and push.

Either of these travels (horizontal or vertical) is accomplished with greater ease if the actions are continuous, because then the loss of momentum is not permitted before the application of the next force. If momentum is lost, each stroke encounters greater inertia (Newton's second law of motion).

MUSCULAR INVOLVEMENT

Some muscular actions in arm-supported and arm-suspended skills are deceptive and obscure. A few generalizations may be helpful to the student attempting to analyze muscular actions.

Stabilization

Stabilization in arm-support positions almost invariably requires contractions of opposing muscle groups in nearly all planes of movement, chiefly because the bone structure of the upper extremities is not designed to bear heavy weight. For example, in the upright arm-support position on the parallel bars, the shoulder-joint flexor and extensor muscles actively oppose each other, but no apparent movement takes place. The abductors and adductors and medial and lateral rotators also act in similar fashion.

Shoulder-Girdle Muscles

It is often difficult to comprehend which muscles acting on the shoulder girdle are bearing the body weight because the muscular actions are often opposite what they appear to be. To illustrate, during a hang from an overhead support, the shoulder girdle is elevated, but the elevators are not contracting. Rather, the depressors contract to hold the girdle from being pulled completely out of position; these muscles oppose the pull of gravity on the body.

If the performer is in an arm-supported position with the body upright and vertical (support positions on various gymnastic apparatus), the depressors are again active. If the body is vertical but inverted (handstand), the shoulder-girdle elevators are contracted. In front support positions (push-ups and various starting stances), the scapular abductors become active.

In all the foregoing instances, the contractions are isometric (static), although the muscles may be either at resting length, elongated, or shortened, depending on the stabilized position of the shoulder girdle.

If we keep in mind the concept of the movable girdle, the nonmoving arms, and the pull of gravity on the body, then muscular actions in the various positions become more clear. When analyzing an arm-support position, it is helpful to think of the body weight being transferred directly through the supporting arms to push the shoulder girdle in that direction.

Contractions Causing Little or No Apparent Movement

Although no movement is observed at a particular joint, it is still important to assess the muscular actions present. A case in point is the action of the elbow flexors during the rope climb. It was pointed out earlier that little flexion or extension of this joint is noticed during skillful climbing. This does not suggest an absence of muscular activity in the elbow. During the time that the weight is supported, the flexors of the bent elbow are highly active to prevent the pull of gravity from forcing the elbow to extend. A similar illustration is the use of the shoulder-girdle elevators in the hand walk.

THE ROLE OF KINESTHESIS IN ARM-SUPPORT BALANCE SKILLS

As a result of the kinesthetic sense and other senses associated with balance activities, such as a handstand, a constant flow of sensory information makes the performer aware of adjustments in muscular contractions that are needed to maintain the balanced position. The result of such information is the addition of nervous impulses to the proper muscles, at the proper time, and of proper intensity to correct the body position and keep the body in equilibrium. A person with a strong kinesthetic sense is acutely aware of the exact positions of body parts, and knows of deviations from the desired positions. This awareness makes it possible to initiate correct adjustments in body position quickly. The muscle contractions which maintain balance are constantly varying for several reasons, the most significant of which is fatigue of active motor units and their replacement by other motor units. This explains loss of balance from expending muscular endurance. The switch must be made from the fatigued motor units to fresh ones, which temporarily changes the kinesthetic information. Eventually, an insufficient number of rested motor units are available, and balance is threatened because of fatigue.

IMPROVING ARM-SUPPORT AND ARM-SUSPENSION SKILLS

For effective performance of arm-supported and arm-suspended skills, two primary qualities are essential. They are (1) *adequate strength and endurance* to support the body in the necessary positions and (2) *ability to shift the body weight quickly* into the correct positions at the right time. The first quality (strength) is dependent upon the three factors which compose it, namely, contractile forces of the mover muscles, ability to coordinate all the muscles involved in the movement, and the mechanical ratios involved. A person who lacks adequate arm and shoulder strength to support the body with ease cannot perform skills effectively in arm-support positions. Therefore, additional strength may be the key to improving performance—up to a certain point. If the skill calls for prolonged or successive contractions, then muscle endurance, in addition to strength, becomes important.

The *second primary quality*, ability to shift the body into correct positions at exactly the right time, depends on the following several specific factors: (1) *Insight into the task to be accomplished.* This requires a vision of the specific movements that must occur and their correct sequence. (2) *Adequate kinesthetic perception.* This is demonstrated by the degree to which one remains aware of the exact position of the body and its parts in space. (3) *Agility.* This is very important because it is the ability to change direction of the body and its parts rapidly. (4) *Fast reactions.* Fast reactions contribute to agility, and the two factors combined contribute greatly to one's ability to make fast adjustments in body position in order to maintain balance and perform desired movements with precision. (5) *Coordination.* Specific neuromuscular coordinations are essential; they may be improved from repeated practice of the specific skill. (6) *Precision and timing.* In arm-supported skills, the specific movements of body segments must be executed with great precision and timing. Any movement made out of sequence or with insufficient quickness and precision will detract from a successful performance.

A training program for improving these kinds of skills should include the following: (1) Exercises to increase strength and endurance of the muscles which carry the heavy loads during the performances and exercises to increase flexibility, especially in the hip, back, and shoulder regions. Much of the muscular-endurance requirements will be obtained from repeated actions of the skills or routines being practiced. (2) When the skill is very complex, it should be broken into parts so that each part may be studied and practiced; then the skill should be put together in total sequence. (It is important not to segment a skill too much, because good performance usually requires a smooth flow of movements throughout the performance.) (3) The skill as a whole should be practiced extensively in order to improve coordination, timing, and form throughout the performance.

STUDENT LABORATORY EXPERIENCES

In order to gain insight into some of the dynamics of arm-support activities, the following questions and problems are posed for the student.

1 Rank in order of difficulty a handstand on the floor, on parallel bars, and on rings.

2 Which muscles at the shoulder joint maintain the iron-cross position, the adductors or the abductors?

3 In the reverse grasp in the horizontal bar pull-up, name the main muscle mover at the shoulder joint.

4 Which balance position has the greatest stability—the headstand or the handstand? Using concepts of mechanics, give two reasons for your answer.

5 What is the centrifugal force of a 60-kilogram gymnast at the bottom of a giant swing on the horizontal bar when her center of gravity is 1.25 meters from the bar and her tangential velocity is 7 meters per second? Would grip strength be adequate? (See formula 50.)

6 How much work* (in meter-newtons) is done by a 75-kilogram gymnast doing a muscle-up (a pull-up from hang to full arm-support position), if he raises his center of gravity 1.25 meters? (See formula 35.)

7 Assume that the tangential velocity of the center of gravity at the bottom of a giant swing with a radius of 1.3 meters performed on a horizontal bar is the same as that achieved in free fall from the diameter distance (2.6 meters). What would be the maximum instantaneous tangential velocity in moving from the top-of-the-bar handstand through the giant swing? (See formula 8.)

Chapter 21

Performance in Water

When we move from a solid surface into water, we experience different problems involving performance. Correct solutions to these problems require special knowledge about such matters as buoyancy, propulsive forces in water, resistive forces in water, and correct mechanics of various swimming strokes.

BUOYANCY

According to Archimedes' principle, "a body emersed in fluid is buoyed up with a force equal to the weight of the displaced fluid." This means that if a body displaces water weighing more than itself, the body will float. A rock displaces water weighing less than its weight; therefore, the rock sinks. A cork displaces water weighing more than it weighs; therefore, a cork floats.

When a body displaces water weighing exactly the same as it weighs, it has a specific gravity of 1. In other words, its density is identical to the density of water. When expressed in a formula:

$$\text{Specific gravity} = \frac{\text{weight of the body}}{\text{weight of displaced water}}$$

If a human body has a specific gravity of less than 1, it will float. If its · specific gravity is 1, the body will sink barely below the surface. The farther the specific gravity is above 1, the deeper the body will sink.

Specific gravity of most human beings is slightly less than 1 (with lungs filled with air), meaning that most people are buoyant. However, a few people are not buoyant. With lungs filled, nearly all adults will float; with lungs empty, almost all adults will sink.

The factor that most influences density of the body, and therefore its buoyancy, is the percentage of weight composed of bone and muscle. Bone and muscle tissues are more dense than other body tissues, such as fat and viscera. On the average, men have a higher percentage of bone and muscle than women; therefore, women are more buoyant. For this reason, children are more buoyant than adults, and fatter people are more buoyant than thinner people.

FLOATS

See Figure 21-1. The best test for buoyancy is either the tuck (jellyfish) or pike float. In these positions, a portion of the upper back protrudes above the water's surface if the body is buoyant. A person who is buoyant in one of these positions can learn to float in either a vertical or supine position with the face out of the water. Whether a person floats in a vertical position or supine position depends on body build, which determines the position of the body's center of gravity. Because the body proportions of

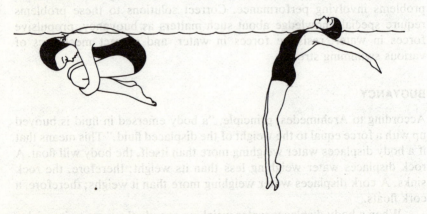

a   *b*

Figure 21-1 Floating positions. (a) Tuck float. (b) Vertical float.

women are typically different from those of men, women float in more of a supine position. Men typically float in a nearly vertical position.

LOCOMOTION IN WATER

Several different strokes and kicks are effectively used to propel the body through water. But regardless of the particular swimming technique used, certain basic facts apply.

Forces Acting

In swimming there are propelling forces and resistive forces. The propelling forces result from the stroke and kick. Resistive forces result from (1) skin resistance (friction), (2) wave-making resistance, and (3) eddy resistance. Skin resistance is by far the most important factor in most cases. In attempting to improve swimming skill, the general objective should be to bring about changes which increase the propelling forces and decrease resistive forces. This can be accomplished by assuming correct body positions and by correctly performing the strokes and kicks with sufficient force.

    Resisting Forces Body position in the water has great influence on resistance to forward progress. The body should be kept near parallel to the water's surface and should present as little body area as possible in the direction of progress. Available evidence from research indicates: (1) The prone position offers less resistance than either the back or side swimming positions. (2) As body rolling action is increased, water resistance increases as a result of friction. (3) At very slow swimming speeds (0.5 meters per second), resistance is greater than at faster speeds 1.5 meters per second), primarily because at the slower speed correct (horizontal) position is not maintained. As speed increases beyond 1.5 meters per second, resistance increases rapidly, because here body position remains essentially the same so the theoretical square law has almost direct application. (4) Tight-fitting suits made of lightweight silk or nylon cause no measurable resistance. The same, however, is not true of cotton and wool suits, although the fit of the suit is more significant than the fabric; loose-fitting suits offer considerably more resistance.

    Incorrect techniques of recovery of the stroke and kick can add greatly to resistance. Recovery should be designed to present as little surface of the arms and legs as possible in the direction of progress. Up-and-down movements of the body increase the wave-making forces, which add to resistance. Therefore, vertical motion of the body should be held to a minimum; in other words, the body should move smoothly in a straight line. The force of inertia can be another source of added resistance if a steady pace is not maintained. Changes in speed result in greatly increased resistance during the acceleration.

Another important source of resistance, although not water resistance, is internal muscle resistance resulting from inability to use a "relaxed" swimming style. Because of the tenseness of some swimmers, the antagonist muscles fail to relax sufficiently to cause free and efficient movement.

Propelling Forces In applying the forces that propel the body through the water, the following guides are important: (1) Almost all the forces should contribute to forward progress, and not to vertical or lateral body movement. (2) A swimmer should seek maximum water resistance against the stroking and kicking movements and minimum resistance against the counter (recovery) movements of the stroke and kick. This means that during the propelling phase, the arms, hands, and feet should present as large a surface as possible to the water, and the arm and hand should *push* against the water, opposite the direction of desired progress. (3) The forces should be applied with speed sufficient to propel the body at an efficient rate; however, the application of forces should not be so great that they are inefficient in terms of energy cost. There is a certain pace for each swimmer which is most efficient, just as there is a certain running pace that is most efficient.

Following are analyses of the four competitive swimming strikes and one utility stroke. Space does not permit analysis of other swimming strokes.

Front Crawl Stroke

See Figures 21-2 and 21-3. It has been observed that excellent crawl-stroke swimmers get at least 70 percent of their propulsion from the arms and 30 percent or less from the legs. However, this ratio varies considera-

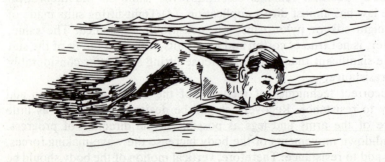

Figure 21-2 Good body position and correct breathing techniques in the crawl stroke.

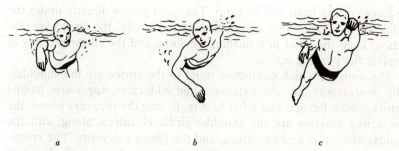

a   b   c

Figure 21-3 Correct mechanics of the crawl stroke (front view).

bly among individuals. Occasionally, a good swimmer is observed who obtains almost all the propulsion from the arm stroke.

To reduce the resistive forces in the crawl stroke to a minimum a swimmer should (1) swim with the head down (face under the water), turning the face to the side only far enough to breathe on every second stroke; (2) keep the whole body near parallel to the surface of the water, thus presenting the smallest body surface possible to the direction of movement; (3) eliminate all actions which move the body up and down or sideward; (4) wear a tight-fitting nylon suit.

The Stroke   To benefit the most from the applied forces in the stroke, the arm and hand should push *backward* against the water's resistance. The counterforce will then be forward and equal to the applied force (Newton's third law). During the early and late phases of the stroke, it is difficult to apply the force directly opposite the direction of progress. When strong force is applied during the early phase, it tends to lift the body, whereas the late phase of the stroke tends to pull the body downward. This problem can be partly eliminated by flexing the wrist at the beginning of the stroke so that the hand "hooks" the water, and hyperextending it during the late phase so that the hand can "push" the water. This causes the palm of the hand to face the desired direction throughout the stroke. However, it still remains that the middle portion of the stroke is by far the most efficient, and the efficiency is the greatest when the arm is in the vertical position (at right angles to the body). Thus the application of force should be maximized during the middle portion of the stroke and minimized during the early and late portions.

The crawl stroke starts with the arm almost fully extended and the hand in front of the shoulder. As the arm begins movement through the water, the elbow flexes slightly, and the wrist flexes enough to cause the hand to pull backward instead of downward against the water. The shoulder dips as it moves backward with the arm. During the middle part of the stroke, medial rotation of the arm is added, which speeds the movement of the hand and forearm. The hand passes directly under the midline of the body. Near completion of the stroke, the wrist hyperextends to keep the hand in a pushing position, and the elbow extends to complete the pushing action.

The muscles which contribute most to the stroke are the shoulder-girdle depressors, shoulder extensors and adductors, upper-arm medial rotators, elbow flexors, and wrist flexors. During the recovery phase, the most active muscles are the shoulder-girdle elevators, along with the shoulder abductors and extensors, and the elbow extensors. The recovery should be ballistic in nature to allow those muscles a brief relaxation period.

The Kick The flutter kick (Figure 21-4) is done faster than the stroke. Good swimmers do between two and four kicks per stroke; this varies at different swimming speeds. At high velocity the flutter kick provides relatively little propulsion, while at slower speeds the kick makes a proportionately greater contribution. Most of the muscular force for the kick comes from the hips, but the follow-through movements of the feet actually cause most of the propulsion. The up-and-down drive from the hips causes the legs to follow through and finally results in a waving (whiplike) movement of the feet. The foot action closely parallels the propelling tail action of a fish. When a fish swims, the driving force comes from movement of the fish's body, which results in slapping-type movements of the tail. The tail movements provide most of the propelling force. The fish's tail moves horizontally, but the swimmer's feet move vertically.

On the down kick, the knee, which has a controlled amount of tension, bends as a result of water force. This bending puts the foot in position so the top pushes downward and backward against the water during the early part of the down stroke, thus propelling the body forward. The ankle must be in a fully extended (plantar flexed) position during the early part of the down kick; at the completion of the down kick, the ankle is partly flexed and the knee is extended. On the up kick, the bottom of the foot provides force against the water in a backward and upward direction. The foot moves from its partially flexed position to full extension at the completion of the kick. The knee remains straight throughout the up kick.

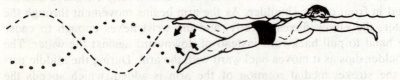

Figure 21-4 Illustration of propelling forces from the flutter kick.

The depth of the kicking action should be 35 to 45 centimeters for adult men, and proportionately less for smaller people. It has been found that increased ankle flexibility will cause more foot action and thus more propulsive force from the flutter kick.

The muscles used most extensively in the flutter kick are the hip flexors and extensors, knee extensors, and ankle flexors and extensors. In addition to the muscles causing the stroke and kick, other muscle groups are used extensively in the crawl stroke. The abdominal and lower back muscles stabilize the pelvic region, and the trunk rotator muscles rotate the trunk in time to the stroking rhythm.

Back Crawl Stroke

The backstroke (Figure 21-5) is somewhat less powerful and less efficient than the front crawl. In the backstroke, a higher proportion of the propelling force comes from the kick (about 35 percent among good swimmers).

The principles relating to resistive forces are the same for the backstroke as those stated earlier for the front crawl. The primary differences between the two swimming methods are (1) the backstroke is performed on the back with the face above the water and the head tilted slightly upward and (2) the stroking action of the backstroke is performed more in the horizontal than in the vertical plane.

The idea of pushing with the hands opposite the direction of progress

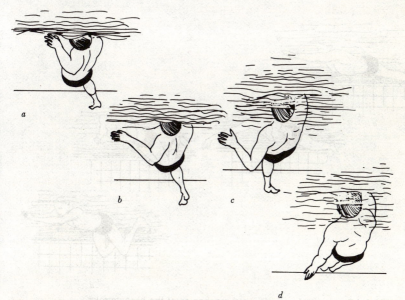

Figure 21-5 Correct mechanics of the back crawl stroke.

is equally as important in the backstroke as in the front crawl. The main muscles involved in this stroke are the shoulder-girdle depressors, shoulder adductors, flexors and medial rotators, elbow flexors, and wrist flexors.

The flutter kick on the back is the same as on the front, except in the reverse direction. The feet should ride high in the water so the toes break the surface at the completion of the up kick. But no part of the kick should be out of the water.

Breaststroke

The main guiding principle for the breaststroke (Figure 21-6), as for every other swimming style, is "maximum efficiency and minimum effort." But it has another basic rule—"symmetry of movement"—which it shares with the fourth stroke to be discussed, the butterfly.

Mechanically, the ideal body position is in the horizontal plane, with the body streamlined. Two factors may cause variation from this position. First, breathing necessitates that the face be clear of the water in the front direction, which is likely to place the body somewhat at an angle. Second, if the body is too horizontal, the feet will break the water's surface and part of the kicking force will be destroyed.

The Stroke   The breaststroke is really only a "half-stroke," performed quickly and forcefully. The pull starts from the glide position with

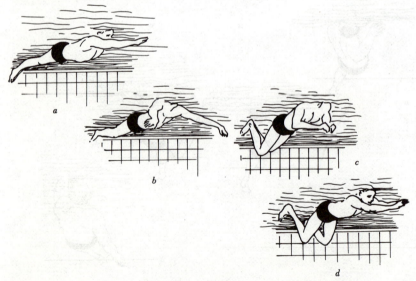

Figure 21-6 Correct body position and mechanics of the breaststroke.

the arms fully extended and the hands in front of the shoulder. The wrists flex to a 45° angle, ready to pull slightly out, down, and forcefully back. As the hands move through the water, the elbows flex slightly and are held high above the hands. The hands move through a sideward-downward arc until the upper arms reach an angle of about 90° to the body. The pull is completed before the arms move past the imaginary perpendicular line extended out from the shoulders. The muscles which contribute most to the pull are wrist flexors, lower-arm medial rotators, elbow flexors, upper-arm medial rotators, shoulder extensors and adductors, and shoulder-girdle depressors.

The arm recovery is no more than a bringing together of the hands underneath the chin, followed by a quick smooth forward thrust of both hands as the swimmer extends into a glide position.

The Kick The "whip kick" (Figure 21-7), which is used in the breaststroke, may contribute more than 50 percent of the total propelling force among good swimmers. In the whip kick, unlike other kicks, the lower legs and knees play a more important part than the hips and thighs.

Beginning from the glide position, the swimmer flexes the knees,

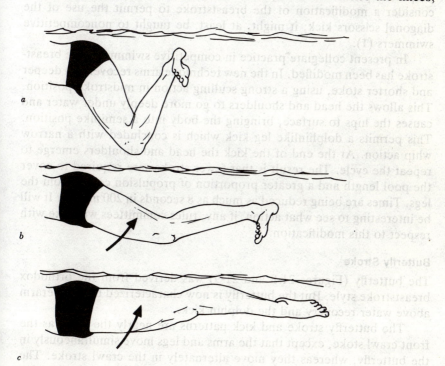

Figure 21-7 Correct mechanics of the whip kick.

bringing the lower legs up and over the knees. The ankles are fully flexed and the feet turned outward (Figure 21-7). While the knees are kept close together, the ankles are separated far apart. The kick is then performed by pushing the feet backward and together in a whiplike motion until the legs are fully extended. The ankles extend and invert during the kick to cause a pushing action with the bottoms of the feet. The hips extend and rotate outward, bringing the ankles together.

During the last half of the stroke, the legs recover from the kick (move to kicking position). As the arms recover from the stroke, the kick is performed, followed by a glide. The complete cycle is stroke-kick-glide.

The muscles used most extensively in the recovery phase of the whip kick are the knee and ankle flexors and the hip flexors and medial rotators. The knee and ankle extensors and hip adductors are the prime contributors to the power phase of the kick.

For recreational swimming a diagonal scissors kick could replace the whip kick in the breaststroke, as it is just as productive in force and efficiency and avoids the frequent trauma called "swimmers knee," which stresses the medial collateral ligaments of the knee in the propulsive phase of the whip kick. Coaches and rules committees could consider a modification of the breaststroke to permit the use of the diagonal scissors kick; it might, at least, be taught to noncompetitive swimmers (1).

In present collegiate practice in competitive swimming, the breast-stroke has been modified. In the new technique arms recover in a deeper and shorter stoke, using a strong sculling action in midstroke position. This allows the head and shoulders to go more deeply under water and causes the hips to surface, bringing the body into a semipike position. This permits a dolphinlike leg kick which is concluded with a narrow whip action. At the end of the kick the head and shoulders emerge to repeat the cycle. The result is that fewer strokes are required to cover the pool length and a greater proportion of propulsion comes from the legs. Times are being reduced as much as 8 seconds in 200 meters. It will be interesting to see what action, if any, rules committees will take with respect to this modification.

Butterfly Stroke

The butterfly (Figures 21-8 and 21-9) was derived from the orthodox breaststroke style. But the butterfly is now characterized by an overarm above water recovery and the dolphin kick.

The butterfly stroke and kick patterns are nearly the same as the front crawl stoke, except that the arms and legs move simultaneously in the butterfly, whereas they move alternately in the crawl stroke. The principles involved and the mechanics of the strokes and kicks are

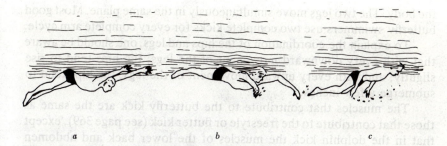

Figure 21-8 Body action during the butterfly stroke.

similar. However, one of the mechanical weaknesses of this stroke is that both arms recover simultaneously, and thus force from the arms is produced intermittently.

The Stroke Refer to page 366 for a description of the crawl stroke. The butterfly stroke differs from that description in only three ways: (1) The arms move simultaneously; (2) the hands pass underneath the shoulders rather than under the midline of the body; and (3) the shoulder does not dip into the stroke.

The Kick The butterfly kick is called the *dolphin kick* because of its resemblance to the movements of the dolphin. The kick is difficult to master because it involves both trunk and leg movements. Also, its timing with the arm pull is difficult. The driving force for the kick begins with an up-and-down movement of the hips. This initiates movements in the spine, and in the hip, knee, and ankle joints, and it results in whiplike movements of the legs and feet. The leg action is similar to that of the flutter kick; but in the dolphin kick the driving force is initiated farther up

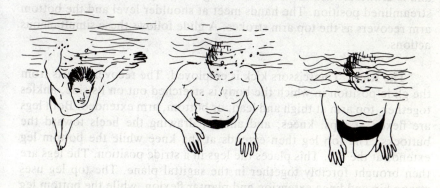

Figure 21-9 Correct mechanics of the butterfly stroke.

the body. The two legs move simultaneously in the same plane. Most good butterfly swimmers use two complete kicks for every complete arm cycle.

To explain the coordination of the hips and legs, one should be aware that with every downward movement of the legs, the hips tend to rise slightly, and with every upward movement of the legs, the hips tend to submerge a few inches.

The muscles that contribute to the butterfly kick are the same as those that contribute to the freestyle or flutter kick (see page 369), except that in the dolphin kick the muscles of the lower back and abdomen become more involved because of the up-and-down movements of the hips.

Sidestroke

The sidestroke is presented here because of its utilitarian value in lifesaving and in recreational swimming. (Less than 5 percent of all swimmers swim competetively; therefore, we devote a few words to the other 95 percent.) The fact that the body lies in the water on the side with the face turned up sufficiently for continuous breathing makes this stroke a comfortable one. The body lies at a slight angle with the horizontal. The hips and legs are below the surface.

The Stroke   The bottom arm uses essentially the same stroke as one arm in the breaststroke, but with the plane of motion rotated 90° due to the side-lying position. The muscles used in stroke and recovery are the same as those used in the breast stroke described earlier in this chapter. The top arm uses the same pattern as is used in the last half of the crawl stroke; again the same musculature as described earlier is involved. The top arm recovers under water (as the bottom arm strokes) and is drawn toward the shoulder along the body's anterior surface in a streamlined position. The hands meet at shoulder level and the bottom arm recovers as the top arm strokes. A glide follows these simultaneous actions.

The Kick   The scissors kick is employed. The recovery starts from the glide position in which the body is stretched out on its side, ankles together, top arm at thigh and lead, or bottom, arm extended. Both legs are flexed at hips, knees, and ankles, drawing the heels toward the buttocks. The top leg then extends at the knee while the bottom leg extends at the hip. This places the legs in a stride position. The legs are then brought forcibly together in the sagittal plane. The top leg uses strong hip and knee extension and plantar flexion, while the bottom leg uses hip flexion, knee extension, and a flexible ankle.

STUDENT LABORATORY EXPERIENCES

Answer the following questions to further fix the concepts and to see quantitative aspects of water activities.

1 List in order the probable buoyancy, ranking from most buoyant to least buoyant: (a) a slender male athlete in training; (b) an overweight woman; (c) an average woman; (d) an average man.

2 In problem #1 would the specific gravity of (a) be greater or less than that of (b)?

3 Would a person with 20 percent body fat have an easier time learning to swim than one with 5 percent body fat, other things being equal?

4 List three basic resistive forces swimmers face.

5 Assume that a racer in the 100-meter freestyle event leaves the blocks 0.3 seconds after the gun with a horizontal velocity of 5 meters per second, enters the water 4 meters from the start, and glides 4 meters, uniformly decelerating to 1.9 meters per second. He then continues to stroke at 1.9 meters per second to the 50-meter bulkhead, where with an efficient flip-turn and push-off at 3.5 meters per second, he slows uniformly to a swimming speed of 1.9 meters per second at 4 meters. What will be his 100-meter time? Is this a world-class time? (See formula **1**, **2**.)

Chapter 22

Summary: How to Improve Performance

It is now appropriate to reintroduce the function of the teacher, coach, and therapist: to help people to increase their ability to perform. This book aims to prepare the reader to give people this kind of help by providing insight into the factors within and outside the body that influence performance. This chapter is a summary of the major factors involved in achieving high-level performance. Five major aspects are involved:

1 Motor development
2 Physiological conditioning
3 Specific skill development
4 Correct application of laws and principles
5 Psychological preparation

Parts of some of these aspects of performance have been covered in detail in previous chapters of this book, and other information is outside the scope of this text. But all the aspects involved in the improvement of performance are covered briefly here in order to give the reader a more complete view.

MOTOR DEVELOPMENT

An individual's general motor ability (general athletic ability) is demonstrated by how well he or she performs skills and demonstrates characteristics which are common to a variety of activities. A person who has a high level of general motor development possesses in large degree the performance characteristics that are useful in numerous situations. These include endurance, strength, agility, power, flexibility, speed, reaction time, and coordination. A person possessing these characteristics to a high degree is said to be a "natural athlete," which is a way of saying that he or she possesses the foundation from which to develop excellence in a number of motor activities.

General motor ability can be increased by developing its various components. Some of the components have rather large potential while others have limited potential for development. The term *general motor ability* does not necessarily mean "inborn." Motor capacity is inborn, but the amount and kind of use greatly influence the level of ability developed within the limits of capacity. A gifted person may possess relatively high levels of ability while others with less endowment display more general motor ability attributable to extensive experience in motor activities.

One important way to develop general motor ability is to participate in a variety of different activities during the formative years. People who are active in a variety of ways develop the characteristics of performance better than those who are not active or those who are active in very limited ways. Another approach is to concentrate specifically on the development of certain components of general athletic ability, such as deliberately increasing strength, endurance, speed, or any of the other components noted above.

It should be noted that general motor ability in itself does not make a person an excellent performer in a particular event, but it does furnish the base from which excellence can be developed by becoming proficient in the skills which are specific to that particular activity, and to elevate the levels of appropriate fitness characteristics.

PHYSIOLOGICAL CONDITIONING

Physiological conditioning is important in all forms of vigorous performance. Conditioning programs are especially designed to bring about positive changes in the functioning of the physiological systems.

Endurance (Circulorespiratory and Muscular)

A large amount of endurance implies that a performer can persist at a given level of exercise. When endurance gives away to fatigue as a result of muscular work, several elements which are important to good performance diminish. Fatigue results in reduction of strength, neuromuscular coordination and timing, speed of movement, reaction time, accuracy, and general alertness. Increased endurance prolongs the time before the onset of fatigue. Therefore, endurance contributes to improved performances in activities where fatigue may be a restricting factor. However, when fatigue is not a restricting factor, this kind of training is of little or no direct value to the performance. In order to increase the endurance of any of the body's systems, that system must be overloaded regularly. The procedure for accomplishing this is explained briefly in Chapter 9.

Strength

The amount of force a person can apply with a particular part of the body is the strength of that part. This definition implies the importance of strength in athletic performance. Even though nearly all human movements are performed against some resistance, athletic movements involve greater resistance than is normal. For instance, in putting the shot, throwing the discus, pole vaulting, gymnastic movements, jumping, running, swimming, leaping, and other such vigorous movements, the body segments apply near-maximum force, and the amount of force that can be applied has strong influence on success. Because strength is so important to athletic performance, let us analyze how it contributes.

It is interesting to note that strength is a basic element in several other components important to performance. Thus strength takes on unusual significance. *Power* is the ability to project the body or an object through space (or to do work against time). Power is basic to jumping activities (projecting the body) and to throwing and putting activities (projecting an object). Power is also the basic element in maximum striking and sprinting. Increased strength causes increased ability to apply force. Therefore, if velocity remains constant, increased strength contributes to power.

Strength is also a contributor to *muscular endurance*. Endurance is the ability to resist fatigue and to recover quickly after fatigue. It enables a performer to persist at a given level of performance. If a weak muscle can perform a movement against a given resistance fifty times, then a stronger muscle can perform against the same resistance with greater ease; therefore, it can repeat the movement considerably more than fifty times. This means that if all else is equal, increased strength aids muscular endurance. Of course, endurance is dependent upon the efficient functioning of several different body systems, but muscular strength is one of the important elements.

Strength contributes to *agility*, which is defined as the ability to change direction of the body and its parts rapidly. Agility is demonstrated in such activities as the dodging shuttle run, zigzag run, and squat thrust. Agility is essential to good performance in field games (such as football, soccer, and hockey) and court games (such as basketball, tennis, volleyball, and badminton). Changing direction requires adequate strength to overcome momentum, which tends to keep the body moving in the same direction. After the direction has been changed, strength (really power, of which strength is a part) is important in regaining momentum in the new direction. Without adequate strength a high level of agility is impossible.

Strength is important to *running speed*, which is basic to performance in many activities. Actually, running speed is closely related to power because running is a series of body projections made alternately from the right and left feet. In running, the body is thrust forward by the force of body levers pushing against a resistive surface. Increased strength will cause increased force, which will improve running speed.

Thus it becomes evident that strength makes a large contribution to many forms of athletics. The coach and performer should give adequate attention to strengthening those muscle groups which contribute directly to the desired movements. Methods of developing strength are explained in Chapter 9.

Even though strength influences performance in several ways, it should not be thought of as a panacea. More strength is not always the answer to improving performance.

Power

The ability to project the body or an object through space is dependent upon power. Obviously, the ability to project the body is important in many performances, including basketball, volleyball, football, some track and field events, gymnastics, dance, and running. The ability to project an object is equally important in track and field throwing events, baseball, softball, basketball, and football. Ability to project the body or an object can be increased by improving one or both of the factors (force and velocity) which contribute to power. The application of force is increased by increasing strength. Velocity is dependent upon the speed of muscular contractions, which can be increased as a result of speed training.

Agility

The ability to make a rapid change in direction of the body or its parts depends on strength, reaction time, speed of movement, and specific coordinations. Agility is important in activities involving dodging and fast starting and stopping, as well as in those requiring a series of quick movements of body segments. In short, agility is a direct result of the degree of acceleration of which a person is capable. It is measurable. Agility in specific movement patterns can be increased by practicing those movements, thereby improving coordinations contributing to the movements. Also, increased strength will increase agility in movements where momentum tends to keep the body in motion in the same direction. Other factors which determine agility, namely, speed of movement and reaction time, may be improved as a result of specific training. But these factors can be influenced only a limited amount. Like power, agility in a specific movement pattern can be favorably influenced by improving coordination in that particular movement, which is accomplished best by correctly practicing the particular movement over and over.

Running Speed

Running is an athletic event by itself and is also important in other athletic activities. To increase running speed, the performer must improve (1) length of stride, or (2) leg speed, or (3) a combination of these. Length of stride can be increased by *increasing power* of the muscle groups which are of prime importance in running (best possibility for improving speed), or by getting the runner to *lengthen the stride* consciously. Also, increased hip flexibility can have a positive effect. Too much lengthening of the stride will have a detrimental effect because the foot is planted too far forward.

The rate with which the legs can be moved while taking full running strides is dependent upon (1) reaction time, (2) coordination of the muscles involved, (3) speed of muscle contractions, and (4) leg strength. If any of these factors is improved, then speed of leg movement will increase. A slight increase can have a significant effect on performance.

A sprinter may sometimes reduce the time by improving parts of the race other than running speed, such as a better starting technique, faster acceleration, improved efficiency, or better finishing technique.

Reaction Time

Reaction time is the time which elapses between the external stimulus and the initial response. It is extremely important in all performances where quick movements are required, and it has special significance in events where individuals defend against each other. Here contestants must respond quickly to each other's movements. Reaction time in specific movements will improve a limited amount as a result of extensive practice of those movements under competitive conditions. For example, practice of starting to a pistol shot will result in faster reactions to that stimulus, and even a small improvement will produce significant results.

Flexibility

Flexibility is influenced by the extensibility of the muscles, tendons, and ligaments. Lack of flexibility restricts full range of motion. However, range of motion may also be restricted by other factors, such as bone structure at the joint, and muscle or other tissue near the joint. Flexibility is important in such performances as modern dance, gymnastics, and diving. In these activities the body parts must bend enough to assume desired positions which are consistent with good form. The pike position, for example, requires great flexibility in the back of the upper legs and the lower back.

Flexibility can be increased by regular stretching of the muscles, tendons, and ligaments. The best approach is to determine the tissues which need to be stretched, place them on stretch, hold the position for a few seconds, and repeat several times. The muscles should be stretched until a stretch pain is felt. This procedure must be followed regularly. Bobbing movements are not recommended; slow stretch is both safer and more effective.

SPECIFIC SKILLS

Specific skills are coordinated movements of throwing, shooting, jumping, swimming, rebounding, and so forth. No one, regardless of other components, will be able to perform well in a particular activity until, through long hours of practice, the skills specific to the performance are developed. For example, endurance, agility, reaction time, power, and speed are general athletic components that are essential in basketball, and they are equally important in other vigorous sports. But shooting, dribbling, passing, and rebounding are specific skills unique to basketball, not needed to the same degree in other sports. In order to play basketball well, a person must develop the skills specific to the game. Likewise, a performer will not do well in tennis, bowling, or soccer without developing the specific skills of those activities.

Essentially, skill improvement amounts to practicing the skill correctly over and over until the movement pattern becomes consistent and effective. Also as a result of correct practice the performer will increase judgment of speed, distance, and time, and insight into the circumstances of the performance.

Accuracy

Accuracy is involved in such skills as shooting in basketball, throwing in baseball, softball, and football, shooting in archery, or rolling a bowling ball. In practicing for accuracy, it is very important for the performer to do so at performance speed. Throwing a baseball accurately at slow speed is different from throwing accurately at a fast speed; performing a lay-up in basketball at slow speed requires different timing and judgments than performing the same skill at high speed. Under competitive conditions, most skills are performed with high speed and maximum effort. Slowing down the performance during practice will aid in analyzing the mechanics of the skill, and improving the movement patterns; but for best results, accuracy skills should be practiced extensively at performance speed and intensity. Accuracy is also dependent upon judgment of speed, distance, and time.

Judgment of Speed, Distance, and Time

Judgment of speed, distance, and time is important to a football player when he throws downfield to a receiver. The passer must judge the distance to the receiver, and also correctly judge the receiver's speed and the speed of the ball.

In shooting a basketball, the player must correctly judge the distance from the basket, then have the skill necessary to put the ball where this judgment indicates it should go. A player passing to a guard cutting in for a lay-up must correctly judge the speed and position of the guard. The guard laying up the shot must correctly judge speed and the rebound of the ball.

Smoothness and Efficiency

Smooth and efficient performances result when (1) superfluous (noncontributing) movements are reduced to a minimum, (2) tension by antagonist muscles is reduced, and (3) correct timing is accomplished. The first factor is accomplished by identifying noncontributing motions and purposely eliminating them. For instance, in swimming, excessive head movement is noncontributing and detrimental. The same can be said about extraneous head, arm, or leg movements while running. The second factor may be accomplished by developing (1) an adequate amount of flexibility in the antagonist muscles, and (2) the neuromuscular coordination necessary to cause these muscles (antagonists) to relax more fully during the desired movements. The third factor can be accomplished only by extensive, correct practice of the movements.

APPLICATION OF LAWS AND PRINCIPLES

Laws and principles influence all motor performances; the influence varies with the nature of the performance. The performer must identify the laws and principles which influence that performance and apply them correctly.

Leverage

The amount of force applied with any body segment and the speed of that segment are partly determined by the relative lengths of the force arm and resistance arm of each lever. Often the relative length may be altered by changing the body position. Correct leverage determines good body mechanics and correct technique (see Chapter 11).

Motion and Force

All performances involve movement of the body, and often motion of an object. Application of force is necessary to cause motion. Therefore, knowledge of how to apply the basic principles of motion and force is essential to improving performance. These principles and their applications are discussed in Chapters 12 and 13.

Balance and Stability

Balance of the body in both static and dynamic positions is important. In certain performances, balance is a prime objective, and the extent to which a person is able to remain in a stable position often determines success. Therefore, the application of the principles of balance and stability becomes basic to good performance. The content of Chapter 15 provides the important information about balance and stability.

Projecting, Spinning, and Rebounding of Objects

Understanding laws and principles relating to the use of implements and how to control them is often a key to better performance. For example, it is necessary to know the optimum angle for projecting a javelin or discus. It is important to know the influence of spin on a volleyball, baseball, or tennis ball. A good performer must have insight into how a handball, basketball, or softball will rebound. Many of these insights are developed through extensive participation, but understanding and applying the basic laws and principles of projection, spinning, and rebounding can be a shortcut to better performance. The application of these laws and principles is discussed in Chapter 14.

PSYCHOLOGICAL PREPARATION

There are two aspects of psychology related to performances; one relates to training and the other to competition. In order to train hard over a period of several months, a person must maintain a positive attitude. Otherwise, the athlete becomes stale and uninterested. The other psychological aspect of performance involves the preparation that the athlete goes through to prepare for each performance.

Audiovisual
Aids

The following audiovisual aids are useful for teachers of kinesiology:

Charts

Large wall charts showing the anatomy of the human body are available from several sources. Charts of the muscular and skeletal systems are of great use in kinesiology, and charts of the nervous, circulatory, and respiratory systems are also helpful. Suggested sources of the charts are:

> Denoyer-Geppert Co., 5235 Ravenswood Ave., Chicago, Ill. 60640.
> Nystron/Division of Carnation Co., 3333 Elston Avenue, Chicago, Ill. 60618.

Models

Of greatest use are models of the muscular and skeletal systems and of specific joints and bones. Following are sources of such models:

> Merck, Sharp & Dohme, West Point, Pa. 19486.
> J. A. Preston Corporation, 60 Page Road, Clifton, N.J. 07012.
> Denoyer-Geppert Company, 5235 Ravenswood Ave., Chicago, Ill. 60640.

Nystron Division of Carnation Co., 3333 Elston Avenue, Chicago, Ill. 60618.

Slides

The following picture slides are very useful:

Slides on the human body by CIBA, Box 195, West Caldwell, N.J. 07006.

Loop Films

Many teachers choose to make their own loop films. Consult your own university film library for useful loops.

Track and field super 8 and 16 mm color films of all events, 1980 Olympics or more recent, *Track & Field News*, P.O. Box 296, Los Altos, Calif. 94022.

Loop films on swimming, volleyball, and several other sports, McGraw-Hill Book Company, 1221 Avenue of the Americas, New York, N.Y. 10020.

Movie Films

The following useful films may be purchased or rented:

Muscle: Chemistry of Contraction, Encyclopaedia Britannica Educational Corp., 425 N. Michigan Ave., Chicago, Ill. 60611.

Muscle: Dynamics of Contraction, Encyclopaedia Britannica Educational Corp., 425 N. Michigan Ave., Chicago, Ill. 60611.

Your Body and Its Parts, Britannica Films, Inc., 425 N. Michigan Ave., Chicago, Ill. 60611.

The Spinal Column, Britannica Films, Inc., 425 N. Michigan Ave., Chicago, Ill. 60611.

The Nerve Impulse, Britannica Films, Inc., 425 N. Michigan Ave., Chicago, Ill. 60611.

Simple Machines, Britannica Films, Inc., 425 N. Michigan Ave., Chicago, Ill. 60611.

Gravity, Britannica Films, Inc., 425 N. Michigan Ave., Chicago, Ill. 60611.

Work of the Heart, Encyclopaedia Britannica Educational Corp., 425 N. Michigan Ave., Chicago, Ill. 60611.

Forces Making Things Move, Encyclopaedia Britannica Educational Corp., 425 N. Michigan Ave., Chicago, Ill., 60611.

Human Body—Skeleton, Coronet Productions, 65 E. South Water Street, Chicago, Ill., 60606.

Human Body—Circulatory System, Coronet Productions, 65 E. South Water Street, Chicago, Ill., 60606.

Consult your own university film library for useful titles connected with any phase of skill in dance, sports, or athletics.

TV Replays

Replayable tapes made of class members in selected movements can also be useful teaching tools.

Slow Motion Film Analysis

The following movie projectors will be useful:

16 mm and super 8 mm stop action and slow motion film analyzers, Lafayette Instrument Co., P.O. Box 5729, Lafayette, Ind. 47903.

Consult your own university audiovisual aids or learning resource center for the above or similar movie projectors.

Appendix B
Glossary

Abduction The movement of any body segment away from the midline of the
  body.

Acceleration Rate of increase in velocity.

Actin A muscle protein which, along the myosin, is responsible for muscle
  contraction and relaxation.

Adduction The movement of body segments toward the midline of the body.

Aerobic Occurring in the presence of oxygen. Aerobic processes occur with
  oxygen present.

Afferent nervous system Also called sensory nervous system. The bodily system
  that directs impulses from sensory receptors toward the spinal cord and
  brain.

Agility The ability to change directions of the body or its parts rapidly.
  Demonstrated in such movements as dodging, zigzagging, stopping, starting,
  and reversing direction of movement.

Agonist muscle A muscle which contributes to the desired movement by its
  concentric contraction.

Alveoli The tiny air sacs in the lungs where external respiration takes place.

Anaerobic Occurring in the absence of oxygen. Anaerobic processes occur with
  no oxygen present.

Anatomical position A stance in which the body is at "military attention" with the palms facing forward.

Antagonist muscle A muscle which acts in opposition to the desired movement.

Anterior Situated before or toward the front.

Appendicular skeleton That portion of the skeleton comprising the upper and lower extremities.

Artery A vessel that carries blood away from the heart.

Autonomic nervous system The bodily system that is involuntary; it cannot be consciously controlled.

Axial skeleton That portion of the skeleton comprising head, neck, and trunk.

Axis A fixed point around which a moving object revolves.

Axon Appendage of the neuron that conducts impulses away from the cell body.

Biomechanics That portion of kinesiology which deals with the quantitative computational aspects of the field. It is, in a sense, the integration of the biological with the mechanical.

Capillary The smallest of the blood vessels.

Capsular ligament A ligament which completely surrounds and encloses a joint.

Cardiac output Volume of blood pumped through the two ventricles in one minute.

Center of gravity The point of intersection of the three primary planes of the body. The exact center of the body. The point around which the body would rotate freely in all directions if it were free to rotate.

Central nervous system (CNS) The bodily system that includes the brain and spinal cord.

Centrifugal force The force that tends to keep a moving object in motion along a straight line. The force that provides resistance to turning movements.

Centripetal force The force that causes a moving object to turn. The force which opposes centrifugal force.

Circumduction Movement in a circular, cone-shaped pattern.

Concentric contraction Shortening of a muscle due to nervous impulses.

Conditioned reflex A reflex pattern which is learned as opposed to being inborn.

Contractile force (muscle) The amount of tension applied by a muscle or group of muscles during contraction.

Coordination The act of various muscles working together in a smooth concerted way. Correct and precise timing of muscle contractions.

Coronary system The body system which includes the blood vessels that service the heart muscle.

Crest (bone) A ridgelike structure upon a bone.

Deceleration Rate of decrease in velocity.

Dendrite The appendage of a neuron which directs impulses toward the cell body.

Diastole The relaxation phase of each heartbeat.

Diastolic pressure The blood pressure during the relaxation of the ventricles.

Distal Farthest from the body midline or point of reference. The hand is at the distal end of the arm.

Dorsiflexion The act of cocking the foot; the act of bringing the top of the foot closer to the tibia.

Dynamic contraction Same as isotonic or phasic contraction.

Dynamic posture The posture or position of the body while in motion.

Eccentric contraction Controlled lengthening of a muscle. The muscle becomes longer as it contracts because the resistance is greater than the contractile force.

Ectomorph An individual who has a slight, or slender, body build.

Efferent system The motor nervous system which directs impulses from the brain and spinal cord to muscles, glands, and organs.

Electrogoniometer A device used to measure and record joint action.

Electromyograph A device used to measure and record the changes in electrical potential of muscles during contraction.

Endomorph An individual who has a fat or heavy body build.

End plate (motor) That portion of a motor neuron which attaches to a muscle fiber.

Endurance Ability to resist fatigue and to recover quickly after fatigue.

Epicondyle (bone) A projection on or above a condyle on a bone which is used for muscle attachment.

Eversion The act of turning the sole of the foot outward.

Extension Movement that increases the angle at a joint, thus straightening the joint.

Extensor thrust reflex An involuntary act caused by pressure on the bottoms of the feet, resulting in a reflex contraction of extensor muscles.

External respiration The exchange of gases at the alveoli in the lungs.

First-class lever A lever arrangement with the axis between the force and the resistance (*F-A-R*).

Flexibility That property of muscles and connective tissue which allows full range of motion.

Flexion Movement that decreases the angle at a joint; the act of bending the joint.

Force The strength or energy exerted to bring about motion or a change in motion.

Fossa A depression in a bone.

Frontal plane An imaginary plane which dissects the body into anterior and posterior halves.

Ganglion A collection or bundle of nerve-cell bodies outside the central nervous system.

Gray matter That tissue in the central nervous system made up of nerve-cell bodies.

Hamstring muscle group Three muscles of the posterior thigh: biceps femoris, semimembranosus, and semitendinosus.

Horizontal extension Extension of a body segment through the transverse (horizontal) plane.

Horizontal flexion Flexion of a body segment through the transverse (horizontal) plane.

Hyperextension Extension of a body segment past the anatomical position.

Hypertrophy An increase in the overall size of a tissue.

Hyperventilation The state caused by hard breathing in which too much air pressure results in dizziness and/or unconsciousness.

Inertia A property of matter by which it remains at rest or in uniform motion in the same straight line unless acted upon by some external force.

Inferior portion The portion of a body that is below, or deeper than, another structure or reference point.

Insertion (of a muscle) Muscle attachment farthest from the midline of the body; the more movable attachment.

Internal respiration The exchange of gases between the circulatory system and the tissues throughout the body.

Internuncial neuron A neuron in the spinal cord that serves as a connection between motor and sensory neurons.

Inversion The act of turning the sole of the foot inward.

Isometric contraction A contraction in which muscle tension increases, but the muscle does not shorten because it does not overcome the resistance.

Isotonic contraction A contraction in which muscle fibers shorten as a result of stimulus.

Kinesthetic sense A sense of awareness, without the use of the other senses, of muscle and joint positions and actions.

Lateral flexion Flexion of the trunk or neck sideward: sideward bend.

Lateral rotation Rotation of a body segment outwardly away from the midline of the body.

Lever (body) A rigid bar comprised of one or more bones which revolves about an axis (joint).

Ligament Tough connective tissue which binds bones together, forming joints.

Locomotion Movement of the body from one point to another by its own power.

Medial rotation Rotation of a body segment inwardly, toward the midline of the body.

Mesomorph An individual who has a husky or muscular body build or a medium-type body build.

Metabolism The sum total of all the chemical processes of the body.

Minute volume (heart) The volume of blood pumped through the left ventricle in one minute.

Momentum The property of a moving body that determines the force required to bring the body to rest. Momentum = mass × velocity.

Motor unit A group of muscle fibers dispersed throughout a muscle and supplied by a single motor nerve fiber.

Movement time The amount of time that it takes to accomplish the movement after the impulse to respond has been received.

Multijoint muscle A muscle that extends over two or more joints.

Muscle boundness A pathological condition brought on by improper training in which the joints lose some of their range of motion due to hypertrophied muscles.

Muscle bundle A group of 20 to 100 muscle fibers, lying parallel to each other and bound together by a connective tissue.

Myosin A muscle protein which, along with actin, is responsible for muscle contraction and relaxation.

Nerve (nerve tract) A cablelike bundle composed of many nerve fibers.

Neuromuscular coordination Coordination which results from nerve impulses reaching the proper muscles, with sufficient intensity, at the correct time.

Neuromyal junction The intersection between the motor end plate of a nerve branch and the muscle fiber.

Neuron A complete nerve cell, including the cell body and all its appendages.

Neutralizer muscle A muscle that acts to equalize the action of another muscle.

Origin (of a muscle) The muscle attachment closer to the midline of the body; the less movable attachment.

Overload The process of demanding more performance from a system than is ordinarily required.

Oxygen debt (deficit) A condition which results when the demand for oxygen is greater than the supply.

Peripheral nervous system The body system which includes all those parts of the nervous system not included in the brain and spinal cord.

Plantar flexion Also known as ankle extension. The act of moving the top of the foot away from the tibia.

Posterior portion Rear or back portion.

Postural muscles Also called antigravity muscles. The muscles used to maintain posture.

Power The product of force × velocity. The ability to apply force at a rapid rate.

Prime-mover muscle A muscle which makes a primary contribution to the desired movement.

Process (of a bone) A prominence or projection on a bone.

Progressive resistance training A muscle-training program in which the amount of resistance is systematically increased as the muscles gain in strength.

Pronation The act of turning the palms of the hands downward.

Proximal Located toward the midline of the body or nearest the point of reference.

Quadriceps muscle group Four muscles of the anterior thigh: rectus femoris, vastus lateralis, vastus medialis, and vastus intermedius.

Range of motion The amount of movement that can occur in a joint, expressed in degrees.

Reaction board A special board used with a scale to determine the location of the center of gravity in a human.

Reaction time That time between the reception of a signal to respond and the beginning of the response.

Reflex An immediate response to a situation in which the thought process is bypassed.

Reflex time Time of nerve impulse travel in a reflex action.

RM (repetition maximum) In weight training, the maximum number of repetitions that can be accomplished against a given amount of resistance.

Rotary motion (angular) The rotation of an object about an axis with each point of the object describing an arc or a circle around the axis.

Rotation Movement of a body segment around its own longitudinal axis.

Sagittal plane An imaginary plane which dissects the body into right and left halves.

Second-class lever A lever arrangement with the resistance between the axis and the force (*F-R-A*).

Segmental method A method of locating the center of gravity in a person by locating the center of gravity of each body segment

Shoulder-girdle depression Lowering of the shoulder girdle.

Shoulder-girdle elevation Raising of the shoulder girdle.

Shoulder-girdle protraction Broadening of the distance between the two shoulder joints.

Shoulder girdle retraction Narrowing of the distance between the two shoulder joints.

6-6-6 A technique in isometric weight training consisting of near-maximum contractions for six seconds and rest for six seconds, repeated six times.

Skeletal muscle Also called striated, motor, and voluntary muscle. A muscle which attaches to and causes movement of the skeleton.

Skill Neuromuscular coordination.

Smooth muscle Also called visceral and involuntary muscle. A muscle located in the internal organs, with the exception of the heart.

Stability Firmness in position. Ability to withstand external force.

Stabilizer muscle Any muscle that acts to stabilize or fix a body segment in order for another segment to move on it.

Static contraction Same as tonic or isometric contraction.

Static posture The posture or position of the body while at rest.

Static work The condition in which no movement occurs when muscular force is applied.

Steady state A condition where the supply of oxygen to the tissues is equal to the demand for oxygen.

Strength The ability to apply force with a segment of the body.

Stretch reflex An automatic reflex to contract in skeletal muscles, brought on by sudden stretching of the muscles.

Stroke volume (heart) The volume of blood pumped out of the left ventricle with each contraction.

Summation wave A sustained muscular contraction caused by high frequency of nerve impulses.

Superior portion A body portion that is above, or over, another body portion or reference point.

Supination The act of turning the palms of the hands upward.

Synapse The intersection (junction) between two or more nerve fibers.

Systole The contracting phase of each heartbeat.

Tendon A tough fibrous tissue that connects muscles to bones.

Third-class lever A lever arrangement with the force between the axis and the resistance (*A-F-R*).

Translatory motion Motion in which an object moves from one point to another point, as opposed to rotary motion. It can occur in either a linear or a curvilinear path.

Transverse plane An imaginary plane which bisects the body into upper and lower halves.

Trochanter   A large projection or prominence upon a bone.
Tuberosity   A large rounded prominence upon a bone.
Turgor   The natural pressure from fluids inside a cell.
Vasomotor tone   The tone of the muscles that line the walls of the blood vessels.
Vein   A vessel that returns blood to the heart.
Velocity   The rate at which an object travels in a given direction.
Viscosity (blood)   The "thickness" of a fluid; the resistance to flow.
Vital capacity   The total amount of air that can be forced out of the lungs after a forced inhalation.
Voluntary nervous system   That part of the nervous system which is consciously controlled.
White matter   That tissue in the central nervous system made up of nerve fibers, not nerve-cell bodies.
Work   A condition occurring when muscles contract. If the muscle contractions cause movement, the work is dynamic; if no movement occurs, the work is static. Also, work = force × distance.

APPENDIX C

Answers to Student Laboratory Experiences

Chapter 3

1 See Figure 3-1 and pages 27–29.
2 See pages 30–34.
3 See your own responses.
4 a Elevation, depression, protraction (abduction), retraction (adduction), upward rotation, downward rotation, anterior lilt
  b Flexion, extension, abduction, adduction, medial rotation, lateral rotation, horizontal flexion (adduction), horizontal extension (abduction), hyperextension, circumduction
  c Flexion, extension, pronation, supination
  d Flexion, extension, ulnar flexion, radial flexion, circumduction
  e Flexion, extension, abduction, adduction, circumduction
  f Flexion, extension, long abduction, short abduction, adduction, circumduction, opponens function
  g Flexion, extension, lateral flexion, rotation
  h Same as g

i Flexion, extension, lateral flexion
j Same as **b**
k Extension; flexion; hyperextension; when knee is flexed, both medial and lateral rotation
l Plantar flexion (foot extension), dorsi flexion (foot flexion)
m Flexion, extension, eversion (pronation), inversion (supination), circumduction
n Flexion, extension, abduction, adduction

Chapter 6

1, **2**, and **3** are subjective.
4 See muscle action table at the end of Chapter 6.

Chapter 7

1 Is subjective.
2 See muscle action table at the end of Chapter 7.

Chapter 8

1, **2**, and **3** are experimental and subjective in nature.
4 See muscle action table at the end of Chapter 8.

Chapter 9

This experience would need to be evaluated by the instructor.

Chapter 11

1 (*a*) A quick heel-raise while not leaning forward. The ball of the foot is the fulcrum, the line of body weight passes through the navicular bone and is the approximate position of resistance. The Achilles tendon attached to the heel bone is the point of application of force. (*b*) The brachioradialis in elbow flexion of the arm with the hand as a fist. Fulcrum is the elbow joint, point of application of effort is the insertion on the distal end of the radius. The resistance is the center of gravity of the forearm and fist, about 10 centimeters above the insertion toward the elbow.
2 (*a*) Elbow extension in the triceps curl, point of force application at the olecranon process of the ulna. Axis at the elbow joint, resistance lower in forearm or hand. (*b*) Head extension from a front flexed position. Weight of the head, the resistance located anterior to the spine. Axis, the atlanto-occipital joint. Point of application of force, the posterior spinal muscles on the occipital bone. (*c*) The tilt of the pelvis by the glutus medius and minimus on the support leg when the opposite leg is raised off the surface. Point of application of force at the midlateral ilium, axis the hip joint, resistance the raised leg. Many other answers are possible.
3 In each case the force application is between the resistance and the axis. Several examples are (*a*) elbow flexion by the biceps, (*b*) knee extension by the quadriceps, (*c*) knee flexion by the hamstrings, (*d*) upper arm abduction

by the deltoid, and (e) horizontal shoulder flexion by the pectoralis major. Dozens more examples could be explored.

4 M.A. is 0.067:1; speed 15:1. It is a first-class lever.
5 M.A. is 2.67:1; it is a force lever and a second-class lever.
6 M.A. is 0.185:1, muscular force is 476.28 newtons. It is a third-class speed lever.

Chapter 12

1 30 meters; the same; linear motion; curvilinear motion
2 (a) 8.33 meters per second; (b) 2.5 meters per second squared (c) 5 meters per second
3 (a) 2 revolutions per second; (b) 12.56 radians per second; (c) 720° per second
4 35.83 meters per second
5 571.42° per second, or 10 radians per second, or 1.59 revolutions per second
6 (a) 17.13 radians per second; (b) 2.73 revolutions per second; (c) 981.18° per second
7 (a) 10.84 meters per second; (b) zero; (c) 83.5 kilogram-meters per second

Chapter 13

1 (a) 294 newtons; (b) 16.33 newtons per square centimeter
2 (a) 1029 newtons; (b) 2206.7 newtons; (c) 2434.9 newtons
3 2205 newtons
4 (a) 37.93 meters per second squared; (b) 275.76 newtons
5 1338 newtons
6 2743.13 newtons
7 1372 meter-newtons
8 (a) 882 meter-newtons; (b) 882 neter-newtons
9 2205 meter-newtons per second
10 279.5 newtons
11 0.839

Chapter 14

1 0.8367
2 2.376 meters
3 (a) 17.85 meters; (b) 3.82 seconds
4 Yes, one at lay-out, three at tuck
5 (a) 20.95°; (b) 0.625 meters; (c) 9.787 meters per second
6 (a) 75.18 meters; (b) 3.28 seconds
7 (a) 5.1 centimeters; (b) θ = 6.43°
8 (a) 6.71 meters per second; (b) 8.29 meters per second; (c) 1.37 seconds; (d) 2.3 meters; (e) 13.87 meters

Chapter 15

1 See instructor for this experience.
2 O'Y' is 75.35 millimeters to the right of OY; O'X' is 64.28 millimeters above

OX. The intersection of *O'Y'* and *O'X'* is the location of the center of gravity.

Chapter 16

See instructor for evaluation of exercises in this chapter.

Chapter 17

1 1800 meters
2 4 meters
3 (*a*) 15 meters per second squared; (*b*) 11.62 meters per second squared; (*c*) 11.23 meters per second squared
4 (*a*) 9.09 meters per second; (*b*) 4.545 strides per second
5 (*a*) 400 newtons; (*b*) 27 °
6 0.557
7 29°
8 (*a*) The degree of the slope; (*b*) the friction between skis and snow; (*c*) gravity; (*d*) air resistance

Chapter 18

1 (*a*) 1.276 meters; (*b*) 1.192 seconds
2 (*a*) 45°; (*b*) 4.24 meters per second; (*c*) 0.46 meters; (*d*) 2.8 meters
3 (*a*) 0.891 meters; (*b*) 1.961 meters
4 (*a*) 9.487 meters per second; (*b*) 18.43°; (*c*) 0.459 meters; (*d*) 7.532 meters
5 19.33 radians per second, or 1107.7° per second, or 3.08 revolutions per second
6 Yes; ω = 1.8 revolutions per second × 1.2 seconds = 2.16 revolutions

Chapter 19

1 (*a*) 22.4 meters per second; (*b*) 73.47 feet per second
2 23.4 meters per second
3 19.4 meters per second
4 (*a*) 63.8 meters; (*b*) 2.47 seconds; (*c*) no
5 (*a*) 22.39 meters; (*b*) 73.44 feet; (*c*) yes
6 (*a*) 218.75 newtons; (*b*) 49.22 pounds

Chapter 20

1 Rings, floor, parallel bars
2 Adductors
3 Latissimus dorsi
4 Headstand; (*a*) larger base area; (*b*) lower center of gravity
5 2,352 newtons or 529.2 pounds; yes
6 918.75 meter-newtons
7 7.14 meters per second

Chapter 21

1 (*a*) A slender male athlete in training; (*b*) an overweight woman; (*c*) an average woman; (*d*) an average man
2 Greater
3 Yes
4 Skin friction, wave-making resistance, eddy resistance
5 50.056 seconds; yes

Appendix D

Natural Trigonometric Functions

Use headings at top of table for degree values in the left column; use headings at bottom of table for degree values in the right column.

Degrees	sin	tan	cot	cos	Degrees
0	.0000	.0000	—	1.0000	90
1	.0175	.0175	57.2900	.9998	89
2	.0349	.0349	28.6363	.9994	88
3	.0523	.0524	19.0811	.9986	87
4	.0698	0699	14.3007	.9976	86
5	.0872	.0875	11.4301	.9962	85
6	.1045	.1051	9.5144	.9945	84
7	.1219	.1228	8.1443	.9925	83
8	.1392	.1405	7.1154	.9903	82
9	.1564	.1584	6.3138	.9877	81
10	.1736	.1763	5.6713	.9848	80
11	.1908	.1944	5.1446	.9816	79
12	.2079	.2126	4.7046	.9781	78
Degrees	cos	cot	tan	sin	Degrees

Degrees	sin	tan	cot	cos	Degrees
13	.2250	.2309	4.3315	.9744	77
14	.2419	.2493	4.0108	.9703	76
15	.2588	.2679	3.7321	.9659	75
16	.2756	.2867	3.4874	.9613	74
17	.2923	.3057	3.2709	.9563	73
18	.3090	.3249	3.0777	.9511	72
19	.3256	.3443	2.9042	.9455	71
20	.3420	.3640	2.7475	.9397	70
21	.3584	.3839	2.6051	.9336	69
22	.3746	.4040	2.4751	.9272	68
23	.3907	.4245	2.3559	.9205	67
24	.4067	.4452	2.2460	.9135	66
25	.4226	.4663	2.1445	.9063	65
26	.4384	.4877	2.0503	.8988	64
27	.4540	.5095	1.9626	.8910	63
28	.4695	.5317	1.8807	.8829	62
29	.4848	.5543	1.8040	.8746	61
30	.5000	.5774	1.7321	.8660	60
31	.5150	.6009	1.6643	.8572	59
32	.5299	.6249	1.6003	.8480	58
33	.5446	.6494	1.5399	.8387	57
34	.5592	.6745	1.4826	.8290	56
35	.5736	.7002	1.4281	.8192	55
36	.5878	.7265	1.3764	.8090	54
37	.6018	.7536	1.3270	.7986	53
38	.6157	.7813	1.2799	.7880	52
39	.6293	.8098	1.2349	.7771	51
40	.6428	.8391	1.1918	.7660	50
41	.6561	.8693	1.1504	.7547	49
42	.6691	.9004	1.1106	.7431	48
43	.6820	.9325	1.0724	.7314	47
44	.6947	.9657	1.0355	.7193	46
45	.7071	1.0000	1.0000	.7071	45

Degrees	cos	cot	tan	sin	Degrees

References

REFERENCES

1 Abendschein, Karol H.: "A Comparative Analysis of the Frog, Scissors, and Whip Kicks Used by Beginning Swimmers," master's thesis, Brigham Young University Press, Provo, 1981.

2 Bangerter, Blauer L., Walter Cryer, and Kathryn Lewis: *A General Kinesiology Laboratory Manual*, Brigham Young University Press, Provo, 1980.

3 Barham, Jerry N., and William L. Thomas: *Anatomical Kinesiology: A Programmed Text*, The Macmillan Company, New York, 1969.

4 Barham, Jerry N., and Edna P. Wooten: *Structural Kinesiology*, The Macmillan Company, New York, 1973.

5 Barnard, James R., et al.: "Histochemical, Biochemical, and Contractile Properties of Red, White, and Intermediate Fibers," *American Journal of Physiology*, vol. 220, pp. 410–414, 1971.

6 Barney, Vernon S., Cyntha Hirst, and Clayne Jenson: *Conditioning Exercises*, 3d ed., The C. V. Mosby Company, St. Louis, 1972.

7 Barrus, A. Ray: "The Application of Scientific Principles to Events in Track and Field," master's thesis, Brigham Young University Press, Provo, 1969.

8 Basmajian, J.V.: "New View of Muscular Tone and Relaxation," *Canadian Medical Association Journal*, vol. 77, p. 203, 1957.

9 Basmajian, J.V.: *Muscles Alive*, The Williams & Wilkins Company, Baltimore, 1962.

10 Berger, R.A.: "Comparison of Static and Dynamic Strength Increases," *Research Quarterly*, vol. 33, pp. 329–333, 1962.

11 Berger, R.A.: "Optimum Repetitions for the Development of Strength," *Research Quarterly*, vol. 33, pp. 334–338, 1962.

12 Bleustein, Jeffrey L., ed.: *Mechanics and Sport*, The American Society of Mechanical Engineers, New York, 1973.

13 Broer, Marion R., and Ronald F. Zernicke: *Efficiency of Human Movement*, 4th ed., W. B. Saunders Company, Philadelphia, 1979.

14 Bunn, John W.: *Scientific Principles of Coaching*, 2d ed., Prentice-Hall, Inc., Englewood Cliffs, N.J., pp. 3–12, 22–92, 1972.

15 Capen, E.K.: "Study of Four Programs of Heavy Resistance Exercises for Development of Muscular Strength," *Research Quarterly*, vol. 27, pp. 132–142, 1965.

16 Chaffee, Ellen E., and Esther M. Greisheimer: *Basic Physiology and Anatomy*, 34th ed., J. B. Lippincott Company, New York, pp. 96–114, 1974.

17 Clauser, Charles E., John T. McConville, and J. W. Young: *Weight, Volume, and Centers of Mass of Segments of the Human Body*, AMRL Technical Report, 1969–70, Wright-Patterson Air Force Base, Ohio, 1969.

18 Cooper, John M., ed.: *Selected Topics on Biomechanics*, The Athletic Institute, Chicago, 1971.

19 Cooper, John M., Marlene Adrian, and Ruth B. Glassow: *Kinesiology*, 5th ed., The C. V. Mosby Company, St. Louis, 1982.

20 DeCoursey, Russell M.: *The Human Organism*, 4th ed., McGraw-Hill Book Company, New York, 1974.

21 DeLorme, Thomas L., and A. L. Watkins: "Techniques of Progressive Resistance Exercise," *Archives of Physical Medicine and Rehabilitation*, vol. 29, pp. 262–273, May 1948.

22 DeVries, Herbert A.: *Physiology of Exercise for Physical Education and Athletics*, 2d ed., W. C. Brown Company Publishers, Dubuque, Iowa, 1972.

23 Dyson, Geoffrey: *The Mechanics of Athletics*, Holmes & Meier Publishers, New York, 1977.

24 Ecker, Tom: *Track and Field Technique through Dynamics*, TAFNEWS Press, Los Altos, 1976.

25 Esch, Dortha, and Marvin Lepley: *Evaluation of Joint Motion: Methods of Measurement and Recording*, University of Minnesota Press, Minneapolis, 1974.

26 Gollnick, P.D., and P.V. Karpovich: "Electrogoniometric Study of Locomotion and Some Athletic Movements," *Report to U.S. Army Medical and Development Command*, Office of Surgeon General, Washington, D.C., 1961.

27 Gowitzke, Barbara A., and Morris Milner: *Understanding the Scientific*

Bases of Human Movement, 2d ed., The Williams and Wilkins Company, Baltimore, 1980.

28 Gray, Henry, and Charles M. Goss: *Gray's Anatomy*, 29th ed., Lea & Febiger, Philadelphia, 1973.

29 Grieve, D. W., et al.: *Techniques for the Analysis of Human Movement*, Princeton Book Company, Princeton, 1976.

30 Grover, Richard, and David N. Camaione: *Concept in Kinesiology*, W. B. Saunders Company, Philadelphia, 1975.

31 Harris, Ruth W.: *Kinesiology: Workbook and Laboratory Manual*, Houghton Mifflin Company, Boston, 1977.

32 Hay, James G.: *The Biomechanics of Sports Techniques*, 2d ed., Prentice-Hall, Inc., Englewood Cliffs, N.J., 1978.

33 Hellebrandt, Frances A.: "Physiological Analysis of Basic Motor Skills," *American Journal of Physical Medicine*, vol. 40, p. 14, 1961.

34 Hellebrandt, Frances A., E.T. Hellebrandt, and Clarence White: "Methods of Recording Movement," *American Journal of Physical Medicine*, vol. 39, p. 5, 1960.

35 Henry, Franklin M.: "Dynamic Kinesthetic Perception and Adjustment," *Research Quarterly*, vol. 24, p. 176, 1953.

36 Hettinger, Theodor: *Physiology of Strength*, Charles C Thomas, Publisher, Springfield, Ill., 1961.

37 Higgins, Joseph R.: *Human Movement: An Integrated Approach*, The C. V. Mosby Company, St. Louis, 1977.

38 Hill, A.V.: "The Design of Muscles," *British Medical Bulletin*, vol. 12, pp. 165–166, 1956.

39 Hill, A.V.: "The Mechanics of Voluntary Muscle," *Lancet*, vol. 261, pp. 947–951, 1951.

40 Hinson, Marilyn M.: *Kinesiology*, 2d ed., Wm C. Brown Company Publishers, Dubuque, Iowa, 1981.

41 Hirt, Susanne: "What Is Kinesiology?" *Physical Therapy Review*, vol. 35, pp. 416–419, 1955.

42 Huxley, A.H., and R.M. Simmons: "Proposed Mechanism of Force Generation in Striated Muscle." *Science*, vol. 233, pp. 533, 538, 1971.

43 Huxley, H.E.: "The Contraction of Muscle," *Scientific American*, vol. 199, p. 67, 1958.

44 Huxley, H.E.: "The Structional Basis of Muscular Contraction," *Proceedings of the Royal Society of London*, vol. B178, pp. 131–149, 1971.

45 Jacob, Stanley W., and Clarice A. Francone: *Structure and Function in Man*, 3d ed., W. B. Saunders Company, Philadelphia, 1974.

46 Jensen, Clayne R.: "Controversy over Warm-up in Athletic Performance," *Athletic Journal*, December 1966.

47 Jensen, Clayne R.: "The Significance of Strength in Athletic Performance," *Coach and Athlete*, January 1966.

48 Jensen, Clayne R., and Garth Fisher: *Scientific Basis of Athletic Conditioning*, 2d ed., Lea & Febiger, Philadelphia, 1979.

49 Jokl, Ernst: "Motor Functions of the Human Brain, A Historical Review," *Medicine and Sport*, vol 6, Biomechanics II, pp. 1–27, Karger, Basel, 1971.

50 Joseph, J.: *Man's Posture—Electromyographic Studies*, Charles C Thomas, Publisher, Springfield, Ill., 1960.

51 Kelley, David L.: *Kinesiology: Fundamentals of Motion Description*, Prentice-Hall, Inc., Englewood Cliffs, N.J., 1971.

52 Krause, J.V., and Jerry N. Barham: *The Mechanical Foundations of Human Motion*, The C. V. Mosby Company, St. Louis, 1976.

53 Kreighbaum, Ellen, and Katharine M. Barthels: *Biomechanics: a Qualitative Approach for Studying Human Movement*, Burgess Publishing Company, Minneapolis, 1981.

54 LeVeau, Barney: *Williams and Lissner: Biomechanics of Human Motion*, 2d ed., W. B. Saunders Company, Philadelphia, 1977.

55 Logan, Gene A., and Wayne C. McKinney: *Anatomic Kinesiology*, Wm.C. Brown Company Publishers, Dubuque, Iowa, 1977.

56 Luttgens, Kathryn, and Katharine E. Wells: *Kinesiology Scientific Basis of Human Motion*, 7th ed., Saunder College Publishing, Philadelphia, 1982.

57 Miller, Doris I., and Richard C. Nelson: *Biomechanics of Sport*, Lea & Febiger, Philadelphia, 1973.

58 Morehouse, Laurence E., and Augustus T. Miller: *Physiology of Exercise*, 4th ed., The C. V. Mosby Company, St. Louis, pp. 30–42, 50–58, 1963.

59 Morehouse, L. E., and P. J. Rasch: *Scientific Basis of Athletic Training*, W. B. Saunders Company, Philadelphia, 1958.

60 Northrip, John W., Gene A. Logan and Wayne C. McKinney: *Introduction to Biomechanics Analysis of Sport*, 2d ed., Wm. C. Brown Company Publishers, Dubuque, Iowa, 1979.

61 O'Connell, Alice L., and Elizabeth B. Gardner: *Understanding the Scientific Bases of Human Movement*, The Williams & Wilkins Company, Baltimore, 1972.

62 Pescopo, John, and James A. Baley: *Kinesiology the Science of Movement*, John Wiley and Sons, New York, 1981.

63 Pipes, Thomas V., and Jack H. Wilmore: "Isokinetic vs. Isotonic Strength Training in Adult Men," *Medicine and Science in Sports*, vol. 7, no. 4, pp. 262–274, 1975.

64 Rasch, Philip J., and Roger K. Burke: *Kinesiology and Applied Anatomy*, 6th ed., Lea & Febiger, Philadelphia, 1978.

65 Reynolds, E., and R. W. Lovett: "Method of Determining the Position of the Center of Gravity in Relation to Certain Bony Landmarks in the Erect Position," *Amer. J. Physiol.*, vol. 24, p. 286, 1909.

66 Sage, George H.: *Introduction to Motor Behavior*, Addison-Wesley Press, Inc., Reading, Mass., 1971.

67 Shepro, David, Frank Belamarich, and Charles Levy: *Human Anatomy and Physiology—A Cellular Approach*, Holt, Rinehart and Winston, Inc., New York, 1974.

68 Spence, Dale W.: *Essentials of Kinesiology: A Laboratory Manual*, Lea & Febiger, Philadelphia, 1975.

69 Terauds, Juris, ed.: *Science in Biomechanic Cinematography*, Academic Publishers, Del Mar, California, 1977.

70 Thompson, Clem W.: *Manual of Structural Kinesiology*, 6th ed., The C. V. Mosby Company, St. Louis, 1976.

71 Tricker, R. A. R., and B. J. K. Tricker: *The Science of Movement*, American Elsevier Publishing Company, Inc., New York, 1967.

72 Vander, Arthur J., James H. Sherman, and Dorothy S. Luciano: *Human Physiology: The Mechanisms of Body Function*, McGraw-Hill Book Company, New York, pp. 209–242, 1970.

73 Vaughan, Janet M.: *Physiology of Bone*, Oxford University Press, Oxford, 1970.

74 Williams, Marian, and H.R. Lissner: *Biomechanics of Human Motion*, W. B. Saunders Company, Philadelphia, 1962.

75 Winter, David A.: *Biomechanics of Human Movement*, John Wiley and Sons, New York, 1979.